A Clinical Guide to

Nutrition Care in Kidney Disease

Edited by
Laura Byham-Gray, PhD, RD, CNSD, and
Karen Wiesen, MS, RD

Renal Dietitians Dietetic Practice Group
of the American Dietetic Association
and the Council on Renal Nutrition
of the National Kidney Foundation

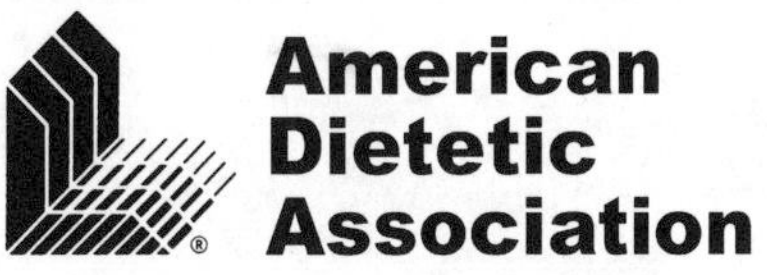

Diana Faulhaber, Publisher
Laura Brown and Kristen Short, Development Editors
Elizabeth Nishiura, Production Editor

10 9 8 7 6 5 4 3 2 1

Library of Congress Cataloging-in-Publication Data

A clinical guide to nutrition care in kidney disease / Laura Byham-Gray, Karen Wiesen, editors; Renal Dietitians Dietetic Practice Group of the American Dietetic Association and the Council on Renal Nutrition of the National Kidney Foundation.— 1st ed.

p. ; cm.
Includes bibliographical references and index.
ISBN 0-88091-344-4
1. Kidneys—Diseases—Nutritional aspects. 2. Kidneys—Diseases—Diet therapy.
[DNLM: 1. Kidney Diseases—diet therapy. 2. Nutrition Therapy—methods. WJ 300 C6385 2004] I. Byham-Gray, Laura. II. Wiesen, Karen. III. American Dietetic Association. Renal Practice Group. IV. National Kidney Foundation. Council on Renal Nutrition.

RC903.C5585 2004
616.6′10654—dc22

2004008704

Contents

Editors and Contributors

EDITORS

Laura Byham-Gray, PhD, RD, CNSD
University of Medicine and Dentistry of New Jersey—School of Health Related Professions
Stratford, NJ

Karen Wiesen, MS, RD
Barnes-Jewish Hospital Dialysis Center at Washington University School of Medicine
St. Louis, MO

CONTRIBUTORS

Patricia DiBenedetto Barbá, MS, RD
Gambro Healthcare
Lincoln, RI

Andrea Bickford, RD
Abbott Laboratories
Winfield, IL

Ronna Biesecker, PhD, RD
Watson Pharmaceuticals
Tucson, AZ

Pamela Charney, MS, RD, CNSD
Dayton, OH

Carolyn C. Cochran, MS, RD, CDE
Dallas Transplant Institute
Dallas, TX

Lori Fedje, RD
Pacific Northwest Renal Services/RCG
Portland, OR

Paula J. Frost, RD, CSR
Lee Street Dialysis
Washington, DC

M. Patricia Fuhrman, MS, RD, CNSD, FADA
Coram Healthcare
St. Louis, MO

Paul Garney, MS, RD
DaVita Med Center Dialysis
Houston, TX

D. Jordi Goldstein-Fuchs, DSc, RD
University of Nevada, School of Medicine
Reno, NV

Janelle Gonyea, RD
Mayo Clinic
Rochester, MN

Jill Lynn Goode, MS, RD
BoneCare International, Inc.
Florence, AL

Kathleen Hunt, RD
Castro Valley, CA

Maria Karalis, MBA, RD
Abbott Laboratories
Winfield, IL

Pamela S. Kent, MS, RD, CSR
Ohio Renal Care Group
Cleveland, OH

Susan C. Knapp, MS, RD, CSR
DaVita Broken Arrow Dialysis
Broken Arrow, OK

Carol Liftman, MS, RD
Franklin Dialysis Center/DaVita
Philadelphia, PA

Linda McCann, RD, CSR
Satellite Healthcare
Mountain View, CA

Maureen P. McCarthy, MPH, RD, CSR
RCG/Pacific Northwest Renal Services
Portland, OR

Lesley L. McPhatter, MS, RD
Lynchburg Nephrology Dialysis, Inc.
Lynchburg, VA

Joni J. Pagenkemper, MS, MA, RD
Creighton University Medical Center
Omaha, NE

Jessie Pavlinac, MS, RD, CSR
Oregon Health & Science University
Portland, OR

Julie Rock, MS, RD
Abbott Laboratories
Abbott Park, IL

Sharon R. Schatz, MS, RD, CSR, CDE
Gambro Healthcare
Cherry Hill, NJ

Donna Secker, MSc, RD
The Hospital for Sick Children
Toronto, Canada

Bruce Smith, MS, RD
DaVita Northstar Dialysis
Houston, TX

Jean Stover, RD
Gambro Healthcare
Philadelphia, PA

Naomi Stuart, MS, RD
East Carolina University
Greenville, NC

Reviewers

Margaret R. Baker, RD, CNSD
Mayo Clinic
Rochester, MN

Julie Barboza, MS, MSN, RD
Elder Service Plan of Worcester
Worcester, MA

Mary Ellen Beindorff, RD
Barnes-Jewish Hospital
St. Louis, MO

Deborah Benner, MA, RD, CSR
DaVita, Inc.
El Segundo, CA

Judith A. Beto, PhD, RD, FADA
Loyola University Medical Center
Maywood, IL

Connie Breach Cranford, MS, RD, CSR
Gambro Healthcare Springfield Central
Springfield, IL

Patricia Edwards-Hare, MPH, RD, CSP
All Children's Hospital
St. Petersburg, FL

Jordi Goldstein-Fuchs, DSc, RD
University of Nevada School of Medicine
Reno, NV

Kathy Hunt, RD
Castro Valley, CA

Barbara A. Hutson, RD
Ozarks Dialysis Services
Springfield, MO

Susan Knapp, MS, RD, CSR
DaVita Broken Arrow Dialysis Center
Broken Arrow, OK

Elizabeth A. Lennon, MS, RD, CNSD
The Cleveland Clinic Foundation
Cleveland, OH

Lisa Murphy, MEd, RD, CSR
Cleve-Hill Dialysis
DaVita, Inc.
Buffalo, NY

Pauline A. Nelson, RD, CSP
Children's Hospital, San Diego
San Diego, CA

Kathy Norwood, MS, RD
Chromalloy American Kidney Center
Washington University School of Medicine
St. Louis, MO

Neha Parekh, MS, RD, CNSD
Cleveland Clinic Foundation
Cleveland, OH

Chhaya Patel, MA, RD, CSR
Walnut Creek DaVita Dialysis
Walnut Creek, CA

Mona Rassi, MSc, RD
Humber River Regional Hospital
Toronto, Canada

Kathy Schiro Harvey, MS, RD, CSR
Puget Sound Kidney Centers
Mountlake Terrace, WA

Jean Stover, RD
Gambro Healthcare
Philadelphia, PA

Alpa Vyas, MS, RD
Olive View—UCLA Medical Center
Sylmar, CA

Kerri L. Wiggins, MS, RD
Cardiovascular Health Research Unit
University of Washington
Seattle, WA

Acknowledgments

The authors for *A Clinical Guide to Nutrition Care in Kidney Disease* recognize the following persons whose assistance was invaluable in the publication of this wonderful resource:

- Denzil F. Frost & children
- Lee Street Dialysis patients
- Satellite Healthcare for their support of Linda McCann's professional activities
- Robert S. Lockridge, Jr, MD
- Polly Nelson, RD and Jean Stover, RD
- Mary P. Anderson, RD
- Sarah Carter, RD, CDE
- Malia Chapman, RD
- Connie Breach Cranford, MS, RD, CSR
- Jennifer Glickman, RD

The editors would like to acknowledge all contributors for the two previous versions of this book, *A Clinical Guide to Nutrition Care in End-Stage Renal Disease,* 1st and 2nd editions.

Foreword

By working closely with the renal health care team to improve the patient's outcomes and quality of life and to decrease comorbid complications, the renal dietitian plays an integral role in the treatment of individuals with chronic kidney disease (CKD). This role continues to expand as more emphasis is placed on the importance of medical nutrition therapy (MNT) and management of comorbidities in the field of nephrology. The National Kidney Foundation Kidney Disease Outcome Quality Initiatives (K/DOQI) reaffirm the significance of nutrition in the care of individuals with CKD. According to these evidence-based guidelines, individuals with pre–end stage renal disease should be referred to a renal dietitian for early MNT intervention, and the nutritional status of maintenance dialysis patients should be monitored monthly (1).

As an outcome of K/DOQI, opportunities for broadening renal dietitians' practices are being reviewed. Key areas where the role of the renal dietitian may expand include the following:

1. The calculation and prescription of diet therapy orders that are in accordance with state and facility regulations and based on biochemical parameter analysis
2. The completion of anthropometric measurements and the subjective global assessment
3. Nutrition-related education of patients and staff and participation in continuing professional education components
4. Assistance in patient care meetings, including the setting of short- and long-term nutrition goals
5. Interpretation of urea kinetic modeling and dialysis adequacy guidelines
6. Management of renal osteodystrophy
7. Management of anemia
8. Continuous quality improvement

MNT is provided to every patient on dialysis. Therefore, appropriate dietitian-to-patient ratios are vital to maximize the patient's nutritional status and improve patient outcomes. The amount of time a dietitian spends in the facility should be determined by the patient load, the patients' levels of acuity for nutrition intervention, and the dietitian's involvement with administrative duties. Staffing patterns need to be continually analyzed so that subsequent recommendations can ensure the achievement of optimal MNT.

As the role of the renal dietitian in the management of individuals with CKD continues to evolve, it is important to have up-to-date and comprehensive references. *A Clinical Guide to Nutrition Care in Kidney Disease* provides the necessary tools and resources to support renal dietitians in their practices.

Susan M. Reams, RD, CSR
Chair, Council on Renal Nutrition of the National Kidney Foundation

Jill Lynn Goode, MS, RD
Immediate Past Chair, Renal Practice Group of the American Dietetic Association

Jennifer C. Smothers, RD
Chair, Renal Practice Group of the American Dietetic Association

REFERENCE

1. National Kidney Foundation. K/DOQI clinical practice guidelines for nutrition in chronic renal Failure. *Am J Kidney Dis.* 2000;35(6 Suppl 2): S1–S140.

Preface

In 1983 the Renal Dietitians Dietetic Practice Group of the American Dietetic Association (ADA-RPG) and the Council on Renal Nutrition of the National Kidney Foundation (NKF-CRN) began an ambitious project to develop a clinical guide intended to assist dietetics professionals who manage the nutrition care of persons diagnosed with kidney disease. At the time, more than 300 renal dietitians were surveyed to determine the guide's content. Respondents identified three key objectives. The clinical guide should be

1. Practical, containing information that is useful in practice and having minimal theoretical information
2. Representative of a consensus formed by clinical practitioners, on the basis of current scientific literature and experience
3. Cognizant of unique patient population characteristics

The two previous editions were written with these objectives in mind. This new book, *A Clinical Guide to Nutrition Care in Kidney Disease,* has considered these initial objectives while expanding the content to keep pace with the rapidly changing field of nephrology. Content areas have been broadened to reflect the widening scope of practice experienced by dietetics professionals employed in dialysis facilities: for example, nocturnal home hemodialysis, acute renal failure, HIV and AIDS, MNT reimbursement, and Internet resources. Unlike the previous editions of the clinical guide, this book aims to assist dietitians preparing to sit for the advanced-level credential Board Specialist in Renal Nutrition (CSR).

Although experienced renal dietitians have contributed to this publication, the audience for *A Clinical Guide to Nutrition Care in Kidney Disease* is much broader. New renal dietitians, clinical dietitians working in acute care facilities, consultant dietitians to long-term care, and dietetics faculty and students will find this book to be a useful resource to guide their learning and experiences within the renal population.

Chapter 1

Overview: Pathophysiology of the Kidney

Janelle P. Gonyea, RD, and
Maureen McCarthy, MPH, RD, CSR

BASIC KIDNEY STRUCTURE AND FUNCTION

The kidneys are located symmetrically on either side of the vertebrae, starting at the 12th thoracic vertebra and extending down to the 3rd lumbar vertebra (1). Each kidney measures approximately 11 to 12 cm long, 6 cm wide, and 3 cm thick. In the adult, each kidney weighs approximately 115 to 170 g, with women's kidneys at the lower end of this range.

Each kidney has two general regions: the cortex, a pale, outer region; and the medulla, a darker inner portion of the kidney. The medulla is divided into cone-shaped regions called the renal pyramids.

Blood is supplied to healthy kidneys through the renal artery, which enters the medulla at a section identified as the renal pelvis. Leading away from the lower portion of the pelvis, the ureters extend for a length of 28 to 34 cm to provide a connection to the bladder.

The basic functional unit of the kidney is the nephron. Each human kidney is comprised of more than 1 million nephrons, which are located in both the cortex and the medulla. Within each nephron, there are several well-known microscopic components, including the following:

1. *The glomerulus/Bowman's capsule/renal corpuscle*. Known as the filtering unit of the kidney, the glomerulus is a network of capillaries surrounded by a narrow wall of epithelial cells. In the glomerulus, approximately 125 mL/min of filtrate is formed. Bowman's capsule, with its basement membrane, holds the glomerulus, and together they are known as the renal corpuscle.
2. *Proximal convoluted tubule*. This is a direct continuation of the epithelium of the Bowman's capsule. Here begins the controlled absorption of glucose, sodium, bicarbonate, potassium, chloride, calcium, phosphate, water, and other solutes. The reabsorption of fluid also takes place in conjunction with active transport of sodium. In addition, ammonia is produced in the proximal tubule.
3. *Loop of Henle*. Urine is concentrated here and may be diluted later as needed. Brenner describes a countercurrent multiplying mechanism, which governs these processes and is not fully understood (1). Water cannot permeate, but sodium can be pumped out. Subsequently, this affects the movement of water in or out of the collecting duct, which is water permeable.
4. *Distal tubule*. This tubule has three parts: a) the thick ascending limb of the Loop of Henle, b) the macula densa, and c) the distal convoluted tubule. There is some active transport of sodium chloride in the thick ascending limb of the Loop of Henle. This region as a whole absorbs approximately 99% of the water that is filtered by the kidneys back into the body. The result is a more concen-

trated urine. Some functions of the thick ascending limb of Henle are governed by hormones, including vasopressin, parathyroid hormone, and calcitonin. In specific sections of the distal tubule, vasopressin stimulates resorption of sodium chloride.

5. *Collecting duct*. The secretion of potassium is a major function of the collecting duct and is regulated by mineralocorticoids (2).

General Function

The major functions of the kidneys can be described as a) excretory, b) acid-base balance, c) endocrine, and d) fluid and electrolyte balance.

The excretory functions of the kidneys include removal of excess fluid and waste products. While approximately 180 L of filtrate pass through the kidneys daily, only 1 to 2 L are removed in the urine each day (3). The remaining fluid is retained in the body to support tissues. Substances removed with the urine include urea; vitamins and minerals consumed in excess of the body's requirements; and metabolites of some drugs and poisons. Of course, if blood levels of any of the former substances are low, the kidneys promote homeostasis, conserving them to maintain blood levels within narrowly defined limits.

Acid–base balance is maintained through a buffer system, which maintains the pH of the blood at approximately 7.4. Bicarbonate carries hydrogen ions to the kidney where they are removed from extracellular fluid in the tubules, to be reabsorbed in the proximal tubule and returned to the bloodstream as needed. In addition, phosphate buffers intracellular fluid and then is concentrated in the tubules as water is removed. Other organic compounds, such as citrate, also support acid–base balance. And finally, metabolites of amino acids may be used to moderate acid or base reactions.

Several hormones are included in the kidneys' endocrine function. 1,25-dihydroxy-vitamin D_3 or calcitriol is produced in the kidney and subsequently enhances calcium absorption. In healthy kidneys, the activation of vitamin D and excretion of excess phosphorus set the stage for maintaining healthy bones. (See Chapter 16 for more detail.)

The anemia of chronic kidney disease is related to altered production of erythropoietin (EPO) in the diseased kidney. Normally, EPO acts on the bone marrow to increase the production of red blood cells, thus enhancing the transportation of oxygen throughout the body's tissues. (See Chapter 17 for more detail.)

The kidney's role in fluid and electrolyte balance is probably its best known function. The antidiuretic hormone (ADH), also known as vasopressin, released from the posterior pituitary regulates the water that is reabsorbed into the body. When fluid volume (blood and/or other fluids) is low, ADH is secreted and reduces urine flow, increasing the absorption of water in the collecting duct. This mechanism maintains the body's osmolality within a very tight range.

When extracellular volume (ECV) decreases, the trio of hormones of the renin-angiotensin-aldosterone system are activated. This leads to less sodium chloride excretion. If ECV increases, the reverse happens.

A person with advanced impairment of kidney function usually experiences edema, uremia (accumulation of waste products in the blood), metabolic acidosis, hypertension, anemia, bone disease, and an increased sensitivity to many drugs.

TYPES OF KIDNEY FAILURE

The onset of renal failure can be sudden, causing acute renal failure (ARF), or progressive, leading to chronic kidney disease (CKD). Each of these forms of kidney failure requires medical nutrition therapy (MNT) intervention.

Patients with ARF will potentially regain their kidney function. Medical management, including nutrition therapy, may control some cases of CKD; for example, several types of glomerulonephritis respond to medical treatment. As CKD progresses, nutrition intervention and dialysis or transplantation are necessary for survival.

Acute Renal Failure

Patients with ARF generally have a rapid onset of symptoms, which occur over a period of hours to days. In the United States, ARF is essentially a hospital-acquired condition because it typically occurs during the course of hospitalization secondary to ischemic events and nephrotoxic injury. It has an associated high degree of morbidity and mortality (4). Symptoms include elevated serum levels of blood urea nitrogen, creatinine, and electrolytes and changes in urine volume (oliguria) or absence of urine output (anuria). When evaluated radiologically, the kidneys and urinary tract appear normal in size (5). Due to structural changes that occur with age, elderly patients are especially at risk for ARF when under physiological stress. Common etiologies of ARF include (6):

- Ischemic injury, which accounts for 50% of all incidence of ARF. This is due to a sudden loss of blood supply to the kidneys secondary to surgical complications, thrombosis, sustained hypotension and hypovolemia as a result of hemorrhage, burns, and trauma.
- Nephrotoxic injury, as a result of medications, contrast medium, chemotherapy, or chemicals such as solvents, heavy metals, and pesticides, accounts for 35% of cases.
- Multiorgan failure, particularly liver failure secondary to the hepatorenal syndrome.
- Sepsis, especially bacterial.
- Obstructive uropathy, secondary to trauma during surgery, an enlarged prostate, or urolithiasis.
- Acute glomerular nephritis.

ARF can occur in previously healthy kidneys. With proper nutrition and dialytic support, such as continuous veno-venous hemodiafiltration (CVVHD), the kidneys can often repair themselves (5). However, quite often ARF can occur superimposed on underlying CKD secondary to diabetes, hypertension, etc. In this scenario, it is hoped that function can return to at least baseline and sustained dialysis is not required. (Refer to Chapter 4 for additional information.)

Chronic Kidney Disease

Recently, a standard for classification of stages of CKD has been outlined by the National Kidney Foundation Kidney Disease Outcomes Quality Initiative (NKF-K/DOQI) guidelines to aid in the treatment of these individuals (7). K/DOQI provides evidence-based clinical practice guidelines that have been developed by physicians and health care providers of the nephrology community and are recognized throughout the world. The K/DOQI project began in 1997 and provides guidelines for all phases of kidney disease. Additional guidelines continue to be developed and existing guidelines are routinely reviewed and updated as needed. The classification for CKD appears in Table 1.1 (7).

It is important to note that some decrease in kidney function is a normal part of aging. Stage 1 and even Stage 2 CKD may be seen in otherwise healthy individuals older than age 60. However, even in older adults, reduced kidney function should be monitored to allow appropriate intervention if the decrease in glomerular filtration rate (GFR) continues into later stages of CKD (8).

As part of a radiologic evaluation, diseased kidneys may appear shrunken as scar tissue replaces functioning nephrons. The exception is cystic disease in which the kidneys appear very large as a result of the growing cysts (3). See Table 1.2 (9).

Patients with CKD experience a permanent loss of GFR that occurs over a period of months to years. In many of the conditions, progression of the disease continues even if the kidney is no longer exposed to the initial trigger (10). Eventually, CKD may lead to Stage 5 CKD, requiring renal replacement therapy such as dialysis or transplantation to sustain life. (Refer to Chapters 3, 5, and 6 for additional information.)

Table 1.1. Stages of Chronic Kidney Disease: A Clinical Action Plan

Stage	*Description*	*GFR (mL/min/1.73m²)*	*Action**
	At increased risk	> 90 with CKD risk factors	Screening. CKD risk reduction
1	Kidney damage with normal or increased GFR	> 90	Diagnosis and treatment. Treatment of comorbid conditions. Slowing progression. CVD risk reduction
2	Mild decrease in GFR	60–89[†]	Estimating progression
3	Moderate decrease in GFR	30–59	Evaluating and treating complications
4	Severe decrease in GFR	15–29	Preparation for kidney replacement therapy
5	Kidney failure	< 15 or dialysis	Replacement, if uremia is present

Abbreviations: CKD, chronic kidney disease; GFR, glomerular filtration rate.

*Includes actions from preceding stages.

[†]May be normal for age.

Source: Reprinted with permission from National Kidney Foundation. K/DOQI Clinical Practice Guidelines on Chronic Kidney Disease. *Am J Kidney Dis.* 2002;39(suppl 1):46.

Table 1.2. Etiologies of Chronic Kidney Disease, Stage 5

Etiology	*Incidence (%)*
Diabetes	40.3
Hypertension	27.1
Glomerulonephritis	12.9
Interstitial disease	4.2
Renal cystic disease	3.4
Tumors	1.7
Other	10.4

Source: Data from reference 10.

NEPHROTIC SYNDROME

Nephrotic syndrome has been described as one of the most serious challenges of clinical nephrology (11). Fundamental alterations of the glomerular basement membrane of the kidney allow persistent losses of large amounts of protein in the urine. These changes in the glomerular filtration barrier allow large molecules to pass into the urine (12). These circumstances are most frequently associated with diabetes mellitus, glomerulonephritis, or amyloidosis. Clinical characteristics include the following:

- Albuminuria (more than 3 g/day urinary albumin losses, with proportionally lesser amounts for children)
- Hypoalbuminemia
- Hypertension
- Hyperlipidemia
- Edema

Because proteinuria (including albuminuria) represents such a high risk for cardiovascular disease and progression of CKD to Stage 5, treatment of nephrotic syndrome must include reduction of urinary losses. Medical intervention may include corticosteroids, immunosuppressants, angiotensin-converting enzyme inhibitors, and/or angiotensin receptor blockers to reduce urinary protein losses and to control blood pressure and fluid balance. Hydroxymethylglutaryl coenzyme A reductase inhibitors are often used for lipid control. With some disorders, particularly focal sclerosing glomerulornephritis, there may be a proteinuric factor, and the removal of this factor may help manage proteinuria (12).

The medical nutrition therapy (MNT) for nephrotic syndome is a moderate protein restriction of 0.8 g/kg standard body weight (13,14). This amount seems to help reduce proteinuria; however, the patient needs to be closely monitored for malnutrition, and, if needed, the diet can be increased to 1 g/kg (13,14). Sodium restriction should be based on fluid status and the need to control edema. Potassium and other electrolytes and minerals need to be monitored and the diet individualized. Dietary therapy for the associated hyperlipidemia may not normalize serum cholesterol levels and pharmacological therapy is generally required (13–15). It is a clinical challenge to add the recommended interventions for nephrotic syndrome to those already in place for the underlying etiology. More research is needed to identify optimal treatment for nephrotic syndrome.

CONCLUSION

This chapter has provided a brief overview of normal kidney function and various consequences of kidney disease, along with the many potential etiologies for compromise in kidney function. More detailed information regarding medical treatment and the MNT required at these various stages will be found throughout the text.

REFERENCES

1. Brenner BM, ed. *Brenner and Rector's The Kidney.* 6th ed. Philadelphia, Pa: WB Saunders Co; 2000:1–67.
2. Massry SG, Glassock RJ, ed. *Massry and Glassock's Textbook of Nephrology.* 4th ed. Philadelphia, Pa: Lippincott Williams & Wilkins; 2001.
3. Koeppen BM, Stanton BA. *Renal Physiology.* 2nd ed. St. Louis, Mo: Mosby-Year Book; 1997.
4. Molitoris BA, Finn WF. *Acute Renal Failure, A Companion to Brenner & Rector's The Kidney.* Philadelphia, Pa: WB Saunders Co; 2001:xi.
5. Brady HR, Clarkson MR. Acute renal failure. In: Schena FP, ed. *Nephrology*. London, UK: McGraw-Hill International Ltd; 2001:409–419.
6. Edelstein CL, Cronin RE. The patient with acute renal failure. In: Schrier RW, ed. *Manual of Nephrology.* 5th ed. Philadelphia, Pa: Lippincott Williams & Wilkins; 2000:132–154.
7. National Kidney Foundation. K/DOQI clinical practice guidelines on chronic kidney disease. *Am J Kidney Dis.* 2002;39(suppl 1):46.

8. Faubert PF, Porush JG. Anatomy and physiology. In: *Renal Disease in the Elderly.* 2nd ed. New York: Marcel Dekker; 1998:1–13.
9. Fisch BJ. The patient with chronic renal disease. In: Schrier RW, ed. *Manual of Nephrology.* 5th ed. Philadelphia, Pa: Lippincott Williams & Wilkins; 2000:155–167.
10. Schomig M, Odoni G, Ritz E. Chronic renal failure. In: Schena FP, ed. *Nephrology*. London, UK: McGraw-Hill International Ltd.; 2001:57–61.
11. Schwarz A. New aspects of the treatment of nephrotic syndrome. *J Am Soc Nephrol.* 2001; 12(Suppl 17):S44–S47.
12. Keane WF. Proteinuria: its clinical importance and role in progressive renal disease. *Am J Kidney Dis*. 2000;35(suppl):S97–S105.
13. Morrison G, Stover J. Renal disease. In: Morrison G, Hark L, ed. *Medical Nutrition and Disease.* Malden, Mass: Blackwell Science; 1999:306–307.
14. Fouqu D. Nephrotic syndrome and protein metabolism. *Nephrologie*. 1996;17:279–282.
15. Kaysen GA. Nutritional management of nephrotic syndrome. *J Renal Nutr.* 1992;2:50–58.

Chapter 2

Nutrition Assessment in Chronic Kidney Disease

Patricia DiBenedetto Barbá, MS, RD, and
Jill Lynn Goode, MS, RD

The initial nutrition assessment of the renal patient evaluates the baseline nutritional status of the patient based on all available subjective and objective data. The nutrition assessment determines a patient's nutrition care plan. Reassessment should be ongoing, especially throughout the first 6 months while the patient adjusts to the new lifestyle and treatment goals. Assessment of the nutritional status of a renal patient involves the evaluation of multiple parameters, including history and physical examination, anthropometric measurements, functional tests, subjective global assessment (SGA), metabolic status, and biochemical and hematologic values. Other areas that will affect the medical nutrition therapy (MNT) of the patient with chronic kidney disease (CKD) include socioeconomic factors and education level. The assessment leads to a plan of achievable goals that are workable and acceptable to the patient. This chapter addresses the use of these parameters as they apply to the adult renal patient. (See Chapter 12 for parameters applicable to children.)

HISTORY AND PHYSICAL EXAMINATION

The patient's history gives a perspective about past and present nutritional status, changes that have been taking place, and areas that need to be addressed in developing a plan of care. Histories provide information concerning comorbid conditions, medications, hospitalizations, adequacy of current intake and any changes in oral intake, gastrointestinal (GI) conditions that interfere with intake, changes in height and weight, economic status, socialization, functional status, as well as information from the physical exam.

Much of the history is obtained by reviewing the medical record and interviewing the patient and, as appropriate, the family or caregiver. The interview is the first opportunity for the patient and dietitian to establish rapport and build trust. Once the relationship has been developed, the patient will be more at ease with sharing information about his or her medical and diet history. Tips for effective interviewing include the following (1):

- Introduce yourself.
- Ensure your posture is receptive and make eye contact.
- Explain why a question is being asked and how the answer will be used.
- Assess prior learning.
- Gear information to the individual's knowledge and education level.
- Ask open-ended questions.
- Use food models and other references to enhance accuracy of patient's responses.
- Acknowledge responses.

- Limit the amount of information reviewed at each session.

The psychosocial history assists with assessment of a patient's ability to obtain, prepare, ingest, and enjoy food, as well as mental status, education level, and functional status. Certain probing questions may inquire about who shops for food and prepares meals and whether economic factors limit meal selections.

The use of the "KAZT Activities of Daily Living, a functional status assessment instrument" or the "Five-Item Instrumental Activities of Daily Living Screening Questionnaire" may be helpful in assessing the patient's functional status (2). Social aspects of a meal may influence intake. It is imperative that the dietitian assess whether the patient is eating alone or with family or friends. Religious and cultural beliefs can affect dietary intake and preferences and need to be assessed (3–5).

Diet histories are reviews of the usual food intake, food intake patterns, and factors that affect intake. Diet histories should assess the "normal" eating habits of the patient and any changes in those patterns. The dietitian should assess the patient's ability to chew, swallow, taste, and smell food, as well as changes in appetite and eating patterns. The use of supplements and alternative or complementary therapies should also be reviewed. Past dietary restrictions and instructions received as well as comprehension of previous counseling sessions should be determined. Food preferences, allergies, and intolerances affect a patient's intake. Lastly, alcohol use and pica should be assessed.

The diet history helps determine adequacy of intake and nutrient content. The reliability and validity of the data depend on the ability of the patient to provide accurate and relevant data and the ability of the interviewer to elicit information from the patient (1,2,5,6). The National Kidney Foundation (NKF) Kidney Disease Outcomes Quality Initiative (K/DOQI) recommends the use of dietary interviews and diaries as "valid and clinically useful for measuring dietary protein, energy, and nutrient intake in maintenance dialysis patients aiding in the identification of any causes of inadequate nutrient intake" (7). The data gathered about dietary intake should be incorporated into the plan of care, inclusive of educational needs and goals. There are three methods for assessing dietary intake:

- Three- or 7-day food records are prospective dietary intake records. The patient will document dietary intake as it occurs for a period of 3 to 7 days. The days should include 1 weekday and 1 weekend day and, for patients on maintenance hemodialysis (MHD), 1 dialysis day and 1 nondialysis day should be included. The clinician will review the food records with the patient and then assess the nutrient intake from the record (6,7). K/DOQI recommends periodic 3-day food records as the preferred method for measuring protein and energy intake for dialysis patients (7).
- Food frequency questionnaires are retrospective. The questionnaire is used to establish how frequently a patient eats certain foods—ie, daily, weekly, monthly. The food frequency is helpful in focusing on the diet in general and specifically on foods that chronic kidney disease patients should limit, but it is not very useful in establishing actual nutrient intake.
- Twenty-four hour food recall is also retrospective. The patient is asked to list specific foods eaten in the previous 24 hours or, possibly, on specific days such as dialysis days vs nondialysis days. The responses are evaluated for nutrient intake (6,7). K/DOQI states that when staffing conditions limit the time available to conduct a more formal assessment of nutritional intake, a 24-hour recall may be substituted for nutritionally stable patients (7).

ANTHROPOMETRIC ASSESSMENT

Anthropometric measurements provide information about adequacy of a patient's weight status; nutritional status; and the distribution of body fat, lean muscle mass, and bone. They can be used to identify nutritional excesses or deficiencies in energy or somatic protein reserves. These measurements also can be used to compare one or more individuals with individuals of other population groups or to record changes in one person over time. In one study, anthropometric standards used for the general population were found to apply to a majority of stable patients undergoing hemodialysis, with the exception of nondiabetic female patients who were significantly thinner (8). K/DOQI states that anthropometric measurements are valid and clinically useful in evaluating protein-energy status in patients on maintenance dialysis. The measures recommended by K/DOQI included percent usual body weight (% UBW); percent standard body weight (% SBW); height; skeletal frame size; body mass index (BMI); skinfold thickness; and mid-arm muscle area, circumference, or diameter. The measurement of these parameters should take place routinely (eg, % UBW monthly; % SBW every 4 months; and height annually) because they provide a clinically useful and valid picture of protein–energy nutritional status (7). There are also some advanced methods of measuring body composition that are worth mentioning, but these may require special equipment and trained personnel, are costly, and are seldom used outside of research facilities. These methods include bioelectrical impedance analysis (BIA), hydrodensitometry, near infrared interactance, and dual energy x-ray absorptiometry (DEXA) (1,5,9).

Body Weight

Body weight can be difficult to determine in CKD patients because as kidney function declines the ability to eliminate excess fluid is lost. The body weight recorded and monitored over time should be the estimated dry weight or "edema-free body weight" (BW_{ef}) as defined by K/DOQI (7). For hemodialysis, this weight should be obtained postdialysis; for peritoneal dialysis patients, it is the weight after drainage of dialysate with the peritoneum empty. For clarity purposes, body weight will be referred to as edema-free body weight for the rest of this chapter. Weight loss should be assessed and provided in terms of percent weight loss (6):

$$\%\text{ Weight Loss} = \frac{\text{UBW} - \text{Actual Body Weight}}{\text{UBW}} \times 100$$

If the patient is just starting dialysis, percent of weight loss due to fluid removal needs to be established. Attempts should be made to determine the patient's UBW prior to developing CKD. Once UBW is established, % UBW should be calculated as follows:

$$\%\text{ UBW} = \frac{\text{Actual Body Weight}}{\text{UBW}} \times 100$$

Percent UBW will indicate if there has been any weight loss, or, if weight is stable, whether there has been a decline in nutritional status (7). Another indicator of nutritional status is percent of standard body weight % SBW. Percent SBW less than 90% indicates malnutrition, between 115% to 130% is considered mildly obese, between 130% and 150% is considered moderately obese, and more than 150% is considered severely obese. The formula for calculating % SBW is as follows:

$$\%\text{ SBW} = \frac{\text{Actual Body Weight}}{\text{SBW}} \times 100$$

SBW can be obtained using the Second National Health and Nutrition Examination Survey (NHANES II) (Tables 2.1–2.4) (10).

Adjusted Body Weight

In very obese or underweight individuals, the use of actual, unadjusted body weight when determining actual nutrient intake or prescribing energy and protein needs can be inappropriate. Therefore, it is important to use adjusted body weight for obese and underweight patients (7). Currently there are a variety of methods and tables to determine adjusted or ideal body weight (11). K/DOQI recommends the use of the NHANES II data (Tables 2.1–2.4) for assessing SBW and % body weight (7). If the patient's body weight is less than 95% or more than 115% of the standard weight as determined by NHANES II data, then "adjusted edema-free body weight" (aBW_{ef}) should be used (1):

$$\text{Adjusted Edema-Free Body Weight} = BW_{ef} + [(\text{SBW} - BW_{ef}) \times 0.25]$$

Table 2.1. Standard Body Weights (kg) for Men Aged 25–54 Years: NHANES II Data

	Frame Size		
Height (cm)	*Small*	*Medium*	*Large*
157	64	68	82
160	61	71	83
163	66	71	84
165	66	74	79
168	67	75	84
170	71	77	84
173	71	78	86
175	74	78	89
178	75	81	87
180	76	81	91
183	74	84	91
185	79*	85	93
188	80*	88	92

*Estimated with linear regression formula.

Source: Data are from Frisancho AR: New Standards of weight and body composition by frame size and height for assessment of nutritional status of adults and the elderly. *Am J Clin Nutr.* 1984;40: 808–819.

Table 2.2. Standard Body Weights (kg) for Men Aged 55–74 Years: NHANES II Data

	Frame Size		
Height (cm)	*Small*	*Medium*	*Large*
157	61	68	77
160	62	70	80
163	63	71	77
165	70	72	79
168	68	74	80
170	69	78	85
173	70	78	83
175	75	77	84
178	76	80	87
180	69	84	84
183	76*	81	90
185	78*	88	88
188	77*	95	89

*Estimated with linear regression formula.

Source: Data are from Frisancho AR: New Standards of weight and body composition by frame size and height for assessment of nutritional status of adults and the elderly. *Am J Clin Nutr.* 1984;40: 808–819.

Table 2.3. Standard Body Weights (kg) for Women Aged 25–54 Years: NHANES II Data

	Frame Size		
Height (cm)	*Small*	*Medium*	*Large*
147	52	63	86
150	53	66	78
152	53	60	87
155	54	61	81
157	55	61	81
160	55	62	83
163	57	62	79
165	60	63	81
168	58	63	75
170	59	65	80
173	62	67	76
175	63*	68	79
178	64*	70	76

*Estimated with linear regression formula.

Source: Data are from Frisancho AR: New Standards of weight and body composition by frame size and height for assessment of nutritional status of adults and the elderly. *Am J Clin Nutr.* 1984;40: 808–819.

Table 2.4. Standard Body Weights (kg) for Women Aged 55–74 Years: NHANES II Data

	Frame Size		
Height (cm)	*Small*	*Medium*	*Large*
147	54	57	92
150	55	62	78
152	54	65	78
155	56	64	79
157	58	64	82
160	58	65	80
163	60	66	77
165	60	67	80
168	68	66	82
170	61*	72	80
173	61*	70	79
175	62*	72*	85*
178	63*	73*	85*

*Estimated with linear regression formula.

Source: Data are from Frisancho AR: New Standards of weight and body composition by frame size and height for assessment of nutritional status of adults and the elderly. *Am J Clin Nutr.* 1984;40: 808–819.

If the patient's BW_{ef} is between 95% and 115% of the median standard weight, the actual edema-free body weight should be used (7). Of the various methods available for deriving ideal body weight or adjusted edema-free body weight, the K/DOQI recommendation of the NHANES II data should be the standard used when assessing the CKD patient. Regardless of what source is used, amputations must be considered and adjustments made (Table 2.5) (11).

Example: Adjusted body weight for one leg amputation at the thigh:

75.5 kg × 10.1% = 7.6 kg

75.5 kg – 7.6 kg = 67.9 kg

Interdialytic Weight Gains

As kidney function diminishes, the body loses its ability to eliminate excess fluid. Patients on hemodialysis

Table 2.5. Amputation Adjustments

Body Segment	*Average Percentage (%) of Total Body Weight*
Entire arm	5.0
Upper arm (to elbow)	2.7
Forearm	1.6
Hand	0.7
Entire leg	16.0
Thigh	10.1
Calf	4.4
Foot	1.5

Source: Reprinted with permission from Wiggins KL. *Guidelines for Nutrition Care of Renal Patients.* Chicago, Ill: American Dietetic Association; 2002:114.

may gain several kilograms of fluid between hemodialysis treatments. This fluid gain is referred to as interdialytic weight gains (IDWG). When assessing the nutritional status of a CKD patient, it is important to assess IDWG. Excessive IDWG, a fluid gain of more than 5% of body weight (11), reflects excessive fluid intake that can potentially cause false laboratory values and lead to hypertension, peripheral edema, ascites, and pleural effusion (1). Low IDWG, fluid gains of less than 2% of body weight (11), reflect minimal fluid and food intake. Low IDWG can also cause laboratory values to be falsely high due to dehydration (1). Adjustments in the estimated edema-free body weight may need to be made after careful inspection of the pre- and postdialysis weights, IDWGs, and treatment course. For example, a patient who gains less than 5% of body weight between treatments, becomes severely hypotensive during their treatments and consistently leaves the unit weighing less than his or her dry weight, may be losing lean body mass due to a suboptimal nutritional intake, and his/her BW_{ef} needs to be adjusted downwardly.

Height

Initial measurement of height is essential. For patients who are unable to stand, recumbent bed height, arm span, or knee height measurements may provide an estimate of stature (11,12). Knee height correlates with stature and may be used to estimate height. A knee-height caliper should be used to measure knee height. Measure the distance from the heal to the top of the knee on the outside of the left leg, then use the following formulas (1):

$$\text{Male Height} = (2.02 \times \text{Knee Height}) - (0.04 \times \text{Age}) + 64.19$$

$$\text{Female Height} = (1.83 \times \text{Knee Height}) - (0.24 \times \text{Age}) + 84.88$$

Where: Height is measured in cm and age is measured in years.

Arm span is approximately equal to height in men and women, with an approximate variation in the results up to 10% (11). Fully extend the arms to the side so that they are parallel to the ground. Measure the distance from the tips of the middle finger on one hand to the tip of the middle finger on the other hand (1). Yearly measurement of height for those who are able to stand is important because decreasing stature may reflect bone disease.

Estimation of Frame Size

Frame size is used with height and weight tables and may be estimated by either wrist circumference or elbow breadth (1). A useful and quick procedure for estimating frame size is having the patient gauge themselves by encircling the nondominant wrist with the thumb and index finger of the dominant hand at the level of the radius and ulnar styloid process (9):

- Small frame: Thumb and index finger overlap.
- Medium frame: Thumb and index finger touch.
- Large frame: Thumb and index finger do not touch.

Body Mass Index

After establishing the edema-free body weight and height, the BMI can be calculated (6). BMIs less than 19 or more than 28 are associated with increased morbidity and mortality (13). BMI can be calculated by (3,6):

$$\text{BMI} = \frac{\text{Weight (kg)}}{\text{Height (m)}^2}$$

or

$$\text{BMI} = \frac{\text{Weight (lb)}}{\text{Height (in)}^2} \times 703$$

Estimates of Body Composition

Skinfold thickness is a well-established clinical method for measuring body fat. Body fat measurements should be taken postdialysis at the following four sites: triceps, biceps, subscapula, and iliac crest (7). Measurement of the body-fat stores help evaluate the patient's energy status, and tracking measurements over time can aid in early detection of malnutrition.

Anthropometric measures of the skinfold also provide an indirect assessment of muscle mass. Estimation of muscle mass is made by measuring mid-arm circumference (MAC), the midpoint of the arm between the acromial and olecranon process (1,7). The MAC and triceps skinfold (TSF) are then used to calculate mid-arm muscle circumference (MAMC) (1):

$$\text{MAMC (mm)} = \text{MAC (mm)} - [3.14 \times \text{TSF (mm)}]$$

Excess fluid and vascular access may affect the anthropometric measurements. It is recommended that measurements be obtained after dialysis in the non-access arm. TSF is often used in the CKD setting because it is a quick, convenient, reliable general indicator of somatic reserves.

Other tools can assist with evaluation of body composition. BIA is used to assess lean body mass, fat reserves, and total body water. Near infrared interactance is used in determining percentage of body fat. Hydrodensitometry (underwater weighing) is used to determine lean body mass. DEXA is used to measure bone, bone mineral content, fat mass, and lean body mass (1).

ENERGY AND NUTRIENT REQUIREMENTS

Nutrient requirements must be individually assessed based on whether the patient is on dialysis, what type of dialysis, cause of kidney disease, and other comorbid conditions. Energy needs are generally established using a kilocalorie per kilogram formula (Table 2.6) (1). Other predictive equations may be used, such as Harris-Benedict with the appropriate stress/injury and activity factors. Wiggins (11) provides a detailed analysis of key methods for determining energy requirements among patients with kidney disease. Protein, potassium, sodium, fluid, phosphorus, and calcium are addressed in each chapter specific for the disease state.

SUBJECTIVE GLOBAL ASSESSMENT

Several nutritional parameters are considered when assessing the nutritional status of a CKD patient. No one parameter by itself is useful in predicting nutritional status or malnutrition. It is important to view several parameters together. Subjective global assessment (SGA) was originally developed to assess the nutritional status of surgical patients (14). SGA provides a nutritional score based on two components, a medical history and a physical assessment. The medical history includes progression of weight loss, eating habits, gastrointestinal (GI) symptoms, physiological functioning, and simple analysis of metabolic stress. The physical assessment includes loss of subcutaneous fat and muscle mass. After evaluation, the patient was scored as either well nourished (A), mild to moderately mal-

Table 2.6. Energy Needs for Individuals With Kidney Disease

Acute (kcal/kg)	*CKD (kcal/kg)*	*Nephrotic Syndrome (kcal/kg)*	*HD (kcal/kg)*	*PD (kcal/kg)*	*Transplant (kcal/kg)*
35–50, depends on stress/nutritional status	30–35 > 60 y 35 ≤ 60 y	35 unless patient is obese; high complex carbohydrates; low cholesterol; < 30% fat	30–35 > 60 y 35 ≤ 60 y	30–35 > 60 y 35 ≤ 60 y, including dialysate kilocalories	30–35, maintain SBW, limit fat to 30% of kcal, < 300 mg cholesterol/d

Abbreviations: CKD, chronic kidney disease; HD, hemodialysis; PD, peritoneal dialysis; SBW, standard body weight.

Source: Adapted from Nutritional assessment charts, tables, and formulas. In: McCann L, ed. *Pocket Guide to Nutrition Assessment of the Renal Patient*. 2nd ed. New York, NY: National Kidney Foundation; 1998:1-1–1-42, with permission from the National Kidney Foundation.

nourished (B), or severely malnourished (C) (7). The SGA has since been validated in a variety of patient populations, including CKD, as a predictor of malnutrition and relative risk of death (7,15). Recently, the point rating system has been adapted to a 7-point scale, instead of an ABC scale, for more accuracy and sensitivity to change. The 7-point scale (7):

- 6 or 7 = very mild nutritional risk to well-nourished
- 3, 4, or 5 = mild to moderately malnourished
- 1 or 2 = severely malnourished

K/DOQI recognizes SGA as a valid and clinically useful measure of protein–energy nutritional status in maintenance dialysis patients (7). K/DOQI recommends using a four-item 7-point scale. The medical history reviews weight change during the previous 6 months, dietary intake, and GI symptoms. The physical exam includes visual assessment of subcutaneous tissue and muscle mass. SGA has been found to be beneficial because it is a cost-effective, reproducible, and validated measure of malnutrition in the chronic kidney failure patient (7).

BIOCHEMICAL PARAMETERS

Many biochemical parameters need to be monitored on an ongoing basis to assess the nutritional status of CKD patients (see Table 2.7) (1). Understanding laboratory results guides the nutrition professional in management of the patient. Protocols must be followed when blood samples are obtained and handled to ensure accuracy. For example, when drawing blood for potassium analysis it is imperative that the blood does not hemolyze or the value will be incorrectly high. Reference ranges are established to indicate when a value for a particular laboratory test is within the range for good health. Values above or below these ranges require further inspection. The clinical staff must determine the cause and take steps to manage the abnormality. The reference ranges for CKD in this book are set by the K/DOQI guidelines. Individual laboratories have their own "normal" reference laboratory values based on their particular procedures and laboratory equipment. The following laboratory tests are key ones that the dietitian evaluates to determine nutritional status in the CKD patient.

Creatinine

Creatinine is the nitrogenous waste product of muscle metabolism. This value is unrelated to dietary protein intake (DPI). It is a more sensitive marker of renal function; ie, the higher the serum creatinine, the greater the loss of renal function. Creatinine is produced on a daily level proportional to body muscle mass (16). Once the dialysis regimen has been established, creatinine values plateau to a steady state. If there is a sudden increase along with a change in blood urea nitrogen (BUN), blood pressure, and/or potassium levels, this may reflect a need to change the dialysis treatment plan. A decrease in creatinine over a period may reflect a loss of lean body mass. It is imperative that residual renal function and changes in treatment plans also be investigated as a possible cause.

Glomerular Filtration Rate

Glomerular filtration rate (GFR) is the amount of filtrate formed per minute (120 to 125 mL/min/1.73 m^2) based on total surface area available for filtration (number of functioning glomerluli) and reflects kidney function. GFR decreases 10% each decade after age 30 years, and the human body can sustain significant decrease in this function before there are any discernable symptoms. As GFR decreases to less than 40 to 50 mL/min/1.73 m^2, there are increasing amounts of toxins in the blood and accumulation in the body tissues. These toxins are responsible for the following symptoms:

- Nausea
- Vomiting
- Itching
- Malaise
- Anorexia
- Bone disease
- Increased blood pressure
- Edema
- Acidosis

A decrease in GFR to 15 mL/min/1.73 m^2 in individuals diagnosed with diabetes and 10 mL/min/1.73 m^2 in nondiabetic patients is a strong indicator for starting dialysis (17).

Serum Proteins

Proteins in plasma and extravascular fluids approximate 3% of total body protein; however, visceral organ

Table 2.7. Summary Table of Biochemical Parameters for Chronic Kidney Disease

Test	*Normal Range*	*CKD Range*
Creatinine	0.5–1.1 mg/dL *F* 0.6–1.2 mg/dL *M*	2–15 mg/dL
Albumin	3.5–5.0 g/dL	WNL for laboratory or > 4.0 g/dL
Transthyretin (prealbumin)	15–36 mg/dL	> 30 mg/dL
C Reactive protein (CRP)	0.8 mg/dL	2–15 mg/dL
Transferrin saturation	15%–50% *F* 20%–50% *M*	WNL
Glucose	70–105 mg/dL	WNL < 200 nonfasting before dialysis; intake has influence
Parathyroid hormone (PTH) (i) intact Biointact (third generation)	 10–65 pg/mL 60–40 pg/mL	 150–300 pg/mL 80–160 pg/mL
Calcium	WNL for laboratory	Normal: 8.4–10.2 mg/dL, preferably at low end (8.4–9.5 mg/dL)
Phosphorus	3.0–4.5 mg/dL	3.5–5.5 mg/dL
Alkaline phosphatase	30–85 ImU/mL	WNL for laboratory
Potassium	3.5–5.0 mEq/L	3.5–6.0 mEq/L
Sodium	135–145 mEq/L	WNL
Cholesterol	< 200 mg	WNL < 150 mg evaluate for nutrient deficit
Triglycerides	35–135 mg/dL *F* 40–160 mg/dL *M*	WNL < 200 mg/dL
Hemoglobin	12–16 g/dL *F* 14–18 g/dL *M*	Variable 11–12 g/dL
Iron	50–170 µg/dL *F* 60–175 µg/dL *M*	WNL
Ferritin	10–150 ng/mL *F* 12–300 ng/mL *M*	≥ 100ng/mL but no known benefit > 800
Blood urea nitrogen (BUN)	10–20 mg/dL	60–80 mg/dL in anuric, well dialyzed, and eating adequate protein
Adequacy HD PD		 Kt/V 1.2 Kt/V 2.0–2.2

Abbreviations: CKD, chronic kidney disease; HD, hemodialysis; PD, peritoneal dialysis; WNL, within normal limits.

Source: Adapted from Laboratory valuesdrug-nutrient interactions. In: McCann L, ed. *Pocket Guide to Nutrition Assessment of the Patient With Chronic Kidney Disease*. 3rd ed. New York, NY: National Kidney Foundation; 2002, with permission from the National Kidney Foundation.

protein constitutes approximately 10%. Because albumin and other plasma proteins are synthesized in the liver, plasma proteins can be thought of as functional indexes of hepatic protein status (11). There are more than 300 proteins identified in human plasma. The following proteins have been determined to be good indicators of nutritional status in spite of the fact that some are acute-phase reactants.

Albumin

Albumin is one measure of total body protein, both muscle and visceral. It is the most frequently used marker of protein status and is the standard recommended by K/DOQI (17). It has a half-life of 21 days and may not give an accurate measure of the patient's actual protein status. Albumin is a negative acute-phase reactant. This means that the production of this protein is negatively influenced by situations that may cause inflammation and stress related situations, including dialysis (18).

Low levels of albumin are found in the following situations (19):

- Protein-losing states such as enteropathies.
- Nephrotic syndrome.

- Liver disease.
- Severe burns.
- Surgery.
- Paracentesis.
- Decreased protein production.
- Redistribution: during sepsis albumin may be lost into the extravascular space due to increased vascular permeability; in ascites albumin is lost into the abdominal cavity.
- Increase peritoneal permeability: a greater loss of albumin occurs across this membrane, protein needs are higher in peritoneal dialysis than in hemodialysis. In the event of peritonitis, the losses are increased as much as 10-fold due to the inflammation, and this condition can continue for few months after the infection resolves.

Eighty percent of oncotic pressure is maintained by albumin, and it is responsible for transport of small molecules such as calcium, unconjugated bilirubin, free fatty acids, cortisol, and thyroxine. When the protein content of plasma is exceptionally low (low oncotic pressure), water can leak into the interstitial spaces causing edema. This process is also referred to as *third spacing* (20).

Elevated serum albumin levels may be a reflection of dehydration. The patient's hydration status must be included into the overall nutrition assessment.

Transthyretin

Transthyretin, also known as prealbumin, is another plasma protein that may be used to assess protein status. It is a transport protein for thyroid hormones and is bound to retinol. Compared with albumin, prealbumin has a much shorter half-life (2 to 3 days), and prealbumin therefore gives a more accurate measurement of the actual protein reserves and response to treatment modalities (17). It is less affected by liver disease or hydration status. In CKD, however, the transthyretin level may be falsely high because the kidney does not excrete the degraded product (21).

C-Reactive Protein

C-reactive protein (CRP) closely reflects the course of an acute-phase response to inflammation. Synthesis and serum concentrations of this protein and other acute-phase proteins (eg, serum amyloid A [SAA], fibrinogen, ferritin) increases during inflammation. This designates them as positive acute-phase proteins. Increases are regulated by the increase in circulating cytokines and tumor necrosis factor-α (20). These markers of inflammation are statistically powerful determinants of albumin level in CKD patients (22,23).

Transferrin

Transferrin serves as an iron-transporting protein (24). Some studies have shown that this protein is also a negative acute-phase reactant and may contribute to poor erythropoietin (EPO) response and anemia (25). This is another marker of protein status in the CKD patient, but this value is influenced by iron pool status and needs to be assessed in conjunction with this value and any iron therapy being administered.

Glucose

Glucose is the principal energy source in the body. The blood level fluctuates with food intake and insulin action. A fasting blood sugar level more than 126 mg/dL may be indicative of diabetes (1). Other factors that may influence glucose include chronic hepatic problems, hyperthyroidism, malignancy, acute stress, emotional distress, burns, diabetic acidosis, and pancreatic insufficiency (1). Low glucose levels may indicate hyperinsulinemia, alcohol abuse, pancreatic tumors, liver failure, pituitary dysfunction, malnutrition, and extreme exercise (1).

RENAL OSTEODYSTROPHY

Parathyroid Hormone

Parathyroid hormone (PTH) is secreted by the parathyroid gland. This hormone is a regulator of bone physiology. It has direct calcium regulatory properties via three target organs: the kidneys, the GI tract, and the bones (26). (Refer to Chapter 16 for more details about renal osteodystrophy.)

Vitamin D helps maintain calcium homeostasis by increasing absorption in the gut. Vitamin D must be in the active form to make this reaction occur. Vitamin D (cholecalciferol) needs two hydroxyl groups added to create the active form 1,25-dihydroxycholecalciferol or calcitriol. One of these comes from the liver and the other from the kidney. In CKD, the kidney loses the ability to activate vitamin D. This in turn causes the body to be unable to absorb calcium in the GI tract.

When the parathyroid gland recognizes a low serum calcium level, the stimuli trigger the parathyroid to secrete its hormone, causing the release of calcium from the bone (26).

Calcium

Calcium is the most abundant mineral in the human body. It comprises approximately 1.5% to 2% of body weight and 39% of all body minerals. Ninety-nine percent of the calcium exists in the bone and teeth. The remaining 1% acts as a cation in the extracellular fluids. Total plasma calcium has three components, protein-bound (47%), ionized (free 43%), and complexed (10%) (27). The extent of protein binding varies with protein concentrations and pH. The calcium in the fluid surrounding muscle fibers regulates muscle contraction. Calcium ions enable nerve conduction and are a factor in the blood-clotting cascade. Calcium is also a cofactor for many enzyme reactions, is a hormone trigger, and also acts in energy-coupling cycles (28). Calcium is bound to albumin. If low serum calcium is noted it is imperative that the albumin be evaluated also. A low serum albumin results in a low serum calcium, without a change in ionized calcium (28). The formula for corrected serum calcium is as follows:

$$\text{Corrected Calcium (mg/dL)} = [(4 - \text{Reported Alb}) \times (0.8)] + \text{Reported Ca}$$

Where: Alb is serum albumin level (g/dL) and
Ca is serum calcium level (mg/dL).

Example: Reported Alb, 2.3 g/dL; reported Ca, 8.6 mg/dL

$$[(4 - 2.3) \times 0.8] + 8.6 = (1.7 \times 0.8) + 8.6 = 9.96 \text{ mg/dL}$$

(Corrected Calcium)

Calcium is discussed in Chapter 16.

Phosphorus

Phosphorus (PO_4) is a mineral. The majority of phosphorus in the body is combined with calcium to form bone tissue. It is vital to energy production and storage and is a component of fats, proteins, and cell membranes (28).

Hyperphosphatemia is a major issue in the assessment of the dialysis patient's overall nutritional status. As renal function decreases, the body loses its ability to adequately filter excess phosphorus into the urine. This mineral then begins to accumulate in the blood. As the level mounts, this triggers a release of PTH that then releases calcium from bone. It is imperative to block the absorption of phosphorus from the gut by dosing phosphate binders at the time of food ingestion. These will form an insoluble complex and the PO_4 will be excreted in the stool (26). Phosphorus clearance is poor in both hemodialysis and peritoneal dialysis and it is imperative that CKD patients be diligent with their binder regimen.

Calcium-Phosphorus Product

Calcium-phosphorous product is the value achieved by multiplying the serum values of both components. If serum albumin is low, the corrected serum calcium must be used in this equation. There is some controversy about the product at which metastatic calcification begins (29). The range can be as low as 55 or as high as 75. When the product reaches these values, there is an increased risk of metastatic calcification of the soft tissues, such as the conjunctivae of the eye, the heart and blood vessels, the lungs, and the extremities. It is thought that this is a result of too much circulating calcium in the serum and its inability to be reabsorbed by the bone (30).

ELECTROLYTES

Potassium

Potassium is the primary intracellular cation. Extracellular potassium influences muscle activity, especially the cardiac muscle (28). Hypokalemia (less than 3.2 mEq/L) or severe hyperkalemia (more than 7 mEq/L) may induce muscle weakness and cardiac arrhythmia. Hyperkalemia may cause cardiac arrest. The kidneys are the chief filters for this ion. When this ability decreases, there is an obvious increase in the serum levels. Other contributing causes include the following:

- Excessive nutritional intake, including nutritional supplements
- Chronic constipation

- Infection
- Gastrointestinal bleeding
- Insulin deficiency
- Metabolic acidosis (low serum CO_2 level)
- Drug content or interactions (ie, the effects of beta-blocking drugs or drugs inhibiting angiotensin-converting enzyme)
- Inadequate dialysis
- Catabolism of malnutrition or cell damage caused by injury or surgery
- Chewing tobacco

It is also wise to check the validity of laboratory values, especially if the blood sample is hemolyzed. If the blood sample were hemolyzed, then there would be lysis of the red blood cells and all the potassium inside the cells would be mixed with the serum, giving a falsely elevated result.

Sodium

Sodium is the principal cation of the extracellular fluids. Functions of sodium include preservation of normal muscle function, maintenance of acid-base balance, osmotic pressure of body fluids, and maintaining permeability of cells (28). Serum sodium level is not a reliable indicator of sodium intake in CKD. Fluid retention (edema) due to decreased urine production can dilute an elevated level making it appear normal. Serum levels must be interpreted in conjunction with the patient's current fluid status.

LIPIDS

Cardiovascular disease is the most common cause of mortality in the CKD population. Therefore, it is imperative that factors affecting this disease process be monitored and modified as much as possible.

Cholesterol

Cholesterol is essential for development of cell membranes and hormones. Low-density lipoprotein (LDL) is often called "bad" cholesterol because too much in blood is thought to contribute to heart disease. High-density lipoprotein (HDL) is often called "good" cholesterol because it removes LDL. (Refer to Chapter 10 for more details concerning dyslipidemias in renal disease.) A low serum cholesterol in CKD is another marker of poor nutrition (22).

Triglycerides

A triglyceride is comprised of three fatty acids joined to a glycerol side chain. Triglycerides are neutral and insoluble (hydrophobic). These neutral fats can be safely transported in the blood and stored in the fat cell (adipocyte) as an energy reserve. Excess levels of these fats in the serum may indicate a metabolic abnormality that can contribute to cardiovascular disease. High triglycerides are often found in patients with diabetes, liver disease, patients on peritoneal dialysis, and those treated with steroids. Low values are seen in malnutrition and malabsorption, pancreatitis, and excessive alcohol use (30).

Chapter 10 gives an in-depth discussion of the application of the National Cholesterol Education Task Force Adult Treatment Panel III guidelines among this unique patient population.

HEMATOLOGICAL PARAMETERS

Hemoglobin

Hemoglobin, a conjugated protein containing four heme groups and globin, is the oxygen-carrying pigment of the erythrocytes (31). In normal circumstances erythrocytes are produced by the bone marrow and released to the circulation, where they survive approximately 120 days. The hormone erythropoietin, produced by the kidney, is one of the main triggers for production of erythrocytes. When this hormone is lacking, production of erythrocytes is diminished. Because erythrocytes carry oxygen to all of the other cells in the body, it is reasonable to assume that as the number decreases the resulting anemia increases and all the signs and symptoms are therefore exacerbated. The development of a synthetic form of recombinant human erythropoietn (rHuEPO) (EPO) has greatly reduced the anemia of dialysis. Following strict protocols, patients receive varying doses of EPO based on blood values of hemoglobin and iron. (Refer to Chapter 17 for a more extensive discussion of this topic.)

Hematocrit

Hematocrit is the volume percentage of erythrocytes in the blood (31). Due to the high fluctuations in fluid volume of the vascular space the reliability of this value to accurately portray the true erythrocyte concentration is questionable. Therefore, hemoglobin is the more reliable marker.

Iron

Iron is a trace mineral that has been recognized as an essential nutrient for more than a century. Iron in the adult human body is found in two major pools: a) functional iron in hemoglobin, myoglobin, and enzymes; and b) storage iron in ferritin, hemosiderin, and transferrin. Iron-deficiency anemia is the world's most common nutritional deficiency disease (28).

Due to the anemia associated with renal failure and the use of EPO, there is an increased need for supplemental iron both orally and intravenously. Oral iron may be used to restore and maintain these stores. If this is not effective, intravenous (IV) iron is the recommended course of treatment unless there is a documented allergic reaction. This is dosed according to a protocol developed by the drug company and the medical team of the dialysis facility.

Oral iron is usually prescribed in three divided doses and is best absorbed on an empty stomach. This is especially true because iron is easily bound to the calcium phosphate binders taken with meals. Therefore, it is recommended that iron supplements should not be taken with meals.

Ferritin

Ferritin is an indicator of iron overload. This sometimes occurs when patients have received blood transfusions. Ferritin is an acute-phase reactant, so elevated levels may be a marker of inflammation rather than iron overload. An elevated ferritin is predictive of EPO resistance (22). For patients using EPO, a ferritin level of 100 to 300 ng/mL is acceptable. Always check with the protocols in effect at the facility before making any recommendations or changes.

Transferrin Saturation

Percent transferrin saturation is another useful tool in the determination of iron availability and the need to dose or not dose with IV iron compounds. The saturation should be at least 25%.

DIALYSIS ADEQUACY

Numerous studies have demonstrated a correlation between morbidity and mortality and the delivered dose of dialysis. Urea kinetic modeling (UKM) measures the adequacy of any single pool treatment, and K/DOQI recommends the UKM form of the Kt/V be done monthly on all maintenance hemodialysis (MHD) patients. An added benefit of this calculation also provides another important tool in the nutrition assessment of the hemodialysis patient: normalized protein catabolic rate (nPCR) (32). This is a mathematical representation of the amount of daily protein intake in MHD. This measure has been shown to be predictive of mortality and morbidity in the MHD population even with Kt/V of 1.2 (30).

Urea is the substance that is most often monitored in clinical practice. This is a readily available solute and is the bulk catabolite of protein, constituting 90% of waste nitrogen accumulated in body water between hemodialysis treatments (29).

Blood Urea Nitrogen

Blood urea nitrogen (BUN) (sometimes referred to as serum urea nitrogen), is the measurement of the nitrogenous waste products of protein. Elevation of this value in CKD may indicate the following:

- High dietary protein intake
- Gastrointestinal bleeding or decreased clearance of dialysis (33)
- Increased catabolism (breakdown of body tissue due to infection, surgery, poor nutrition, or glucocorticoid usage)

Decreased BUN may indicate:

- Low dietary protein consumption
- Loss of protein due to emesis or diarrhea
- Protein anabolism or overhydration (15,28)

Due to this multifaceted picture, BUN cannot be used exclusively to assess adequacy of nutrition status or adequacy of dialysis. The Centers for Medicare and Medicaid Services (CMS) has a recommended range of reduction between pre- and post-dialysis BUN values (urea reduction rate [URR] > 65%). If this value is not achieved, this is a strong indication that ineffective dialysis may be a contributing cause of this finding.

Kt/V

Kt/V is best described by K/DOQI as "the fractional clearance of urea as a function of its distribution volume" (17). *K* represents the dialyzer clearance measured in liters per minute plus residual renal clearance unless the patient is anuric, and *t* is the treatment time (in minutes). The volume of the distribution of urea is *V*. The following are formulas for calculating single pool Kt/V and nPCR (34):

$$Kt/V = -Ln[R - (0.008 \times t)] + [4 - 3.5 \times R)] \times (UF/Wt)$$

Where: Ln is the natural logarithm; R is the ratio of postdialysis to predialysis BUN; t is time of dialysis in hours; UF is the amount of ultrafiltration (liters); Wt is the postdialysis weight (kg).

$$nPCR = \frac{\text{Pre - BUN}}{\left[a + b(Kt/V) + \left[\frac{c}{Kt/V}\right]\right]} + 0.168$$

Where: Pre-BUN = blood urea nitrogen level before hemodialysis treatment (mg/dL); Kt/V = Kt/V calculated from predialysis and postdialysis BUNs.

In the nPCR formula, the coefficients a, b, and c are determined by how frequently dialysis is given and the day of the week that predialysis BUN is drawn. See Tables 2.8 and 2.9 for coefficients.

These calculations are done by the laboratory and are cited here for reference purposes only. Monthly measurement of the daily dose of dialysis is recommended to ensure that the patient is receiving the prescribed and most adequate dose of dialysis for his condition, body size, and residual renal function. If a Kt/V of 1.2 or more is not achieved, then adjustments in treatment plan must follow. Adequacy in peritoneal dialysis as determined by K/DOQI is based on modality, and the Kt/V can range from 2.0 to 2.2 (refer to Chapter 6).

Table 2.8. Coefficients for Thrice-Weekly Dialysis

	a	*b*	*c*
Beginning of the week	36.3	5.48	53.5
Midweek	25.8	1.15	56.4
End of the week	16.3	4.30	56.6

Table 2.9. Coefficients for Twice-Weekly Dialysis

	a	*b*	*c*
Beginning of the week	48.0	5.14	79.0
End of the week	33.0	3.60	83.2

Urea Reduction Rate

Urea reduction rate (URR) is a simple measure of the change in urea concentration between pre- and post-dialysis blood tests. It has been shown to be a statistically significant predictor of mortality (17). However, it does not account for the ultrafiltration factor in the final delivered dose of dialysis and does not allow for determination of nPCR (17). The following formula allows for calculation of the URR:

$$URR = \frac{\text{Pre-BUN} - \text{Post-BUN}}{\text{Pre-BUN}}$$

REFERENCES

1. McCann L, ed. *Pocket Guide to Nutrition Assessment of the Renal Patient*. 2nd ed. New York, NY: National Kidney Foundation; 1998.
2. *Chronic Kidney Disease (Non-dialysis) Medical Nutrition Therapy Protocol*. Chicago, Ill: American Dietetic Association; 2002:appendixes 3,8, 10,11.
3. Charney PJ. Nutritional screening and assessment. In: Skipper A, ed. *Dietitian's Handbook of Enteral and Parenteral Nutrition.* 2nd ed. Gaithersburg, Md: Aspen Publishers; 1998:3–20.
4. McGinnis C. Parenteral nutrition focus: nutrition assessment and formula composition. *J Infus Nurs*. 2002;25:54–64.
5. Goldstein DJ. Assessment of nutritional status of renal disease. In: Mitch WE, Klahr S, eds. *Handbook of Nutrition and the Kidney*. 3rd ed. Philadelphia, Pa: Lippincott-Raven; 1998:45–84.
6. DeHoog S. The assessment of nutritional status. In: Mahan LK, Escott-Stump S, eds. *Krause's Food, Nutrition, and Diet Therapy*. 9th ed. Philadelphia, Pa: WB Saunders Co; 1996:361–385.
7. National Kidney Foundation. K/DOQI clinical practice guidelines for nutrition in chronic renal failure. *Am J Kidney Dis*. 2000;35(suppl):S27–S86.

8. Nelson EE. Anthropometry in the nutritional assessment of adults with end-stage renal disease. *J Ren Nutr*. 1991;1:164.
9. Page CP, Hardin TC, Melnick G. Nutritional assessment. In: Page CP, Hardin TC, Melnick G, eds. *Nutritional Assessment and Support: A Primer*. 2nd ed. Philadelphia, Pa: Williams and Wilkins; 1994:10–23.
10. Frisancho AR: New Standards of weight and body composition by frame size and height for assessment of nutritional status of adults and the elderly. *Am J Clin Nutr.* 1984;40:808–819.
11. Wiggins KL. *Guidelines for Nutrition Care of Renal Patients*. 3rd ed. Chicago, Ill: American Dietetic Association; 2002:113–116.
12. Grant A, DeHoog S, eds. Anthropometric assessment. In: *Nutritional Assessment and Support*. 4th ed. Seattle, Wash: Grant and DeHoog; 1991:9–86.
13. Chumlea WC. Anthropometric assessment of nutritional status in renal disease. *J Ren Nutr.*1997; 7:176–181.
14. Detsky A, McLaughlin J, Baker J. What is subjective global assessment of nutritional status? *JPEN J Parenter Enteral Nutr.*1987;11:8–13.
15. McCann L. Subjective global assessment as it pertains to the nutritional status of dialysis patients. *Dial Transplant.* 1996;4:190–198.
16. *Study of Renal Disease and Dietary Implications.* Hines, Ill: Hines Veterans Administration Hospital; 1975.
17. National Kidney Foundation. NKF-DOQI clinical practice guidelines for hemodialysis adequacy. *Am J Kidney Dis.* 1997;3(Suppl 2):S15–S66.
18. Albumin, general information. SydPath Web site. Available at: http://www.sydpath.stvincents.com.ass/tests/albumin.htm. Accessed April 30, 2003.
19. Neyra NR, Hakim RM, Shyr Y, Ikizler A. Serum transferrin and serum prealbumin are early predictors of serum albumin in chronic hemodialysis patients. *J Ren Nutr.* 2000;10:184–190.
20. Beck FK, Rosenthal TC. Prealbumin: a marker for nutritional evaluation. *Am Fam Physician.* 2002;65:1575–1578.
21. Zazra JJ. Interpreting laboratory values in the renal patient. *Renal Nutr Forum.* November, 2000.
22. Kaysen, George A. C-reactive protein: a story half told. *Semin Dial.* 2000;13:143–146.
23. Mehrotra R, Kopple JD. Nutritional management of maintenance dialysis patients: why aren't we doing better? *Ann Rev Nutr.* 2001 21:343–379.
24. Jacobsson S. Clinical value of serum transferrin measurements. *EJIFCC* [online journal of International Federation of Clinical Chemistry].vol 13, no 2. Available at: http://www.ifcc.org/ejifcc/vol13no2/1301200126.htm. Accessed April 7, 2004.
25. Grunnell J, Yeun J, Depner TA, Kaysen GA. Acute-phase response predicts erythropoietin resistance in hemodialysis and peritoneal dialysis patients. *Am J Kidney Dis.* 1999;33:63–72.
26. *Your Kidneys, Your Bones and You.* North Chicago, Ill: Abbott Laboratories Renal Care; 1995.
27. Jacobs D, Oxley D, DeMott W. *Jacobs & DeMott Laboratory Test Handbook: With Key Word Index.* Hudson, Ohio: Lexi-Comp; 2001:131.
28. Mahan LK, Escott-Stump S, eds. *Krause's Food, Nutrition, and Diet Therapy.* 10th ed. Philadelphia, Pa: WB Saunders Co; 2000:112,116,117, 125,156,157,384,781.
29. National Kidney Foundation. K/DOQI clinical guidelines for bone metabolism and disease in chronic kidney disease. *Am J Kidney Dis.* 2003;42(Suppl 3):S1–S202.
30. Block G, Port FK. Calcium phosphate metabolism and cardiovascular disease in patients with chronic kidney disease. *Semin Dial.* 2003;16: 140–147.
31. Lim VS, Flanigan MJ. Protein intake in patients with renal failure: comments on the current NKF-DOQI guidelines for nutrition in chronic renal failure. *Semin Dial.* 2001;14:150–152.
32. Schneider HA, Anderson CE, Coursin DD, eds. *Nutritional Support of Medical Practice.* New York, NY: Harper & Row; 1977:367.
33. Scantibodies Clinical Laboratory. The clinical benefit of CAP™ and the CAP/CIP™ ration for secondary hyperparathyroidism. Available at: http://www.scltesting.com/ Accessed April 8, 2004.
34. Wiggins KL. *Renal Care: Resources and Practical Applications.* Chicago, IL: American Dietetic Association; 2004:74–75.

Chapter 3

Nutrition Management in Early Stages of Chronic Kidney Disease

Lori Fedje, RD, and
Maria Karalis, MBA, RD

The role of nutrition in the care of pre-end stage renal disease (pre-ESRD) patients is vital. The nutritional status of the patient at the start of dialysis is a clinically significant risk factor for subsequent clinical outcomes on dialysis (1,2). Chronic kidney disease (CKD) has been defined as either "kidney damage or glomerular filtration rate (GFR) < 60 mL/min/1.73 m^2 for ≥ 3 months" where kidney damage is defined as "pathologic abnormalities or markers of damage including abnormalities in blood or urine tests or imaging studies" (3). The National Kidney Foundation (NKF) Kidney Disease Outcome Quality Initiatives (K/DOQI) Clinical Practice Guidelines for Chronic Kidney Disease classified CKD into terms and stages that would "improve communication between patients and providers, enhance public education, and promote dissemination of research results" (3).

The level of CKD is determined by a combination of evidence of kidney damage and level of kidney function as indicated by GFR. Operationally, GFR is estimated using an equation that considers age, sex, and body weight on creatinine generation. More recently, a modified equation such as the Modification of Diet in Renal Disease (MDRD) formula has been found to be the "standard of measurement" because it incorporates the effects of age, gender, and race plus three biochemical measures (rather than one). These biochemical measures are serum creatinine, serum albumin, and serum urea nitrogen. This modified GFR equation can be found in the K/DOQI Nutrition Guidelines (4,5).

The primary goal for nutrition management in the early stages of CKD is to prevent protein-energy malnutrition. Other goals include: a) minimize uremic toxicity and delay the progression of renal disease, b) prevent secondary hyperparathyroidism, and c) ameliorate metabolic acidosis.

Deteriorating kidney function affects nutritional status and thus clinical management of pre-ESRD patients. The interrelationships between renal pathology and nutritional intake are complex and must be evaluated together. Altered kidney function will warrant some type of nutrition intervention. The questions remain: what type of intervention and when should it be instituted? Ultimately, left untreated, deteriorating kidney function may cause edema, uremia, metabolic acidosis, hypertension, anemia, bone disease, hyperphosphatemia, hyperkalemia, and muscle wasting (6–10).

LITERATURE REVIEW

Control of protein intake may delay the progression of kidney failure and ameliorate the aforementioned effects of excessive accumulation of nitrogenous wastes. In rats with CHF, a high-protein diet may lead to increased proteinuria and renal damage, whereas a restriction of dietary protein may lead to improvement in these parameters (11). Early intervention with a low-protein diet in humans with chronic renal failure may decrease clinical uremic symptoms by decreasing formation of nitrogenous compounds. A high protein intake orally or via total parenteral nutrition has been demonstrated to increase the workload on the kidney in rats and humans, respectively (12). Proposed mechanisms of action for decreased renal function include increased glomerular perfusion and intraglomerular capillary pressures once a critical decrease in renal mass occurs (6).

Unfortunately, clinical studies are not as clear (4,12–14). Two large studies, the Modification of Diet in Renal Disease (MDRD) Study and the Diabetes Control and Complications Trial (DCCT), have produced results that are inconclusive, but they affect the nutritional care in CKD.

MDRD Study

The MDRD Study was a randomized, multicenter trial involving 840 patients in varying degrees of nondiabetic renal failure (4). This 2.2-year study was one of the largest that examined whether controlling dietary protein and phosphorus would slow down the progression of renal disease.

The MDRD study divided subjects into two groups based on the level of renal function; within each of these groups subjects were randomly assigned to treatment regimens that varied in the quantity and source of dietary protein. Study A patients (GFR of 25–55 mL/min/1.73m^2) were assigned to two different dietary protein levels. The two dietary levels consisted of a) usual protein (around 1.3 g/kg BW) and usual phosphorus (16–20 mg phosphorus /kg/day), and b) low protein (0.55 g/kg/day), low phosphorus (5–10 mg phosphorus/kg/day). Study B patients (GFR of 13–24 mL/min/1.73m^2) assigned to the low-protein diet or to a very-low-protein diet (0.28 g/kg/day) with supplemental ketoacid supplements of 0.28 g/kg/day and very-low-phosphorus diet (4–9 mg phosphorus/kg/day). Intensive counseling and frequent follow-up visits with medical, nursing, and nutrition staff were an important part of the study. The use of carefully trained registered dietitians and the frequency of self-monitoring resulted in excellent dietary adherence.

Prior research has suggested that control of dietary protein and phosphorus can delay the onset of chronic kidney disease. However, the results of the MDRD Study were not conclusive in this regard. There has been speculation that the study ended before a significant separation between the different levels of dietary protein was observed. The MDRD Study did demonstrate slower progression of renal disease when blood pressure was better controlled. It also demonstrated that with careful follow-up, nutritional status can be maintained on a modified-protein diet.

DCCT Study

The DCCT was another large multicenter study following subjects with insulin-dependent diabetes mellitus (IDDM) for 6.5 years (15). Subjects were randomly assigned one of two treatment groups: conventional treatment (2 insulin injections/day, occasional blood glucose checks); or intensive treatment (3 or more injections with frequent glucose monitoring). In the intensive group, albuminuria and microalbuminuria (defined as 20–200 μg/minute) were seen at 54% and 39%, respectively, of the incidence observed in the conventional group. This is significant because microalbuminuria is a marker in the progression into diabetic nephropathy. Overall, the incidence of diabetic nephropathy in intensively treated subjects was reduced by more than 50%. As with the MDRD Study, the involvement of dietitians in DCCT was crucial to the study design and success.

An important limitation of the DCCT was the exclusion of subjects with non-insulin-dependent diabetes mellitus (NIDDM). In these patients the incidence of diabetic nephropathy seems to equal or exceed that seen in IDDM (15). The results from the DCCT cannot be directly generalized to the NIDDM population, but the American Diabetes Association supports the application of the DCCT findings as a beneficial strategy until clearer information is known (16).

In addition to a variety of comorbid factors (diabetes, cardiovascular disease, hypertension, liver disease) affecting nutritional needs, the various stages of kidney failure will also impact these requirements. For example, the kidneys do a remarkable job of compensating and it is not until the creatinine clearance decreases to less than approximately 50 mL/min/1.73m^2 that azotemia and mild anemia occur (17). These factors will affect patient appetite and thus overall dietary intake. Depending on the level of kidney function, if excessive protein is consumed, the problems of high blood urea nitrogen (BUN) levels, anorexia, nausea, vomiting, weakness, taste changes, confusion, lethargy, and generalized itching may be compounded (6). Once creatinine clearance decreases to 10 to 15 mL/min/

1.73m^2, fatigue, nausea, vomiting, loss of appetite, metabolic acidosis, and hyperphosphatemia generally occur (17).

Thus far, no studies have proven that a protein restriction will completely stop the progression of chronic kidney disease. For the most part, a protein restriction does seem to minimize some of the metabolic consequences of uremia. While dietary modifications may be warranted in some patients, the risk of inducing malnutrition and thus increasing morbidity and mortality should be carefully evaluated.

RECOMMENDED DIET PRESCRIPTION

Patients with GFR less than 60 mL/min/1.73m^2 should "undergo assessment of dietary protein and energy intake and nutritional status" (3). Additionally, patients with "decreased dietary intake or malnutrition should undergo dietary modification, counseling and education or specialized nutrition therapy" (3). A decrease in appetite is one of the most significant markers of uremia and kidney failure. A spontaneous decrease in protein and calories begins when the GFR falls below 60 mL/min/1.73m^2 (3). For patients with a GFR or more than 60 mL/min/1.73m^2, it is appropriate for patients to maintain their weight and nutritional status by consuming a heart-healthy diet such as that outlined in the National Cholesterol Education Program Adult Treatment Panel III (ATP III) recommendations (18). (See Table 3.1 for those guidelines and Chapter 10 for further information on dyslipidemia.)

There have been discrepancies in the literature regarding which body weight measurement to use when determining protein and calorie requirements. According to K/DOQI Nutrition Guidelines, it is recommended that standard body weight (SBW) be used based on the Second National Health Nutrition Evaluation Survey (NHANES II) (5). (See Chapter 2 for further description.)

K/DOQI Nutrition Guidelines suggest 0.6 g of protein per kilogram per day for those with GFR less than 25 mL/min/1.73m^2, which corresponds approximately to CKD Stages 4–5 (3,5). The MDRD Study found no evidence of a beneficial effect from dietary protein intake more than the Recommended Dietary Allowances (RDA) of protein for normal adults of 0.75 g/kg/day. (RDA has now been replaced by Dietary Reference Intakes [DRIs] and recommends 0.8 g per kg body weight per day.) As such, it seems prudent to prescribe this level of protein for those patients in CKD

Table 3.1. Nutrient Composition of the Therapeutic Lifestyle Changes (TLC) Diet

Nutrient	*Recommended Intake*
Saturated fat*	< 7% of total calories
Polyunsaturated fat	Up to 10% of total calories
Monounsaturated fat	Up to 20% of total calories
Total fat	25%–35% of total calories
Carbohydrate†	50%–60% of total calories
Fiber	20–30 g/d
Protein	Approximately 15% of total calories
Cholesterol	< 200 mg/d
Total calories‡	Balance energy intake and expenditure to maintain desirable body weight/prevent weight gain

**Trans* fatty acids are another LDL-raising fat that should be kept at a low intake.

†Carbohydrates should be derived predominantly from foods rich in complex carbohydrates including grains, especially whole grains, fruits, and vegetables.

‡Daily energy expenditure should include at least moderate physical activity (contributing approximately 200 kcal/d).

Source: Reprinted from Executive Summary of the Third Report of the National Cholesterol Education Program (NCEP) Expert Panel on Detection, Evaluation and Treatment of High Blood Cholesterol in Adults (Adult Treatment Panel III). *JAMA.* 2001;285:2486–2497.

Stages 1–3. In all cases, the clinician should carefully assess for evidence of malnutrition and individualize the dietary prescription (3,5).

At least 50% of the dietary protein should be of high biological value. However, inadequate energy intake may mitigate the potential benefit of a low-protein diet because ingested protein (as well as somatic protein stores) may be catabolized for energy (5,19–21).

Calorie needs of CKD patients parallel those of normal healthy individuals (5). However, unlike the general population, CKD patients tend to have inadequate dietary intakes and may become malnourished by the time dialysis is initiated. The daily calorie intake for individuals with GFR less than 25 mL/min/1.73m^2 (which corresponds to CKD Stages 4–5) is 35 kcal/kg/day for those younger than 60 years old and 30 to 35 kcal/kg/day for those 60 years or older (3,5). Obese patients typically require fewer kilocalories, at 20 to 30 kcal/kg/day adjusted body weight. Underweight (or catabolic) patients require more calories, at 45 kcal/kg/day adjusted body weight. The goals for this energy level include: a) maintain neutral nitrogen balance, b) promote higher serum albumin levels, and c) maintain or improve anthropometrics (3).

Energy requirements are most difficult to meet in CKD. Studies have shown that even with extensive counseling, adequate calorie intake is seldom achieved. Kopple et al have shown that 35 to 40 kcal/kg/day were needed to achieve positive nitrogen balance in patients with chronic renal failure (CRF) (22). It has been suggested that higher energy intake leads to more efficient utilization of nitrogen. As such, calorie needs for the CKD Stages 1 through 3 will depend on the nutritional status of the patient and presence or absence of clinical signs of protein-energy malnutrition.

The DCCT recommended the usual level of 25 kcal/kg/day be increased to 35 kcal/kg/day for people with diabetes (15). However, for the overweight individuals with type 2 diabetes, exercise remains an important component for controlling weight and blood sugars. Recently, strong evidence has shown that sucrose and sucrose-containing foods do not need to be restricted in people with diabetes but rather substituted for other carbohydrate sources. The newly released evidence-based recommendations by the American Diabetes Association state that the total amount of carbohydrate in meals and snacks is more important than the source (starches or sugars) or type (glycemic index) (16). Although the diet may be more liberal, tight glycemic control is recommended and may require intensive insulin therapy as utilized in the DCCT. Refer to Table 3.2 for the stages of chronic kidney disease and corresponding nutrient recommendations (3,5,11, 20,23).

Although there is not clear evidence that control of dyslipidemias help prevent kidney disease progression, we know that CKD patients are at a high risk for atherosclerotic cardiovascular disease (ACVD) (3,24,25).

Table 3.2. Stages of Chronic Kidney Disease and Corresponding Nutrient Recommendations

Stage	*Description*	*GFR (mL/min/ 1.73m²)*	*Protein (g/kg/d)*	*Calories*	*Sodium (g/d)*	*Potassium (g/d)*	*Phosphorus (g/d)*	*Calcium (g/d)*	*Vitamins*
1	Kidney damage with normal or increasing GFR	= 90	0.75	Based on energy expenditure	Varies from 1–4 to no added salt, depending on comorbidities	Usually no restriction unless serum level is high	Monitor and restrict if serum levels > 4.6	1.2–1.5; maintain serum Ca on lower end	DRI
2	Kidney damage with mild decreasing GFR	60–89	0.75	Based on energy expenditure	Same as stage 1	Same as stage 1	Same as stage 1	Same as stage 1	DRI
3	Moderate decreasing GFR	30–59	0.75	Based on energy expenditure	Same as stage 1	Same as stage 1	8–12 mg/g protein or 800–1000 mg/d	Same as stage 1	B complex and C: DRI Individualize vitamin D, zinc, and iron
4	Severe decreasing GFR	15–29	0.6	30–35 kcal/kg/d	Same as stage 1	Same as stage 1	Same as stage 3	Same as stage 1 but not to exceed 2000 mg/d	Same as stage 3
5	Kidney failure	< 15 or dialysis	0.6–0.75	30–35 kcal/kg/d	Same as stage 1	Same as stage 1	Same as stage 3	Same as stage 4	Same as stage 3

Abbreviations: DRI, dietary reference intake; GFR, glomerular filtration rate.

Source: Data are from references 3,5,11,20.

For this reason, it is prudent for patients to follow the National Cholesterol Education Program ATP III recommendations (18). This document will not encompass all of the recommendations but will refer to only the diet guidelines. The level of low-density lipoprotein cholesterol (LDL) along with other risk factors determines when to start therapeutic lifestyle changes, which include the diet guidelines. (See Table 3.2 for exact recommendations.)

Dietary phosphorus has also been implicated in the progression of renal disease, although research is not conclusive. The modified protein diet limits total dietary phosphorus, but further restriction of some high-phosphorus foods may be important to prevent renal osteodystrophy. Changes in phosphorus/calcium balance begin at an early stage in renal disease. Early phosphorus control (maintaining serum levels at the lower end of normal) may delay renal bone disease.

The diet should be limited to 8 to 12 mg phosphorus/kg/day (800–1,000 mg/day) (23). This is effective only in patients with moderate renal failure (GFR 30–60mL/min/1.73m^2, which corresponds to CKD Stages 2 and 3) (26). As renal failure advances, diet alone will not control serum phosphorus; therefore, other measures such as phosphate binding medications, will be needed. Phosphate binder therapy should be initiated when serum phosphorus reaches upper limits of normal, but care should be taken to prevent phosphorus depletion because low serum phosphorus can aggravate other types of bone disease. (Refer to Chapter 16 for more specific information about bone disease.)

When the diet is limited in protein and phosphorus, dietary calcium intake will also be low. Changes in the activation of vitamin D-3 alter intestinal absorption of calcium in renal insufficiency. Altered absorption and low dietary intake can precipitate negative calcium balance and bone demineralization. Calcium intake of 1.2 to 1.5 g/day may be reasonable for patients with a GFR of 10 to 40 mL/min/1.73m^2 (which corresponds to CKD Stages 3 through 5). Patients with advanced renal failure (GFR < 10 mL/min/1.73m^2, which corresponds to CKD Stage 5) may need a calcium intake of 1.5 to 2.0 g/day (26). With current research addressing vascular calcification, it may be prudent to monitor laboratory data closely and remain current with scientific literature regarding levels of total calcium intake in CKD patients (27,28). The NKF K/DOQI guidelines recommend that total elemental calcium from diet and binders not exceed 2,000 mg/day as patients advance to Stages 4 and 5 (23).

Fluid and electrolyte balance may be altered in CKD. If indicated, sodium modification should be based on blood pressure and fluid balance. Other disease states, such as congestive heart disease, nephrotic syndrome, or advanced liver disease may increase the need for sodium restriction. The recommended intake of sodium is 1 to 4 g/day. It should be noted that reduced sodium intake has been associated with further renal impairment in some renal diseases (29). Monitoring body weight will help determine when a fluid restriction is needed. As requirements for sodium and fluid vary markedly, each patient will need to be managed individually.

Dietary potassium is rarely restricted until urine output decreases to less than 1,000 mL/day or serum levels are above normal. Other than excessive intake of potassium, other causes of hyperkalemia should be evaluated, such as the use of angiotensin-converting enzyme inhibitors or beta-receptor blockers, hypoinsulinism or acidosis (30). As serum levels increase to more than 5.0 mg/dL, a mild potassium restriction of 3 to 4 g/day may be needed.

Vitamin and mineral requirements are not well defined in CKD, but nondialyzed patients treated with a controlled-protein diet may need some vitamin supplementation. Vitamin preparations should contain the DRI for the water-soluble vitamins including folate (31). Vitamin C supplementation should not exceed 100 mg/day because it plays a role in the formation of oxalosis. Fat-soluble vitamins should be avoided as renal function declines, especially vitamin A, which is elevated in renal failure (32). Vitamin D supplementation is individualized based on nutritional deficiency as measured by serum 25-hydroxyvitamin D levels or according to the treatment of bone disease. Mineral supplementation, including trace minerals, is not recommended in this population. Iron supplementation should be individualized and iron stores monitored closely, especially if recombinant human erythropoietin is used to treat anemia. Patients should be counseled to avoid over-the-counter dietary supplements and medications unless approved by their physician.

MONITORING

Ongoing monitoring to prevent and/or treat malnutrition is the most critical aspect in the nutrition care of the CRF patient. Evaluation should include changes in medical status (ie, medications, surgery), review of dietary intake and biochemical parameters, anthropometrics, measurement of urea nitrogen appearance, protein equivalent of nitrogen appearance (PNA), and protein catabolic rate (5,19).

Close monitoring of dietary protein intake (DPI) is critical in the prevention of malnutrition. Dietary recalls are useful but are not always the most accurate way to determine if the patient is complying with protein requirements. PNA can be used to estimate DPI and should be normalized with desirable body weight. This measurement requires a 24-hour urine collection for urine urea and protein analysis. PNA can be calculated as follows (33):

$$\text{PNA(g/day)} = \{6.25 \times [\text{Urinary Urea N (g/day)} + 0.031\ \text{Weight (kg)}]\} + \text{Urinary Protein Losses (g/day)}$$

Additionally, it is recommended that serum albumin *and* edema-free actual body weight or percent standard body weight (NHANES II) *or* subjective global assessment be measured. Refer to Table 3.3 for frequency of these monitoring parameters (5).

The K/DOQI Clinical Practice Guidelines for Nutrition address the treatment plan for patients not meeting protein and energy requirements (5). It states:

> In patients with chronic renal failure (eg, GFR <15 to 20 mL/min) who are not undergoing maintenance dialysis, if protein-energy malnutrition develops or persists despite vigorous attempts to optimize protein and energy intake and there is no apparent cause for malnutrition other than low nutrient intake, initiation of maintenance dialysis or a renal transplant is recommended.

Table 3.3. Recommended Measures for Monitoring Nutritional Status in CKD Patients With GFR <20 mL/min/1.73 m^2

Recommended Measure	*Frequency*
Serum albumin levels	Every 1 to 3 mo
Edema-free actual body weight, % standard body weight, or SGA	Every 1 to 3 mo
nPNA or dietary interviews and diaries	Every 3 to 4 mo

Abbreviations: GFR, glomerular filtration rate; nPNA, normalized protein nitrogen appearance; SGA, subjective global assessment.
Source: Data are from reference 5.

MEDICAL NUTRITION THERAPY

As of January 2002, Medicare began providing payment for medical nutrition therapy (MNT) for non-dialysis kidney disease. MNT services are defined in statute as "nutritional, diagnostic, therapy and counseling services for the purpose of disease management which are furnished by a registered dietitian or nutrition professional . . . pursuant to a referral by a physician" (34). The ultimate goal of MNT is to reduce the burden of nutrition-related illnesses on the patient, payor, and the entire community. Those eligible for reimbursement include patients with GFR 15 to 50 mL/min/1.73m^2. This equates to patients in CKD Stages 3 and 4 or Stage 5 who are not yet on dialysis (3). (More specific information about MNT can be found in Appendix A.)

CONCLUSION

Although it is not absolutely proven that protein-controlled diets delay the progression of renal disease, the diet can be beneficial in minimizing the uremic symptoms. The question of whether these diets promote protein-energy malnutrition has been addressed in the literature (31,35–36). The MDRD research showed that with close monitoring, nutritional status and patient compliance can be maintained on protein-restricted diets. The renal dietitian makes an important contribution as part of the health care team caring for this population. The dietitian's special nutritional assessment skills, understanding of changing renal function, ability to tailor the nutrition plan to the individual's needs, and the expertise to monitor nutritional status, can make nutrition intervention a successful option for the treatment of early kidney disease. Additionally, with the recent MNT Medicare reimbursement, registered dietitians can play an active role in preventing protein-energy malnutrition and ultimately improving patient outcomes.

REFERENCES

1. Hakim RM, Lazarus JM. Initiation of dialysis. *J Am Soc Nephrol.* 1995;6:1319–1328.
2. Holland D, Lam M. Predictors of hospitalization and death amongst pre-dialysis patients: a retrospective study. *Nephrol Dial Transplant.* 2000; 15:650–658.
3. National Kidney Foundation. K/DOQI clinical practice guidelines for chronic kidney disease:

evaluation, classification, and stratification. *Am J Kidney Dis.* 2002;39:S128–S129.

4. Klahr S, Levey AS, Beck GJ, Caggiula AW, Hunsicker L, Kusek JW, Stricker G, and the MDRD Study Group: The effects of dietary protein restriction and blood pressure control on the progression of chronic renal disease. *New Engl J Med.* 1994;330:877–884.
5. National Kidney Foundation. K/DOQI clinical practice guidelines for nutrition in chronic kidney disease. *Am J Kidney Dis.* 2000;35(6 suppl 2): S1–S140.
6. Goldstein DJ, McQuiston BD. Nutrition and renal disease. In: Coulston AM, Rock C, eds. *Nutrition in the Prevention and Treatment of Disease*. San Diego, Calif: Academic Press; 2001:617–636.
7. Shaver MJ. Chronic renal failure. In: Carpenter G, Griggs R, Loscalzo J, eds. *Cecil Essentials of Medicine*. Philadelphia, Pa: WB Saunders; 2001: 291–300.
8. Yousri M, Barri H, Sudhir S. Approach to the patient with renal disease. In: Carpenter G, Griggs R, Loscalzo J, eds. *Cecil Essentials of Medicine*. Philadelphia, Pa: WB Saunders; 2001:232–237.
9. Zawada E. Initiation of dialysis. In: Daugirdas J, Blake P, Ing T, eds. *Handbook of Dialysis*. Philadelphia, Pa: Lippincott Williams & Wilkins; 2001:3–11.
10. Karalis M., McQuiston B. Nutrition management in the Pre-ESRD patient. *Nephrol News Issues*. 2002;16:44–51.
11. Mitch WE. Influences of diet on the progression of chronic renal insufficiency. In: Kopple JD, Massry SG, eds. *Nutritional Management of Renal Disease*. Baltimore, Md: Williams & Wilkins; 1997: 317–340.
12. Brenner BM, Meyer TW, Hostetter T.H. Dietary protein intake and the progressive nature of kidney disease: the role of hemodynamically mediated glomerular injury in the pathogenesis of progressive glomerular sclerosis in aging, renal ablation, and intrinsic renal disease. *New Engl J Med.* 1982;307:652–659.
13. Klahr S. Effects of protein intake on the progression of renal disease. *Annu Rev Nutr.* 1989;9:87–108.
14. Levey AS, Adler S, Caggiula AW, England BK, Greene T, Hunsicker LG, Kusek JW, Rogers NL, Teschan PE. Effects of dietary protein restriction on the progression of advanced renal disease in the Modification of Diet in Renal Disease Study. *Am J Kidney Dis.* 1996;27:652–663.
15. DCCT Research Group. The effect of intensive treatment on the development and progression of long-term complications in insulin-dependent diabetes mellitus. *New Engl J Med.* 1993;329:977–986.
16. American Diabetes Association. Evidence-based nutrition principles and recommendations for the treatment and prevention of diabetes and related complications (Position Statement). *Diabetes Care.* 2002;25:202–212.
17. Blachley J, Knochel J. The biochemistry of uremia. In: Brenner B, Stein J, eds. *Chronic Renal Failure.* New York, NY: Churchill Livingstone; 1981:28–45.
18. Grundy SM, Becker D, Clark LT, Cooper RD, Denke MA, Howard WJ, Hunninghake DB, Illingworth DR, Luepker RV, McBride P, McKenney JM, Pasternak RC, Stone NJ, VanHorn L. Executive summary of the Third Report of the National Cholesterol Education Program (NCEP) expert panel on detection, evaluation, and treatment of high blood cholesterol in adults (adult treatment panel III). *JAMA.* 2001;285:2488–2497.
19. Wiggins K. *Guidelines for Nutrition Care of Renal Patients*. 3rd ed. Chicago, Ill: American Dietetic Association; 2002.
20. McCann L. *Pocket Guide to Nutrition Assessment of the Patient with Chronic Kidney Disease*. 3rd ed. New York, NY: National Kidney Foundation; 2002.
21. Pre-End-Stage Renal Disease. In: *Manual of Clinical Dietetics*. 6th ed. Chicago, Ill: American Dietetic Association; 2000:487–499.
22. Kopple JD, Monteeon RJ, Shaib JK. Effect of energy intake on nitrogen metabolism in nondialyzed patients with chronic renal failure. *Kidney Int.* 1986;29:734–742.
23. National Kidney Foundation Kidney Disease Outcomes Quality Initiative. Clinical practice guidelines on bone metabolism and disease in chronic kidney disease. *Am J Kidney Dis.* 2003:42(suppl 3):S1–S140.
24. National Kidney Foundation. Kidney Disease Outcomes Quality Initiative Clinical Practice Guidelines Cardiovascular Disease in Dialysis Patients (draft version). In press 2004.
25. Levey AS, Beto JA, Coronado BE, Eknoyan G,

Foley RN, Kasiske BL, Klag MJ, Mailoux LU, Manske CL, Meyer KB, Parfrey PS, Pfeffer MA, Wenger NK, Wilson PW, Wright Jr JT. Controlling the epidemic of cardiovascular disease in chronic renal disease: what do we know? What do we need to learn? Where do we go from here? National Kidney Foundation Task Force on Cardiovascular Disease. *Am J Kidney Dis.* 1998;32:853–906.

26. Massry SG, Kopple JD. Requirements for calcium, phosphorus and vitamin D. In: Mitch WE, Klahr S, eds. *Nutrition and the Kidney.* 2nd ed. Boston, Mass: Little Brown and Company; 1993: 96–113.
27. Goodman WG, Goldin J, Kuizon BD, Yoon C, Gales B, Sider D, Wang Y, Chung J, Emerick A, Greaser L, Elashoff RM, Salusky I. Coronary artery calcification in young adults with end-stage renal disease who are undergoing dialysis. *New Engl J Med.* 2000;342:1478–1483.
28. Block GA, Port FK. Re-evaluation of risks associated with hyperphosphatemia and hyperparathyroidism in dialysis patients: recommendations for a change in management. *Am J Kidney Dis.* 2000;35:1226–1237.
29. McCarron DA, Bennett WM, Reusser ME. Adverse effects of sodium restriction with concurrent medication use. *J Ren Nutr.* 1995;5:108–115.
30. Beto J, Bansal VK. Hyperkalemia: evaluating dietary and nondietary etiology. *J Ren Nutr.* 1992; 2:28–29.
31. Kopple JD. Nutritional management of nondialyzed patients with chronic renal failure. In: Kopple JD, Massry SG, eds. *Nutritional Management of Renal Disease.* Baltimore, Md: Williams & Wilkins; 1997:497–531.
32. Smith AS, Goodman DS. The effects of diseases of the liver, thyroid, and kidneys on transport of vitamin A in human plasma. *J Clin Invest.* 1971; 50:2426.
33. Maroni BJ, Steinman TI, Mitch WE. A method for estimating nitrogen intake of patients with chronic renal failure. *Kidney Int.* 1985;27:58–65.
34. Williams ME, Chianchiano D. Medicare medical nutrition therapy: legislative process and product. *J Ren Nutr.* 2002;12:1–7.
35. Kopple JD, Berg R, Houser H, Steinman T, Teschan P. Nutritional status of patients with different levels of chronic renal insufficiency. MDRD Study Group. *Kidney Int.* 1989;36(suppl): S184–S194.
36. Maroni BJ: Requirements for protein, calories, and fat in the predialysis patient. In: Mitch WE, Klahr S, eds. *Nutrition and the Kidney.* 2nd ed. Boston, Mass: Little Brown and Co, 1993:185–212.

Chapter 4

Nutrition Management in Acute Renal Failure

Andrea Bickford, RD, and
Sharon R. Schatz, MS, RD, CSR, CDE

OVERVIEW OF ACUTE RENAL FAILURE

Acute renal failure (ARF) is the rapid, often reversible, deterioration of renal function. Defined by a sudden decline in glomerular filtration rate (GFR) over hours to days, ARF is typically characterized by the retention of nitrogenous waste products, fluid overload, acid-base disturbance, electrolyte imbalance, and hemodynamic instability (1,2). ARF can be present in all settings but is most predominant during hospitalizations, in as many as 5% of all patients and approximately 30% of intensive care unit (ICU) admissions (1,3–6). It is associated with major in-hospital morbidity and mortality that is independent of initiating dialysis. Varying factors that influence prognosis include age, severity of underlying illnesses, number of failed organs, and other serious complications.

Mortality rates range from 7% to 80%, with highest incidence associated with sepsis or shock with a poor or nonfunctioning gastrointestinal tract, cardiorespiratory complications, and hepatic failure as defined by both jaundice and coagulopathy (2,3,7,8). Infection co-exists in 50% to 90% of the cases (1). Preexisting or hospital-acquired malnutrition, frequently seen in patients with ARF, is an important and independent contributor to these higher mortality rates and can be compounded by the catabolic effects of underlying illnesses (9). The increasing size of the elderly population and corresponding comorbid conditions in this group have also affected the incidence and mortality rate of ARF (8,10). Despite advances in clinical support and technologies, the survival rate has not significantly improved during the past 20 years (8,11). Discharged patient survival probability after 5 years for ARF is 50% (12).

ETIOLOGY AND PATHOLOGY

ARF is associated with various conditions such as cancer, pregnancy, pulmonary-renal syndrome, liver disease, nephrotic syndrome, and HIV infection, in addition to trauma, cardiac surgery, and postrenal transplantation. ARF can be classified into three categories: prerenal, postrenal, and intrinsic or parenchymal (Box 4.1). When identified and treated aggressively, prerenal and postrenal ARF are usually reversible with minimal long-term harm and require limited nutrition intervention. If not quickly corrected, both can cause damage to the kidney parenchyma, leading to intrinsic ARF.

Prerenal Causes

Prerenal azotemia is the most common cause of ARF, accounting for approximately 50% to 60% of all cases (11,13). Prerenal ARF is associated with reduction in renal blood flow as with intravascular volume deple-

Box 4.1. Causes of Acute Renal Failure

Prerenal ARF

Intravascular volume depletion

- Hemorrhage, vomiting, diarrhea, surgical drainage, burns, fever, third-spacing, diuretic use, inadequate fluid replacement, hyperemesis of pregnancy, septic abortion, hypoadrenalism

Decreased cardiac output

- Congestive heart failure or cardiomyopathy, valvular heart disease, pulmonary hypertension
- Sepsis syndrome, cirrhosis, hepatorenal syndrome
- Drugs: nonsteroidal anti-inflammatory agents (NSAIDs), angiotensin converting enzyme inhibitors (ACE-I), cyclosporin or tacrolimus, radiocontrast agents, amphotericin B, cocaine, herbs

Postrenal ARF

- Benign prostatic hypertrophy or prostate cancer, cervical cancer, colorectal cancer, intraluminal bladder or pelvic mass, retroperitoneal disorders, neurogenic bladder, urethral strictures, intratubular deposition and obstructions (uric acid and oxylate, sulfonamides, acyclovir, methotrexate)

Intrinsic or Parenchymal ARF

Vascular disease

- Atheroembolic disease, thrombotic thrombocytopenic purpura, hemolytic uremic syndrome, post partum ARF, renal artery occlusion, thrombosis, vasculitis

Interstitial nephritis

- Allergic reactions (antibiotics, allopurinol, NSAIDs, diurectics, ACE-I), acute pyelonephritis, infiltrative diseases (lymphoma, leukemia, sarcoidosis), infections (cytomegalovirus or candidiasis)

Glomerular disease

- Glomerulonephritis and vasculitis (systemic lupus erythromatosis), small vessel vasculitis (Wegener's granulomatosis), IgA nephropathy, postinfection, radiation nephritis, scleroderma, hemolytic uremic syndrome, toxemia of pregnancy

Acute tubular necrosis

- Ischemia: major surgery, hypotension, cardiogenic, septic or hypovolemic shock, obstetric complications
- Nephrotoxicity: acyclovir, aminoglycoside antibiotics, amphotericin B, acetaminophen, NSAIDs, radiocontrast agents/dyes, chemotherapy agents (cisplatin, cyclosporin/tacrolimus), organic solvents (ethylene glycol and toluene), heavy metals, pigments, cocaine
- Intratubular deposition and obstruction: myeloma proteins, uric acid, oxylates, acyclovir, methotrexate, sulphonamides

Source: Data are from references 1,3,11,13,16.

tion, decreased cardiac output, sepsis syndrome, cirrhosis, hepatorenal syndrome, or drug interactions (3, 5,14). Each can lead to a decline in urine and sodium output and a buildup of nitrogenous waste products. Diagnostic signs include a low urinary sodium level of less than 10 mEq/L, high urine osmolality of more than 350 to 500 mOsm/kg, and a blood urea nitrogen (BUN) to creatinine ratio of more than 20:1 (1,3,11,13). Prerenal ARF has high prevalence in the elderly population due to general decline in renal function; use of multiple medications; and increased risk of dehydration associated with decreased urine concentration, impairment in thirst regulation, and reduced sodium retention (15). Early diagnosis and restoration of circulating blood volume to the kidneys is essential. Prerenal azotemia should reverse within 1 to 2 days after renal perfusion is restored, but recovery may be delayed in those with substantial decline in baseline renal function (3). Limited nutrition intervention is necessary if the underlying cause is corrected and volume status is promptly restored.

Postrenal Causes

Postrenal ARF results from an obstruction of the urine flow and accounts for approximately 5% to 15% of all cases (5,14). This may be caused by prostate, gynecological, or bladder cancers; benign prostate hyperplasia; calculi; or blood clots or strictures (3,5). The elderly and young are most commonly affected (11,15). Often, patients with severe oliguria (urine volume of <400mL/day) or anuria (urine volume of <50 mL/day) are more likely to have postrenal ARF (16). Other diagnostic signs may include urine osmolality of more than 400 mOsm/kg early and approximately 300 mOsm/kg late with a BUN to creatinine ratio of 10:1 to 20:1 (11). Azotemia usually resolves by correcting the obstruction and resuming normal hydration. Again, minimal nutrition management is typically needed.

Intrinsic or Parenchymal Causes

Intrinsic ARF is associated with actual tissue damage to the renal parenchyma and accounts for 20% to 30% of all cases (14). Frequently, the patient will present with increased azotemia, marked electrolyte disturbances including hyperkalemia and hyponatremia, urine sodium concentrations of more than 30 to 40 mEq/L, a urine osmolality of less than 350mOsm/kg, and BUN to creatinine ratio of 10:1 to 20:1 (1,3,11,13). The kidney's four compartments can classify causes: vascular (renal artery occlusions, atheroembolisms), interstitial (allergic interstitial nephritis), glomerular (glomerulonephritis, systemic disorders), and tubular (ischemic or nephrotoxic acute tubular necrosis [ATN]) (11,16). ATN, the most common cause, is associated with prolonged systemic hypotension, prerenal hypoperfusion, or damage associated with pharmacologic agents or poisons (11). Atherosclerotic vascular disease in the aging population, widespread use of vasoactive drugs, and frequency of invasive vascular procedures have also led to increased incidence (11,15). ATN is usually associated with oliguria and acute onset or worsening of azotemia, even after withdrawal of the causative agent and replacement of adequate fluid (13).

The clinical course of ATN occurs in three phases (1,16):

- Initiating phase:
  - Period between onset and established renal failure.
  - Usually reversible by treating the underlying disorder or removing the offending agent.
  - Time frame: hours or days.
- Maintenance phase:
  - Epithelial cell injury.
  - Urine output is at its lowest and complications associated with uremia, fluid overload, and electrolyte imbalance (decreased sodium, increased potassium levels) can occur.
  - Time frame: 10 to 16 days in oliguric patients and 5 to 8 days in nonoliguric patients.
- Recovery phase:
  - Defined by tubule cell regeneration and gradual return of GFR.
  - BUN and creatinine levels return to near normal.
  - May be complicated by marked diuresis, dehydration, and fluid and electrolyte imbalance (increased sodium, decreased potassium levels) if not closely monitored.
  - Time frame: days to months.

METABOLIC ALTERATIONS

ARF is associated with substantial alterations in protein, carbohydrate, and lipid metabolism in addition to disturbances in fluid and electrolyte balance, divalent cation homeostasis, and urinary acidification mechanisms. Metabolic changes cannot solely be attributed to the uremic state and loss of excretory function. Consideration needs to be given to underlying causes, accompanying catabolism in the critically ill, and treatment modality and frequency. These contributors should not be viewed as separate issues when addressing the patient's nutrition care. It is important to understand the metabolic mechanisms and how they impact one another. Nutrient requirements for the metabolic alterations of ARF need to be met instead of just adapting for those of chronic renal failure (CRF) (17).

Protein Catabolism

The distinctive characteristic of ARF's metabolic alterations is the accelerated protein breakdown that cannot be effectively suppressed by providing exogenous nutrient substrates (18). Renal failure is responsible for increasing the severity and duration of the catabolic phase leading to stronger consequences. Starvation can potentiate this response. Several kilograms of muscle may be lost, resulting in a reduction of lean body mass (19). Immune response and physiological defense against infection may also be compromised.

There are causes other than uremic effects. Insulin resistance in ARF is the main trigger of the muscle catabolism (17). The maximal rate of protein synthesis that is stimulated by insulin is depressed, and protein degradation is increased (17). Other hormonal derangements, including a concomitant increase in insulin and insulin counter-regulatory hormones such as glucagon, catecholamines, and cortisol, can further exacerbate these metabolic alterations. Acidosis, which acts by a glucocorticoid-dependent pathway, is an important mediator of muscular protein breakdown, resulting in negative nitrogen balance (6,17,20). In addition, increased secretion of parathyroid hormone can promote protein catabolism in uremia, enhancing amino acid release from muscle tissue and decreasing tissue responsiveness to insulin through inhibition of insulin secretion by pancreatic beta cells (6,17,21). Protein degradation is increased and anabolism is decreased by abnormalities in the growth hormone/insulin-like growth factor (21,22).

Carbohydrate Metabolism

Hyperglycemia often develops due to peripheral insulin resistance early in the course of ARF. Glucose uptake by skeletal muscles can decrease by 50% (17). In uremia there may be a defect in insulin action with a decrease in both insulin clearance and secretion (6,21, 23). Increased hepatic gluconeogenesis from amino acids is insensitive to the negative feedback normally induced by a glucose load and further increases blood sugar levels and possibly insulin requirements. Coexistence of diabetes or medications such as corticosteroids or immunosuppressants may also play a role here. Hyperglycemia raises the metabolic rate, and fat synthesis and deposition in the liver, leading to hepatic dysfunction, carbon dioxide production, minute ventilation, and insulin and catecholamine secretion (24). High blood glucose levels are associated with impaired wound healing, higher risk of infection, delayed weaning from mechanical ventilation, and abnormalities in cellular functions related to catabolism (25). Glucose, an osmotically active agent, can lead to fluid and electrolyte disturbances such as intracellular dehydration, hyperosmolar coma, hyponatremia, and dehydration.

Lipid Metabolism

Altered lipid metabolism and clearance can be linked to impaired lipolysis and can occur within 48 to 96 hours of renal deterioration (14). Activities of peripheral lipoprotein lipase and hepatic triglyceride lipase are reduced to less than half of normal during ARF. Metabolic acidosis and insulin resistance may inhibit the action of lipoprotein lipase (20). Total cholesterol and high-density lipoprotein (HDL) levels are frequently decreased (17,23,26). Observed elevated triglycerides can be linked to higher very-low–density lipoprotein (VLDL) and low-density lipoprotein (LDL) concentrations related to an increased rate of synthesis by the liver and decreased clearance due to inhibition of lipoprotein lipase (26). Long- and medium-chain triglyceride clearances are reduced 50% to 60% during ARF, although this can be partially reversed by the administration of amino acids and glucose (14,23). Intravenous infusion of lipid emulsions has delayed clearance where the elimination half-life is doubled (20). Despite the decreased lipolytic activity, endogenous lipids are well metabolized and can be used depending on the individual's tolerance to them (26).

Acidosis

ARF is commonly complicated by metabolic acidosis. This may be severe due to endogenous production of hydrogen ions by diabetic or fasting ketoacidosis, lactic acidosis complicating generalized tissue hypoperfusion, liver disease, sepsis, and metabolism of ethylene glycol or methanol (1).

Other Complications

Anemia develops rapidly in ARF. This is multifactorial and could be due to impaired erythropoiesis, hemolysis, bleeding, hemodilution, and decreased red blood cell survival time (1). The patient's underlying illness or recent surgery may also be a factor. Mild gastrointestinal bleeding occurring in 10% to 30% of the patients due to stress ulceration of gastric or small intestine mucosa may also contribute to anemia (27). In contrast to CRF, treatment with erythropoetin and/or iron replacement is typically not initiated with ARF and can be contraindicated with acute illness.

Uremic syndrome may be due to unidentified toxins that are possibly urea or other products of nitrogen metabolism (1). Symptoms include nausea, vomiting, pericarditis, pleuritis, mental status changes, cardiac tamponade, and ileus (1,3). Neuropsychiatric disturbances in ARF include lethargy, confusion, stupor, coma, agitation, psychosis, asterixis, myoclonus, hyperreflexia, and restless leg (1). Gastritis, stomatitis or gingivitis, parotitis, or pancreatitis may occur. Cardiac complications may also be present.

IMPLICATIONS OF DIALYSIS

Initiation of renal replacement therapy is frequently recommended for patients with pronounced azotemia, electrolyte imbalance, volume overload, severe acidosis that is resistant to conservative measures, or when significant symptoms of uremia are present (11). There is no consensus about when to start dialysis, but it is used in 85% of the patients with oliguric ARF and in 30% of those with nonoliguric ARF (8). The purpose of initiating dialysis is not only to correct or treat these complications but also to provide adequate renal support to maintain the essential functions of other organs (28). Conventional hemodialysis remains the standard treatment if the patient is hemodynamically stable (28,29).

Due to the risk of hypotension and wide swings in body weight, use of slower, ongoing methods for the removal of fluid and solutes through continuous renal replacement therapies (CRRT) has become more frequently used in patients with unstable cardiovascular status or severe volume overload (30). With CRRT, blood is slowly removed from the body, passed through a hemofilter, and then returned to the patient. Access can either be arteriovenous (AV), which relies on the patient's mean arterial pressure to drive the process, or venovenous (VV), which requires a pump-driven circuit to maintain control of blood flow. Types of continuous therapies include the following (30–33):

- *Continuous hemofiltration (CAVH, CVVH):* Clearance occurs through convection or movement of fluid across a membrane where solute transfer is a consequence of transmembrane pressure gradient or "solute drag."
- *Continuous hemodialysis (CAVHD, CVVHD) or sustained low-efficiency dialysis (SLED):* Ultrafiltration volume may be replaced with alternative fluid, which is similar in composition to plasma. Clearance occurs through diffusion as with conventional hemodialysis in which molecules in a solvent move from a region of higher concentration to that of a lower concentration. Provides continuous hemodialysis with slower blood and dialysate flow rates.
- *Continuous hemodialfiltration (CAVHDF, CVVHDF):* Clearance occurs through a mix of both convection and diffusion as noted previously.
- *Slow continuous ultrafiltration (SCUF):* Clearance is limited purely to ultrafiltration.

Peritoneal dialysis (PD) is another modality choice for ARF, although it is used less often in the United States than hemodialysis or continuous renal replacement therapies. PD may have advantages regarding reduced incidence of septicemia and hypotension, in addition to decreased need for systemic anticoagulation, but it may be contraindicated when large volume or solute clearances are needed (1,30,32,34). It is most frequently used in pediatric patients or those with severe coagulopathy, and possibly in remote rural areas where access to technology is more limited (1,32,34).

Regardless of the modality chosen, all renal replacement therapies (RRT) have nutritional implications. Protein or amino acid losses can average 5 to 15 g per day with HD and CRRT but may be reduced with glucose containing dialysate (14,23). Protein losses can be higher in PD, averaging 10 to 20 g per day (14). Changes in glutamine metabolism have been associated with CVVHD, with as much as a 33% decrease upon initiation, and supplementation may be indicated during the first few days of use or in selected ICU patients (23,35). Potential exposure to excessive amounts of lactate from CRRT solutions may contribute to protein catabolism, especially in acute and chronic liver failure or in conditions with increased lactate formation such as circulatory shock, septic shock, or hypoxia (36). Biocompatible membranes have been recommended to deter activation of inflammatory agents to reduce rates of catabolism, although the nutritional advantage has not been proven (4,8,26).

Carbohydrate absorption from dextrose-containing solutions and lactate must be considered, especially with provision of parenteral nutrition. Failure to account for these additional kilocalories may result in overfeeding (23,37). Dextrose-free dialysate promotes glucose loss during continuous hemodiafiltration, but the loss is small and predictable (24). Use of dextrose-containing ultrafiltrate replacement fluid results in significant increase in glucose; however, glucose losses in effluent is less predictable (24). Glucose absorption can approach 35% to 45% from dialysate or replacement fluids equivalent to 140 to 355 g glucose/day (24). The estimated absorption rate for each liter of dialysate infused per hour is as follows (23):

Dialysate glucose concentration (%)	*Absorption (g/hr)*
1.5	5.8
2.5	11.4
4.25	14.9

Dialysate solutions (1.5%) can be infused at 2 liters per hour with an estimated absorption rate of 9.6 g per hour (23). Solutions containing 45 mmol/L of lactate can provide additional calories: approximately 12 kcal/L (23).

With CVVHD, the blood flow is controlled, and therefore the rate of glucose transfer across the dialysis membrane should be relatively constant, allowing for a single measure to estimate glucose transfer over longer periods of time (Box 4.2).

The amount transferred is dependent on several interacting variables, including the glucose concentration of the dialysate solution, dialysate flow rate, blood flow rate, ultrafiltration rate, and the patient's blood glucose. Substitution fluid used in CRRT should contain glucose in a concentration of 100 to 180 mg/dL to maintain a zero glucose balance (36).

With continuous hemodiafiltration, phosphorus clearance can be achieved and maintained more rapidly with increased risk of hypophosphatemia if not monitored closely (38). Losses of calcium, water-soluble vitamins, and carnitine have also been demonstrated (23,36,39). Removal of antioxidant nutrients during CRRT can contribute to profound impairment of the oxygen radical scavenger system that is present in the critically ill (23,36). CRRT replacement fluids are typically magnesium-free, resulting in significant losses of magnesium and negative nitrogen balance (39). Losses of vitamin C, copper, and chromium in ultrafiltrate have been detected, but the clinical significance is unclear (40).

Box 4.2. Glucose Absorption in CVVHD

Use the following formula to calculate glucose absorption from CVVHD:

$$\text{Glu Added} = (\text{Glu In} - \text{Glu Out}) \times \text{BFR} \times k$$

Where: Glu out = blood flowing from patient to dialyzer; Glu in = blood returning to the patient; BFR = blood flow rate; k = conversion factor = 0.0144

Source: Data are from reference 25.

NUTRITION ASSESSMENT

Close monitoring of the patient's nutritional status through physical assessment, including subjective global assessment (SGA), anthropometrics, laboratory values, and strict intake and output (I&Os), is essential throughout the disease process. (Refer to Chapter 2 for additional information.) Classic nutrition assessment parameters are not always appropriate in patients with ARF, especially for those in the ICU.

Anthropometrics

Anthropometric evaluation should include height, edema-free body weight, percent of ideal or standard body weight, and percent change in body weight (2). Use of actual body weight needs to be interpreted with caution because it typically reflects changes in fluid status. It is not uncommon for postoperative ARF patients to have as much as 10 L of fluid overload due to fluid replacement during surgery. Weight gains of more than 0.5 to 1 kg per day usually represent fluid retention, not tissue synthesis. Interdialytic weight changes must also be considered when evaluating daily weights. Comparing pre-illness usual body weight with edema-free body weight is advantageous to determine fluid status and identify changes or wasting of lean body mass (2). Checking for complications associated with hypovolemia and fluid overload such as edema, bibasilar lung rales and crackles, increased jugular venous pressure, pleural effusion, and pulmonary edema should be part of the ongoing assessment (1–3,21). Triceps skinfold and mid-arm muscle circumference measurements may be helpful, but may be distorted by fluid retention. To be beneficial, serial measurements are needed and they should be performed after dialysis when the patient is at dry weight. Although limited data are available on its use in the critically ill population, SGA successfully identified patients with malnutrition at admission and was shown to be an independent predictor of in-hospital mortality (9). Benefits of bioelectrical impedance have not been demonstrated in the critically ill, and this is typically used exclusively in research facilities (20,21).

Laboratory Assessment

Patients with ARF have changes in serum proteins similar to those seen in nonrenal malnutrition or during acute illness. Albumin concentrations may be falsely low due to fluid overload, intravascular fluid shifts (third-spacing), or liver damage, or may be elevated with use of exogenous albumin infusions (2,23). Changes in response to catabolism or nutritional supplementation may not occur until late in the acute disease process (21). Prealbumin may be more sensitive to immediate changes in visceral protein status; however, because it is cleared by the kidneys, it may be falsely elevated in ARF (21). Insulin growth factor-1 (IGF-1) is a newer parameter that has shown a positive response to nutrition support in renal patients diagnosed with infections; this indicates that IGF-1 may be used as a specific marker for malnutrition in hemodialysis. (21,41).

BUN and creatinine levels during ARF are more related to changes in kidney function and less reflective of nutritional status (2,21). Together, these indices are useful in assessing nutritional status and are predictive of morbidity and mortality. They should be routinely drawn and evaluated. The patient's baseline levels prior to the original insult or development of ARF should be used to determine preexisting nutrition risk status.

The standard method for determining nitrogen balance requires a creatinine clearance of more than 50 mL/min/1.73m^2 for accurate interpretation (42). In patients with ARF, urea nitrogen appearance (UNA) is a more appropriate method for determining nitrogen balance and may assist in determining adequate delivery of protein and calories. However, this calculation is tedious and infrequently used in the clinical setting (2,14). Due to increased catabolic rates with any type of critical illness, PCR should not be used as a reliable index of protein intake (21).

UNA is defined as the amount of urinary urea nitrogen plus the change in the urea nitrogen pool. It is calculated as follows:

$$\text{UNA (g)} = \text{UUN} + [(\text{BUN2} - \text{BUN1}) \times 0.6 \times \text{BW1}] + [(\text{BW2} - \text{BW1}) \times \text{BUN2}]$$

Where: Net protein breakdown = UNA × 6.25; UUN = urinary urea nitrogen (g/24 hr); BUN1 = initial collection of blood urea nitrogen, postdialysis (g/L), BUN2 = final collection of blood urea nitrogen, predialysis (g/L); BW1 = postdialysis weight (kg); BW2 = predialysis weight (kg).

A UNA of less than 6 indicates mild stress; a UNA of 6 to 10 indicates moderate stress; and a UNA of more than 10 indicates severe stress (2,6). Frequent complications in ARF include hyponatremia, hyperkalemia, hyperphosphatemia, hypocalcemia, hypermagnesemia, and metabolic acidosis. These complications have implications for nutrition care planning (1,3). Given the nature of ARF and its treatment, the patient's metabolic status is subject to change, necessitating alterations in nutrition therapy. Serum electrolytes should be monitored daily during ARF to prevent or correct any imbalances. Mineral levels of calcium, magnesium, and phosphorus should be checked weekly with the frequency varying per patient stability, more so with CRRT.

Additional considerations in laboratory assessment include sodium, potassium, phosphorus, calcium, magnesium, vitamins, and trace elements.

Sodium

Hyponatremia can occur with excess ingestion of water or excessive provisions of hypotonic saline or isotonic dextrose during or after medical and/or surgical procedures and as renal replacement fluid, especially while urine output is impaired (1,36).

Hypernatremia can occur if water losses via hypotonic urine are not replaced or are inappropriately replaced by hypertonic solutions (27). Risk of hypernatremia is heightened during the diuretic phase of ARF.

Potassium

Although hypokalemia occurs infrequently, it can be a result of extracellular to intracellular shifts. This is seen with carbohydrate delivery within the first few days of initiating nutrition support or in anabolism if potassium replacement is insufficient (2,37). Magnesium deficiency may cause hypokalemia that may be resistant to potassium supplementation (37).

Hyperkalemia may be exacerbated by metabolic acidosis and may be severe in rhabdomyolysis, hemolysis, and tumor lysis syndrome (1,3,43). Elimination of potassium supplements or drugs in a potassium salt form, use of insulin and intravenous (IV) glucose, IV administration of sodium bicarbonate or calcium gluconate, potassium-binding resins such as sodium polystryrene sulfonate, diuretics, and dialysis may be recommended to restore normal potassium levels (1,3).

Phosphorus

Hypophosphatemia can develop with CRRT if not monitored closely. Most RRT solutions do not contain phosphorus, and this can aggravate hypophosphatemia (36). Concomitant use of phosphorus-free parenteral nutrition can also increase risk of phosphate depletion (36). Excessive or inappropriate use of phosphate binders, especially as renal function recovers, can contribute to lower phosphorus levels, too. Refeeding syndrome can also contribute to hypophosphatemia.

Hyperphosphatemia is an anticipated consequence of ARF (27). Mild hyperphosphatemia (5–10 mg/dL) is common; but it may be severe (10–20 mg/dL) in highly catabolic patients (1). Initiation of phosphorus binders may be necessary to correct or prevent further elevations.

Calcium

Hypocalcemia can be a result of tissue resistance to the action of parathyroid hormone and lower levels of 1,25-dihydroxy vitamin D over time or metastatic deposition of calcium phosphate in soft tissues with elevated calcium-phosphate products (27,39). It may also be due to inadequate supplementation especially with CRRT. Patients with hypocalcemia are often asymptomatic but may be more symptomatic with rhabdomyolysis, acute pancreatitis, or after treatment of acidosis with bicarbonate. Magnesium deficiency may also cause a calcium deficiency.

Hypercalcemia can develop as a result of excessive calcium supplementation, immobilization, fractures, or various disease states. Late-onset hypercalcemia can develop with hyperparathyroidism (39).

Serum total calcium should be corrected for hypoalbuminemia. Refer to Chapter 2 for the equation for calculating corrected calcium.

Magnesium

Mild asymptomatic hypermagnesemia may occur with oliguric ARF and reflects impaired excretion of ingested magnesium from the diet or magnesium-containing laxatives or antacids (1). It may be due to drugs injuring the loop of Henle (1).

Hypomagnesemia is generally seen in 20% to 44% among the critically ill, even when patients are monitored for total parenteral nutrition (TPN). This could reflect the acute-phase response to illness rather than magnesium status.

Vitamins and Trace Elements

Vitamin status in ARF has not been extensively studied and may differ from that seen in CRF. Serum levels of vitamins A, C, D, and E have shown to be decreased beyond the losses in CRRT (17,23,26,40,44). Vitamin K levels are either normal or elevated (17). Antioxidants are likely decreased due to oxidative stress, but the ARF may also contribute to the depletion (23,40).

Metabolism of trace elements in ARF represents unspecific alterations within the spectrum of an acute-phase reaction and do not reflect effects induced by ARF (20). Selenium concentration in plasma and erythrocytes is decreased (17,23,26,30,40). There was no difference in this depletion when patients undergoing CRRT were compared with others in the ICU (40). Zinc levels may also be decreased, but this is not consistently shown (39,40). Iron levels in plasma are lower, while those of copper are increased (20).

NUTRITIONAL NEEDS

Nutritional needs must be based on the patient's clinical condition, degree of catabolism, laboratory values, fluid status, and type and frequency of dialysis. Estimated needs should be continually reevaluated because overall status, renal function, dialysis therapy, and stress levels may change (Table 4.1).

Energy

Calories should be provided to meet energy requirements and minimize protein degradation without in-

Table 4.1. Daily Dietary Recommendations for Adult ARF

Nutrient	*Recommendations*
Energy	Basal energy expenditure (BEE) × stress factor (1.2–1.3) or 25–35 kcal/kg
Protein	0.8–1.2 g/kg noncatabolic, without dialysis 1.2–1.5 g/kg catabolic and/or initiation of dialysis
Fluid	24–hour urine output + 500 mL for insensible losses (Approximately 750–1500 mL) Increase fluid to prevent dehydration during diuresis, with CRRT, and as needed for increased insensible loss as with fever, sepsis or burns.
Sodium	2.0–3.0 g (87–130 mmol) Needs may increase to replace additional losses with diuresis.
Potassium	2.0–3.0 g (50–80 mmol) Requirements depend on lab values and degree of hyperkalemia. Needs may increase with dialysis, diuresis/return of kidney function, and anabolism.
Phosphorus	8–15 mg/kg (0.25–0.48 mmol/kg) May need to include phosphate binders Requirements may increase with CRRT/daily dialysis, return of kidney function, and anabolism.

Source: Data are from references 6,17,18,46.

creasing the risk of overfeeding. Energy requirements should be based on the underlying disease state or complications because ARF has limited effect on energy expenditure (45). Additional energy requirements are minimal with ARF because there is a 10% energy savings with the absence of normal kidney metabolism. If, however, intermittent dialysis is initiated, metabolic rates can increase slightly by 15% to 20% (6,26,37). Even in hypermetabolic conditions, such as sepsis or multiple organ failure, energy expenditure rarely exceeds 130% of calculated basal energy expenditure (6,45). Indirect calorimetry, when available, should be used to help estimate energy needs and determine substrate utilization, especially when potential for overfeeding exists. Typical recommendations for energy needs are based on the Harris-Benedict equation for predicted basal energy expenditure (BEE) with a stress factor of 1.2 to 1.3, or 25 to 35 kcal/kg/day (6,17). Use of ideal/standard body weight vs actual dry weight to determine energy needs continues to be debated. Current nutrition guidelines typically are based on use of ideal body weight; however, in instances such as morbid obesity, significant underweight status, or amputations, use of actual or usual weight may be more appropriate (46). Adjusted body weight has also been used for the obese. Overfeeding can result in fatty degeneration of the liver, increased release of stress hormones, elevated body temperature, and carbon dioxide production, which may delay weaning from ventilator (45). Although underfeeding can result in further negative nitrogen balance, complications may be less deleterious than with overfeeding.

Protein

Recommendations for optimal allowance of protein are still somewhat controversial. Protein or amino acid requirements for noncatabolic patients should not be restricted to less than 0.8 g/kg/day unless renal insufficiency will be brief and dialysis is not necessary (17). To compensate for amino acid losses during RRT, daily protein intake can be increased by 0.2 to 0.3 g/kg/day (18,39). Patients undergoing RRT should receive at least 1.2 g/kg/day with additional protein as needed for repletion (6). Intakes more than 1.5 g/kg/day have been ineffective at further ameliorating negative nitrogen balance and may enhance the formation of urea and other nitrogenous waste products (4,18). It may not be possible to force protein synthesis in ARF by increasing amino acid intake as the metabolic pathways for protein and insulin are defective (39).

Micronutrients

Additional dietary modifications may involve sodium, potassium, and phosphorus; however, the diet should be liberalized as much as possible to promote adequate oral intake. Requirements should be continually reevaluated as needs may change with the routine assessment of oral intake, recovery of kidney function, use of dialysis, and anabolism.

Vitamin recommendations are not well defined and are typically based on healthy subjects or patients with chronic renal failure and do not necessarily apply to patients in ARF (44). Additional water-soluble vitamins including 1 mg/day of folate and 1 mg/day of pyridoxine are suggested (14). To prevent oxalate deposition, vitamin C doses should not exceed 100 to 200 mg/day (14,17,37). Further study is needed regarding whether vitamin D supplementation for ESRD applies to ARF (44). Routine supplementation of vitamins A and E may be needed (44). Dietary Reference Intakes (DRIs) of vitamin K have been regarded as safe, as no toxicities have been reported with low-dose supplementation (44).

The actual micronutrient requirements for CRRT are unknown (23). In critically ill patients selenium replacement improved clinical outcome and reduced the incidence of ARF requiring CRRT (17).

NUTRITION SUPPORT CONSIDERATIONS

The goals of nutrition support for ARF are similar to those of other catabolic diseases. Multiple routes of nutrition delivery may be initiated during the course of ARF. The decision to start nutrition support is based on the patient's nutritional status, tolerance to feedings, gastrointestinal impairment, type and severity of underlying disease, and degree of catabolism (20).

Oral Intake

The oral route is always the preferred mode of feeding; however, this may not be possible with acutely ill, hypercatabolic patients (17). In addition to previously stated factors that may negatively impact food intake, the following need to be considered: treatment schedules and testing; the experience of being in the hospital, especially in an ICU environment; physical ability to eat and possible need for feeding assistance; and constraints of the hospital foodservice system and provision of food that differs from the patient's preferences. The dietitian will need to interface medical, physical, and psychosocial influences in trying to achieve adequate food consumption. Nutrition supplements may be needed to augment intake. Choice of product will depend on hospital formulary, product composition as it compares with the patient's individual nutritional and fluid needs, and of course, patient acceptance. (See Chapter 13.)

Tube Feeding

Nutrition therapy should not be delayed due to the risk of renal failure, but nutrition intervention is only indicated after the acute phase of shock has been managed (8,26,47). Enteral feeding may actually improve renal function as fewer amino acids (AA) perfuse the kidney due to their hepatic metabolism that is not needed for the parenteral route (48). Tube feedings may be used in conjunction with an oral diet to achieve adequate intake (2). Parenteral nutrition can be used simultaneously because even a small amount of nutrients supplied via the gastrointestinal tract has a major role in enterocyte metabolism (2,26).

At present, there are a few formulas that are specific for ARF; products with only essential amino acids (EAAs) are incomplete and not indicated (17). Ready-to-use renal formulas for hemodialysis may offer a reasonable alternative (17). However, these may be unable to meet the high protein needs of a hypercatabolic patient without the addition of more modular protein. Choice of product and prescription recommendations should not only be based on provision of energy and protein, but also on total fluid and electrolyte and mineral content. Determination of feeding rate should consider the number of hours that it can actually infuse given the demands of therapies including dialysis and other interruptions, especially in the ICU. Enrichment by glutamine, arginine, nucleotides, or n-3 fatty acids for immune function might exert beneficial effects; but more studies are needed (17,26). (Refer to Chapter 13 for additional information on enteral supplementation.)

Parenteral Nutrition

When initiating total parenteral nutrition (TPN), the metabolic consequences and alterations in nutrient balances that are induced by RRT must be considered (17). Solutions containing both EAA and nonessential amino acids (NEAA) should be used in ARF. The use of EAA to synthesize NEAA has no advantage and wastes energy (18). Several NEAAs, such as histidine, arginine, tyrosine, serine, and cysteine, may become indispensable in patients with ARF (17). Hyperammonemia and metabolic encephalopathy can occur when EAA are used for more than 2 to 3 weeks (49). NEAAs including arginine, ornithine, and citrulline need to be supplied in renal failure to enable detoxification of ammonia via the Krebs urea cycle (49). Deficiency of NEAAs may disrupt normal protein synthesis (37). In light of these concerns, EAAs should be used solely in cases of very-low protein catabolism, no need for dialysis, no wasting, and for periods of time less than 2 weeks (6). Use of specific AA solutions is not supported by clinical studies (26). There is no persuasive evidence that AA solutions rich in branched chain amino acids (BCAA) promote anabolism in ARF (18).

Although the metabolism of lipids is impaired, this should not prevent their use in TPN (17,26). Lipids remain a predominant substrate for oxidation in ARF as shown by a low respiratory quotient (26). Advantages of using medium-chain triglycerides in ARF have not been substantiated (20,26).

Hyperglycemia impacts glucose use in TPN. Lower glucose loads may be needed if the patient is absorbing a significant amount from dialysate or ultrafiltrate replacement (24). Calories received from CRRT must be considered in order to prevent overfeeding (23).

Volume of fluid delivery should be adjusted against the patient's fluid status, adjusted based on urine output, dialysis and RRT, and need of fluid replacement. Dextrose concentrations of 70%, lipid emulsions with 20% or 30%, and amino acid concentrations of 10% to 15% can be used to reduce the nutrition to a smaller volume (37).

Electrolyte content is dependent on the patient's status and is subject to change. To prevent expensive waste of inappropriate solutions, TPN should not be used to attempt electrolyte corrections (14). Additional IV supplementation may be needed for sodium, potassium, calcium, phosphorus, and magnesium. Zinc in IV bolus is not required, and may even be toxic during CRRT (39). The exact required amounts for trace elements and vitamins in ARF are unknown (17,37). Recommendations for trace elements range from two to three times per week. (See Chapter 14.)

Monitoring

Monitoring of nutrition care in ARF patients is similar to that for other patients. Early detection of feeding complications can hasten changes in feeding regimens to improve tolerance (14). Any exaggerated protein or amino acid intake results in a high BUN (20). Due to fluctuations in electrolyte balance, especially with CRRT, closer follow-up may be indicated with lab data being checked twice per day. When feeding is first initiated, the glucose, phosphorus, and potassium levels are particularly prone to change and require close attention (20). Glucose and potassium may be obtained one to six times per day in unstable patients (20). Ammonia, transaminases, and bilirubin should be checked twice weekly in unstable patients and weekly in stable patients (20). Precise intake and output data is required given the contributions from multiple sources of fluid including nutrition, medications, all IVs, and replacement fluid for CRRT. Caloric intake from all possible origins needs to be assessed to make appropriate adjustments with estimated goals compared to what was actually received (14). The critically ill patient with ARF will require daily intervention by the dietitian.

Nutrition is often inadequately supervised because it is only one facet of life-supporting procedures, monitoring tasks, and therapies that competes for access to the patient with ARF (39). The dietitian can play a key role here because collaboration is needed with the health care team to foster care plans for optimal nutrient delivery (14).

CONCLUSION

ARF is extremely complex, without consensus about the most appropriate course of treatment. Although nutrition support has not been demonstrated to improve outcomes consistently, it is possible that the absence of nutrition support could have further deleterious effects. Malnutrition is an obvious consequence given the severity of the catabolism, metabolic alterations, and complications that occur in ARF. Compounding this is the patient's loss of appetite and inability to eat due to a myriad of reasons; nutrient losses via RRT also contribute to the problem. Patients often die from the severity of the underlying disease and complications (23). Nutrition support requires an integrated, overall view of energy, protein, fluid, and electrolyte metabolism (23). By being aware of all of these components, dietitians better serve patients by developing nutrition care plans that encompass all aspects of their needs. It therefore remains a challenge that requires a breadth of skills and knowledge.

REFERENCES

1. Brady HR, Brenner BM, Clarkson MR, Lieberthal W. Acute renal failure. In: Brenner B, ed. *The Kidney*. Vol 1. 6th ed. Philadelphia, Pa: WB Saunders; 2000:1201–1262.
2. Butler B. Nutritional management of catabolic acute renal failure requiring renal replacement therapy. *ANNA J*. 1991;18:247–254.
3. Mindell JA, Chertow GM. A practical approach to acute renal failure. *Med Clin North Am*. 1997;81:731–748.
4. Bozfakioglu S. Nutrition in patients with acute renal failure. *Nephrol Dial Transplant*. 2001;16(Suppl 6):21–22.
5. Nally J. Acute renal failure in hospitalized patients. *Cleve Clin J Med*. 2002;69:569–574.

6. Riella MC. Nutrition in acute renal failure. *Ren Fail.* 1997;19:237–252.
7. Block CA, Manning HL. Prevention of acute renal failure in the critically ill. *Am J Respir Crit Care Med.* 2002;165:320–324.
8. Star R. Treatment of acute renal failure. *Kidney Int.* 1998;54:1817–1831.
9. Fiaccadori E, Lombardi M, Leonardi S, Rotelli CF, Tortorella G, Borghetti A. Prevalence and clinical outcome associated with preexisting malnutrition in acute renal failure: a prospective cohort study. *J Am Soc Nephrol.* 1999;10:581–593.
10. Van de Noortgate N, Verbeke F, Dhondt A, Colardijn F, Van Biesen W, Vahnolder R, Lameire N. The dialytic management of acute renal failure in the elderly. *Semin Dial.* 2002;15:127–132.
11. Albright RC. Acute renal failure: a practical approach. *Mayo Clin Proc.* 2001;76:67–74.
12. Morgera S, Kraft AK, Siebert G, Luft FC, Neumayer HH. Long-term outcomes in acute renal failure patients treated with continuous renal replacement therapies. *Am J Kidney Dis.* 2002;40: 275–279.
13. Guzman NJ, Peterson J. Acute renal failure. In: Tisher CC, Wilcox CS, eds. *Nephrology.* 3rd ed. Baltimore, Md: Tisher Williams & Wilkins 1995;69–82.
14. Rodriguez D, Lewis S. Nutritional management of patients with acute renal failure. *ANNA J.* 1997;24:232–242.
15. Pascual J, Liano F, Ortuno J. The elderly patient with acute renal failure. *J Am Soc Nephrol.* 1995; 6:144–153.
16. Agrawal M, Swartz R. Acute renal failure. *Am Fam Physician.* 2000;61:2077–2088.
17. Druml W. Nutritional management of acute renal failure. *Am J Kidney Dis.* 2001;37(1 suppl 2): S89–S94.
18. Druml W. Protein metabolism in acute renal failure. *Miner Electrolyte Metab.* 1998;24:47–54.
19. Leblanc M, Garrett W, Cardinal J, Pichette V, Nolin L, Ouimet D, Geadah D. Catabolism in critical illness: estimation from urea nitrogen appearance and creatinine production during continuous renal replacement therapy. *Am J Kidney Dis.* 1998;32:444–453.
20. Druml W. Nutrition support in acute renal failure. In: Mitch WE, Klahr S, eds. *Handbook of Nutrition and the Kidney.* 4th ed. Philadelphia, Pa: Lippincott Williams & Wilkins; 2002:191–213.
21. Ikizler TA, Himmelfarb J. Nutrition in acute renal failure. *Adv Renal Replace Ther.*1997;4(2 supp 1):54–63.
22. Saadeh E, Ikizler A, Yu S, Hakim RM, Himmelfarb J. Recombinant human growth hormone in patients with acute renal failure. *J Ren Nutr.* 2001;11:212–219.
23. Marin A, Hardy G. Practical implications of nutritional support during continuous renal replacement therapy. *Curr Opin Clin Nutr Metab Care.* 2001;11:219–225.
24. Frankenfeld DC, Reynolds HN, Badellino MM, Wiles CE. Glucose dynamics during continuous hemodiafiltration and total parenteral nutrition. *Intensive Care Med.* 1995;21:1016–1022.
25. Kaufman DC, Haas CE, Spencer S, Veverbrants E. Adjustment of nutrition support with continuous hemodiafiltration in a critically ill patient. *Nutr Clin Pract.* 1999;14:120–123.
26. Leverve X, Barnoud D. Stress metabolism and nutritional support in acute renal failure. *Kidney Int.* 1998;53(suppl 66):S62–S66.
27. Schor N. Acute renal failure and the sepsis syndrome. *Kidney Int.* 2002;61:764–776.
28. Mehta R. Indications for dialysis in the ICU: renal replacement vs. renal support. *Blood Purif.* 2001; 19:227–232.
29. Sasaki S, Gando S, Kobayashi S, Nanzaki S, Ushitani T, Morimoto Y, Demmotsu O. Predictors of mortality in patients treated with continuous hemodialfiltration for acute renal failure in an intensive care setting. *ASAIO J.* 2001;47:86–91.
30. Murray P, Hall J. Renal replacement therapy for acute renal failure. *Respir Crit Care Med.* 2000; 162:777–781.
31. Ahmad S. Continuous therapies. In: *Manual of Clinic Dialysis.* London: Science Press; 1999: 53–64.
32. Ronco C, Brendolan A, Bellomo R. Continuous renal replacement techniques. *Blood Purif.* 2001; 19:236–251.
33. Marshall MR, Golper TA, Shaver MF, Chatoth DK. Hybrid renal replacement modalities for the critically ill. *Blood Purif.* 2001;19:252–257.
34. Ash SR. Peritoneal dialysis in acute renal failure of adults: the safe, effective, and low-cost modality. *Blood Purif.* 2001;19:210–221.
35. Novak I, Sramek V, Pittrova H, Rusavy Z, Tesinky P, Laciogova S, Eiselt M, Kohoutkova L, Vesela E, Opatrny K Jr. Glutamine and other amino acid

losses during continuous venovenous hemodiafiltration. *Artif Organs.* 1997;21:359–363.

36. Druml W. Metabolic aspects of continuous renal replacement therapies. *Kidney Int.* 1999;56(suppl 72):S56–S61.
37. Barco K. Total parenteral nutrition for adults with renal failure in acute care. *Support Line.* 2002;24: 22–28.
38. Tan HK, Bellomo R, M'Psis DA, Ronco C. Phosphatemic control during acute renal failure: intermittent hemodialysis versus continuous hemodiafiltration. *Int J Artif Organs.* 2001;24:186–191.
39. Klein CJ, Moser-Veillon PB, Schweitzer A, Douglass LW, Reynolds HN, Patterson KY, Veillon C. Magnesium, calcium, zinc, and nitrogen loss in trauma patients during continuous renal replacement therapy. *JPEN J Parenter Enteral Nutr.* 2002;26:22–93.
40. Story DA, Ronco C, Bellomo R. Trace element and vitamin concentrations and losses in critically ill patients treated with continuous venovenous hemofiltration. *Crit Care Med.* 1999;27:220–223.
41. Moore LW, Acchiardo SR, Smith SO, Gaber AO. Nutrition in the clinical care setting of renal disease. *Adv Renal Replace Ther.* 1996;3:250–260.
42. Bajpai S. Nutrition in acute renal failure. *Renal Nutr Forum.* 1998;17:1–7.
43. Brady H, Brenner B. Acute renal failure. In: Fauci A, ed. *Harrison's Principles of Internal Medicine.* 14th ed. New York: McGraw-Hill; 1998: 1504–1513.
44. Druml W. Fat-soluble vitamins in patients with acute renal failure. *Miner Electrolyte Metab.* 1998;24:220–226.
45. Druml W. Nutritional considerations in the treatment of acute renal failure in septic patients. *Nephrol Dial Transplant.* 1994;9:219–223.
46. Renal disease. In: *Manual of Clinical Dietetics.* 6th ed. Chicago, Ill: American Dietetic Association; 2000:449–454.
47. Bergstrom J. Nutrition in renal failure: the role of enteral feeding. *Nestle Nutrition Workshop Series Clinical and Performance Program.* 2000;3:247–256.
48. Mouser J, Hak E, Kuhl D, Dickerson R, Gaber L, Hak L. Recovery from ischemic acute renal failure is improved with enteral compared with parenteral nutrition. *Crit Care Med.* 1997;25:1748–1754.
49. American Society of Parenteral and Enteral Nutrition Board of Directors. Guidelines for the use of parenteral and enteral nutrition in adult and pediatric patients. *JPEN J Parenter Enteral Nutr.* 2002;26(Suppl):78SA–80SA.

Chapter 5

Nutrition Management of the Adult Hemodialysis Patient

Ronna Biesecker, PhD, RD, and
Naomi Stuart, MS, RD

Patients begin dialysis when their blood contains a higher than normal range of electrolytes and waste products. This occurs when the glomerular filtration rate (GFR) reaches approximately 10 mL/min/1.73 m^2 in someone without diabetes and 15 mL/min/1.73 m^2 in someone with diabetes. Some of the signs and symptoms of uremia are hyperpigmentation, ammonia-like breath, prolonged bleeding time, pericarditis, tremors, nausea, vomiting, loss of appetite, fatigue, and altered mental status.

The hemodialysis process removes concentrated molecules and excess fluid from a patient's blood through the mechanisms of diffusion and ultrafiltration. By removing small molecules (<300 daltons) such as electrolytes and urea, but not larger molecules such as albumin and red blood cells, the patient's blood is partially cleansed of toxins, and uremic symptoms are reduced (1). The major components of hemodialysis are the artificial kidney (dialyzer), the mechanical device (dialysis machine), and the dialysis bath (dialysate). Patient-specific modifications can be made to the major components, as well as to the blood flow rate, ultrafiltration rate, hydraulic pressure, length of time, and frequency of treatments and anticoagulation therapy (1). This chapter will cover the dialyzer and dialysate, emphasizing nutritional concerns rather than the mechanics of dialysis.

ARTIFICIAL KIDNEYS AND THE DIALYSIS BATH

Three types of hemodialysis currently used in the United States are based primarily on ultrafiltration efficiency: conventional (lowest clearance of molecules), high-efficiency (increased clearance of molecules), and high-flux (greatest clearance of molecules and fluid) (1). Dialysis works on the principle that blood components are altered by exposure to the dialysate by a semipermeable membrane through diffusion and ultrafiltration (2). Diffusion is the transfer of particles through a semipermeable membrane, the speed of which depends on the concentration gradient and the size of both the particle and membrane pore. Ultrafiltration is the movement of water through a membrane driven by hydrostatic or osmotic pressure.

During hemodialysis, blood flows in one direction through the inside of the hollow fibers filling the dialyzer while the dialysate flows in the opposite direction on the outside of the fibers. This counter-current flow maximizes the concentration gradient; additional pressure can be adjusted across the membrane to vary the resistance (2). Hollow-fiber semipermeable membranes are constructed from various materials: cellulose, substituted cellulose, cellulosynthetic, or synthetic material (3). Unsubstituted cellulose membranes activate the complement system more readily than other membrane types, resulting in neutropenia and deleterious effects on the immune system, and are prescribed less frequently than other types (3).

Thickness of the semipermeable membrane and pore size can be adjusted to increase efficiency (the higher the surface area the greater the ability to remove urea) and flux (the larger the pore size the greater the large molecule and water clearance) (3). Smaller molecules, such as urea, creatinine, glucose, and potassium, are cleared more readily than larger molecules such as vitamin B-12, while large molecules such as albumin and red blood cells do not pass through semipermeable membranes (3). Dialyzer clearances (KoA) can be found in the product information sheets included with each dialyzer and are reported as blood flow rates: the lower the number, the less efficient (2).

Reuse, the process of chemically cleaning and removing germicide from hollow fiber dialyzers for multiple uses, was the standard of care because it was more economical than single-use dialyzers. Although reusing dialyzers reduces costs and "first use" (anaphylactic) responses, there are reports of increasing complications from disinfecting agents, risk of transmission of infectious agents, and potential for decreased dialyzer performance (4). Additionally, substantial albumin is lost when bleach is used in dialyzer reprocessing (5).

Sodium, calcium, and potassium are the main components of the dialysis bath, along with magnesium, chloride, bicarbonate, and dextrose in a highly purified (deionized) water base. Most dialysis units purchase commercial formulations or concentrates, which may be delivered through a centralized system to the individual machines. A wide variety of liquid formulations are available as well as powder to reconstitute. Dialysate components vary in concentration, with potassium concentration ranging from 0 to 5 mEq/L, calcium concentration ranging from 2.0 to 3.5 mEq/L, sodium from 135 to 145 mEq/L, bicarbonate concentrations from 30 to 40 mEq/L, and magnesium from 0.5 to 0.75 mEq/L (3). Some components can be adjusted within narrow ranges on newer dialysis machines. The composition of the dialysate influences "protein and carbohydrate metabolism, systemic vasomotor tone, cardiac contractility and rhythm, pulmonary gas exchange, and bone turnover" and is therefore a critical issue in hemodialysis (1).

HEMODIALYSIS ACCESS

To initiate hemodialysis, access to the patient's blood is essential. This access can be for temporary or permanent use. There are various types of vascular access, each with their own advantages and disadvantages.

Temporary accesses include catheters inserted in the femoral, internal jugular, or subclavian veins. When the need for dialysis is projected to be short, the femoral vein is usually chosen (6). The internal jugular vein is preferred for extended use and is associated with lower infection risks, but it may present problems with neck mobility once the catheter is in position (6). The subclavian vein is commonly used as a last option due to higher incidences of insertion-related complications and risk of vein stenosis (6).

Permanent accesses include the cuffed venous catheter, the arteriovenous (AV) fistula, and the AV graft, and are located in the lower arm, forearm, or upper leg. The AV fistula and AV graft surgically connect an artery to a vein that creates a loop for dialysis and results in reduced blood flow to the limb below the access (6).

The AV fistula is known to be the safest and most advantageous permanent vascular access (6). The National Kidney Foundation's Kidney Disease Outcomes Quality Initiative (K/DOQI) guidelines recommend using the AV fistula as the preferred access for patients undergoing hemodialysis (7). It has low rates of complications and exceptional patency. However, it can take several months for the fistula to mature, and it may fail to develop adequately to support the prescribed blood flow rate (6).

The AV graft is used when an AV fistula cannot be formed (7). A tube, made from synthetic material, is used to form an AV connection (6). The advantages of the AV graft are the short maturation time and a larger surface area provided by the tube, enabling better ability to achieve sufficient blood flow (6).

The cuffed venous catheter is an option for patients who need a temporary access or are unable to have accesses placed arteriovenously. The K/DOQI guidelines do not recommend the cuffed venous catheter as a permanent access (7). One of the problems noted with this type of access is the inability to achieve adequate blood flow rates (6).

SETTINGS

Hemodialysis is performed in a variety of settings. Daily hemodialysis and home hemodialysis allow the greatest flexibility in treatment schedules enabling patients to maintain more independent lifestyles.

Daily Home Hemodialysis or Nocturnal Hemodialysis

Although not reimbursed by the Centers for Medicare and Medicaid Services (CMS) at this time, daily home hemodialysis is received by a limited number of patients in the United States. Hemodialysis is performed 6 nights a week in the home setting using a low blood flow rate for a period of 8 to 10 hours. Initial studies in the United States have concluded that compared with any other form of dialysis, nocturnal home dialysis reduces the need for many medications and dietary restrictions, requires phosphorus supplementation instead of binding, helps normalize blood pressure and fluid control, and improves quality of life (8). (For further information, refer to Appendix D.)

Home Hemodialysis

Home dialysis describes traditional thrice-weekly hemodialysis in the home. A hemodialysis machine is installed in the home after electrical wiring and water are assessed for adequacy. This setting allows more personal choice in treatment time, although a trained adult helper is required and personal water and electricity costs are increased.

Self-Care Hemodialysis

Self-care dialysis is performed in the hemodialysis unit. Patients are taught to perform their own dialysis with minimal staff assistance, which allows more independence.

In-Center or Staff-Assisted Hemodialysis

The most frequent mode of hemodialysis is performed in a hemodialysis unit or hospital, and the staff performs all aspects of the treatment. This setting allows for the least personal choice in time and treatment scheduling and requires the most medical supervision.

NUTRITION CONSIDERATIONS

Malnutrition is one of the greatest concerns observed among patients undergoing hemodialysis. Nutrient intake is often suboptimal, which could be a result of poor appetite produced by uremic conditions. Increased levels of leptin and inflammation were also found to decrease intake and lead to the progression of protein-energy malnutrition (PEM) (9). Other causes of malnutrition include metabolic acidosis, diabetes or insulin resistance, and the dialysis procedure itself (10). Patients who have been on hemodialysis for several years may be at greater risk for becoming malnourished (11). Many patients beginning dialysis have various comorbid conditions that may also contribute to increased risk of malnutrition (12).

It is important to adequately assess patients that are at risk for PEM. Nutrition therapy should be individualized based on various factors such as residual renal function, laboratory analysis, and overall nutritional status. Liberalization in dietary restrictions may be indicated for malnourished patients. Nutrition therapy should be reevaluated periodically according to the changing status of the patients.

Additional factors that contribute to the overall determination of the patient's nutrition therapy include the dialysis prescription as determined by the nephrologist. This includes the dialysis and blood flow rates, the length of treatment time, the dialysate bath, and the type of artificial kidney required for each individual patient.

PROTEIN

Protein recommendations are designed to compensate for the 10-g to 12-g free amino acid loss per treatment during dialysis (13). Greater amino acid losses occur when glucose-free dialysate (14) and high-flux dialyzers are used (3). Other factors related to diminished albumin levels and the need for increased dietary protein recommendations are: abnormalities in protein metabolism; altered albumin turnover; metabolic acidosis, which increases amino acid degradation and catabolism related to surgery; inflammation; and infection. Recovery of albumin losses due to infection and hospitalization was shown to take at least 3 months (15).

K/DOQI guidelines recommend 1.2 g protein/kg standard body weight per day with at least 50% of the dietary protein as high biological value—meats, poultry, game, fish, eggs, soy, and dairy products (14). Although protein recommendations have been consistent for the past 20 years, more than 50% of hemodialysis patients report dietary protein intakes less than

1.0 g/kg/day, and malnutrition is common (14). The resulting impaired nutritional status, as reflected in daily dietary protein intakes of less than 1.2 g/kg and hypoalbuminemia, is associated with a higher incidence of morbidity and mortality in retrospective studies (16,17). See Table 5.1 for recommended levels of individual nutrients (18–23).

ENERGY

For adult patients younger than 60 years of age, K/DOQI guidelines recommend daily energy levels of 35 kcal/kg of standard body weight . Adults older than 60 years of age or those who are obese may benefit from a daily energy level of 30 to 35 kcal/kg of body weight (24,25). (Refer to Chapter 2.)

Energy expenditure has been found to be similar in hemodialysis patients as compared with normal healthy individuals (24). Achieving energy intake at this level has been shown to provide neutral nitrogen balance (24). The lower calorie level suggested for older adults reflects a more sedentary lifestyle and an overall loss in lean body mass (24). Higher energy levels may be indicated for patients who have extremely high activity levels, patients who are underweight, or for patients who have catabolic stress (26).

There is concern, however, about whether patients can ingest this amount of calories daily. Intake should be evaluated and, if intake is insufficient, high-calorie supplements may need to be initiated. The actual energy intake reported in studies of hemodialysis patients is less than recommended in all age ranges (27). Participants in the Hemodialysis (HEMO) study had average daily intakes of 23 kcal/kg and 76% of the participants had daily energy intakes less than 28 kcal/kg (28).

Hemodialysis patients are at risk for disorders of lipid metabolism. Therefore, it is recommended that calories from fat be less than 30% and less than 10% from saturated fat. Daily cholesterol intake should also be less than 300 mg, and attempts should be made to achieve a daily fiber intake of 20 to 25 g (29), which may be difficult due to the potassium and phosphorus content of high-fiber foods. However, hemodialysis patients who have high cholesterol levels may not necessarily benefit from further dietary restrictions because total energy intake will decrease and may lead to malnutrition (30). For further information on cardiovascular disease in relationship to kidney failure, please refer to Chapter 10.

Among patients receiving dialysis, a decrease in mortality has been evident for patients following an exercise regimen, relative to those who do not exercise (31). Improved cardiac fitness is one benefit of a well-designed exercise program during hemodialysis (32). Promoting exercise and achievement of ideal body weight is recommended. In addition, treatment with various lipid-lowering medicines has also been shown to be beneficial in reducing low-density lipoprotein cholesterol and increasing high-density lipoprotein cholesterol (33).

Table 5.1. Daily Recommended Nutrient Intakes for Adults on Hemodialysis

Nutrient	*Daily Recommendation for Adults on Hemodialysis*
Protein	1.2 g/kg average weight (50% high biological value)
Energy	
Adults < 60 y	35 kcal/kg
Adults > 60 y or obese	30–35 kcal/kg
Sodium and fluid	
≥ 1 L fluid output	2–4 g Na and 2 L fluid
≤ 1 L fluid output	2 g Na and 1–1.5 L fluid
Anuria	2 g Na and 1 L fluid
Potassium	40 mg/kg IBW or SBW
Phosphorus	800–1000 mg or < 17 mg/kg IBW or SBW
Calcium	Individualized
Magnesium	0.2–0.3 g
Iron	Individualized
Zinc	8–11 mg
Vitamin A	700–900 µg
Vitamin D	5–15 µg
Vitamin E	15 mg
Vitamin K	90–120 mg
Thiamine	1.1–1.2 mg
Riboflavin	1.1–1.3 mg
Biotin	Unknown
Pantothenic acid	Unknown
Niacin	Unknown
Folic acid	800–1000 µg
Vitamin B-6	1.3–1.7 mg
Vitamin B-12	2.4 µg
Vitamin C	75–90 mg

Abbreviations: IBW, ideal body weight; SBW, standard body weight.

Source: Data are from references 18–23.

SODIUM AND FLUID

Sodium and water restrictions must be individualized to accommodate historical fluid gains, blood pressure control, and residual renal function. With fluid output greater than 1 L per day, mild sodium and fluid restrictions are recommended to keep intradialytic fluid gain to less than 5% of the patient's dry weight (25). This corresponds to approximately 2 to 4 g sodium per day (87 to 174 mEq) and 2 L (2,000 mL) fluid intake per day (25). If fluid output is less than 1 L per day, sodium intake of 2 g/day (87 mEq) is recommended with a fluid intake of 1 to 1.5 L (1,000 to 1,500 mL) per day (25). With anuria or no urine output, it is recommended that daily sodium intake be limited to 2 g (87 mEq) with fluid intake no more than 1 L (1,000 mL) per day (25).

POTASSIUM

As the GFR declines, the excretion rate of potassium increases both by urinary and by fecal excretion. However, as kidney failure continues to worsen this response becomes less efficient, and eventually potassium retention and hyperkalemia will occur (34). The potassium allowance for a patient undergoing hemodialysis varies depending on urine output. Generally, a minimum of 2.5 g of potassium is well tolerated by most patients receiving hemodialysis (34). However, hyperkalemia may occur at this level in patients who are anuric or have constipation. A stricter potassium allowance may be indicated if the patient has insulin deficiency, metabolic acidosis, is treated with beta blockers or aldosterone antagonists, or is in a hypercatabolic state (34). Individual requirements for potassium are approximately 40 mg per kg of edema-free body weight (35).

Mild hyperkalemia occurs at serum levels greater than 5.5 mEq/L. Moderate to severe hypokalemia occurs at levels less than 3.5 mEq/L (34). Measures to avoid hyperkalemia include limiting high-potassium food sources. A detailed list of these foods can be found in the National Renal Diet (18, 36).

Nutrition counseling about avoiding high-potassium food sources can help patients with chronic hyperkalemia reduce potassium levels. Oral administration of a sodium polystyrene sulfonate resin is also used as a therapy to treat hyperkalemia for short-term use when dialysis may not be available (36). The patient may also benefit from a lower potassium dialysate bath (less than or equal to 1.0 mEq/L) if serum potassium levels remain chronically elevated (29). The use of 0 mEq/L potassium baths are primarily used in acute-care settings where the patient can be closely monitored.

In anuric patients, hyperkalemia may occur due to causes other than dietary intake or problems with dialysis (37). Increasing the sodium concentration in the dialysate may be associated with a significant increase in plasma potassium within the initial 2 hours after treatment. Therefore, reducing the sodium concentration in the dialysate may help prevent hyperkalemic rebound after dialysis and would help prevent hyperkalemia interdialytically (38,39).

VITAMIN D

Activation occurs with enzymatic hydroxylation in the kidney. As kidney function declines, calcitriol (the active vitamin D-3 molecule) levels fall, calcium absorption is diminished, phosphorus excretion is impaired, and parathyroid hormone levels increase to compensate. These metabolic alterations can lead to changes in bone histology before dialysis is initiated (40). Vitamin D therapy suppresses parathyroid hormone production and enhances calcium absorption, thus helping to suspend or delay progression of renal bone disease, but may inadvertently cause hypercalcemia. Vitamin D products include the active form of vitamin D-3, plus active and inactive vitamin D-2 analogs. These products should only be taken under the supervision of a nephrologist. Over-the-counter vitamin supplements do not contain the active form of vitamin D and are thus are not effective in hemodialysis patients.

PHOSPHORUS

Hyperphosphatemia generally does not occur until the GFR decreases to between 20 and 30 mL/min/1.73 m^2 and the serum level varies depending on dietary intake (40). NKF K/DOQI guidelines state that patients with GFRs less than 60 mL/min/1.73 m^2 may require some dietary intervention or monitoring (41). Restriction of dietary phosphorus may have been instituted prior to hemodialysis initiation, but this is unlikely. To maintain serum albumin levels at 4.0 mg/dL in hemodialysis patients, protein consumption is encouraged and, untreated, the corresponding high phosphorus intake leads to hyperphosphatemia.

Treatment for hyperphosphatemia consists of dietary phosphorus restriction, use of phosphate binders, and clearance of phosphorus through dialysis. Phosphorus accumulation in the plasma occurs even when phosphorus intake is restricted. Although phosphate binders absorb 50% of dietary phosphorus, the remaining phosphorus cannot be cleared with current dialyzers (25). Hemodialysis clears phosphorus at a rate of 500 to 1,000 mg per treatment, mainly during the first 60 to 90 minutes of hemodialysis (25,40). There is very little additional clearance of phosphorus as the concentration in the blood is reduced, and the movement of phosphorus into the plasma from other body compartments occurs slowly. Because hyperphosphatemia alone was linked to increased morbidity and mortality in a retrospective review (19), dietary phosphorus control and binder adherence remain an important part of dialysis therapy.

Recommendations from the K/DOQI Work Group on Bone Metabolism and Disease in Chronic Kidney Disease are a dietary phosphorus intake of 800 to 1,000 mg phosphorus per day, or less than 17 mg/kg ideal body weight or standard body weight (41). Dietary counseling about high-protein/low-phosphorus food choices and the appropriate timing and dose of phosphate binders is standard practice in dialysis clinics. (Refer to Chapter 16 for more information.)

CALCIUM

Balance in hemodialysis patients is determined by dietary calcium intake, use of calcium supplements and calcium-based phosphate binders, dialysate calcium levels, and vitamin D therapy. Dietary intake of calcium is frequently decreased to approximately 500 mg per day, in part due to the limitation of high-phosphorus dairy foods in the hemodialysis diet (40). If hypocalcemia occurs, calcium supplementation between meals or at bedtime may be required, along with adjusting of dialysate calcium levels to maintain appropriate plasma calcium levels. Additional calcium may be obtained from calcium-based phosphate binders. Vitamin D therapy enhances calcium absorption in the gut.

Complications occur when elevated serum calcium and phosphorus precipitate, leading to soft tissue calcifications and acceleration of cardiovascular-related complications in hemodialysis patients compared with healthy subjects (42,43). A serum calcium × phosphorus product of 55 or less and a serum phosphorus less than 5.5 mg/dL are associated with improved outcomes based on retrospective analysis (44); however, it is difficult for patients to achieve that level. Calcium, phosphorus, and parathyroid levels should be monitored closely and calcium supplements, binders, vitamin D, and dialysate calcium adjusted as needed.

MAGNESIUM

The kidneys are the main organs responsible for the excretion and maintenance of magnesium metabolism. However, hypermagnesemia is not as common as hyperphosphatemia or hyperkalemia in hemodialysis patients because the magnesium content of most foods is less than the amount of potassium and phosphorus found in many foods (29). The gastrointestinal absorption of magnesium can be decreased. Therefore, magnesium concentration is usually normal to elevated in hemodialysis patients. However, patients with hypermagnesemia usually have only mildly elevated levels (<1.5 mEq/L) and are usually without clinical symptoms (45).

The reference range for magnesium is 1.4 to 2.3 mEq/L, the same as for nondialysis patients (46). Total recommended intake of magnesium is 0.2 to 0.3 g and is generally not supplemented in hemodialysis patients (25). Green leafy vegetables are the main dietary source of magnesium (45).

Hypomagnesemia may be seen in patients with diabetic ketoacidosis, hypercalcemia, alcohol abuse, diarrhea or malabsorption, pancreatitis, malnutrition, refeeding syndrome, and with use of some diuretics (46). Hypomagnesemia can cause cardiac arrhythmia and can block the release and action of parathyroid hormone (47).

Hypermagnesemia is seen with excessive intake (eg, from drinking water or in over-the-counter medications). Hypermagnesemia may also appear in dehydration or from too much magnesium in the dialysate (46). Hypermagnesemia can cause hypertension, weakness, and bradyarrhythmias. Chronic hypermagnesemia may result in adynamic bone disease by suppressing parathyroid secretion (48). Discontinuing the use of magnesium-containing compounds rectifies the problem. Hemodialysis is also effective in reducing serum magnesium levels (47) as long as a lower magnesium dialysate is used. The dialysate solution usually contains 0.75 to 1.5 mEq/L of magnesium (47,49).

IRON

Dietary iron absorption is less efficient in uremic patients and varies with inflammation status, age, sex, iron stores, and concomitant medications. Dietary iron intake is often decreased in predialysis diets and many patients were shown to have severe iron deficiency at initiation of hemodialysis (50). Yearly iron losses are estimated to be approximately 3 g in hemodialysis patients. This can be estimated from whole blood losses in dialysis tubing and dialyzers, gastrointestinal bleeding, frequent blood draws, surgical losses, and menstrual losses (50).

Oral iron supplements (200 mg elemental iron, two to three times a day) may be prescribed to correct iron deficiency and support erythropoiesis (51). Oral iron preparations are complexed with fumarate, gluconate, and sulfate salts and polysaccharide. Their varying side effects, such as diarrhea, constipation, cramping, and black stools, can hamper patient acceptance and compliance. In initial studies, a new oral product made from heme iron appears to be more bioavailable than traditional iron supplements with a reduced incidence of side effects (20). Because maximal absorption of iron occurs in the duodenum and upper jejunum, use of enteric (timed-release) preparations is not appropriate because iron may be released beyond the preferred site (52).

Although oral iron may support erythropoiesis when blood loss is limited, hemodialysis patients have difficulty maintaining sufficient iron stores with oral iron. This was clearly demonstrated in a study of hemodialysis patients receiving recombinant human erythropoietin (EPO) and randomized to take one of four oral iron preparations for 6 months (53). Although weekly pill counts and education improved compliance and the hematocrit remained stable, albeit low, more than 85% of the patients had serum ferritin levels of 100 or less ng/mL and transferrin saturations of 20% or less at the end of the study, indicating iron deficiency (53).

Several factors may contribute to the inability to correct the anemic condition using oral preparations alone. First, as mentioned previously, many patients are severely iron deficient when they start hemodialysis. Second, EPO has become the standard treatment of the anemia of renal disease. EPO increases iron utilization, which exceeds the body's ability to mobilize sufficient iron from storage to incorporate into the newly formed red blood cells (54). Third, another study measured normal absorption of oral iron in hemodialysis patients but found delayed incorporation of iron into the red blood cells, as compared with healthy patients (55).

Intravenous (IV) iron can be administered during dialysis and generates fewer gastrointestinal side effects while maintaining more consistent hemoglobin levels than oral iron (56). Compared with oral supplements of iron, IV iron complexed with dextran generates less frequent although more severe side effects, such as anaphylaxis (57), whereas newer iron preparations complexed with sodium gluconate and sucrose have fewer severe side effects of hypotension, nausea, and vomiting (58,59). The recommended intake of dietary iron is difficult to establish; thus, iron intake and supplementation must be determined individually as an adjunct to EPO therapy using currently recommended laboratory measures of iron status. (See Chapter 17 for more information.)

ZINC

Serum zinc has been found to be either normal or less than the reference range in hemodialysis patients (60). Low levels of serum zinc may be a result of increased zinc removed from the dialysis procedure along with low levels in the dialysate (29). Decreased serum zinc levels could also result from deficient intake of total energy or malnutrition resulting in insufficient dietary intake of zinc (29).

The recommended intake of zinc for patients on hemodialysis is the same as that recommended for the general population. The dietary reference intake is 8 to 11 mg/day. Decreased levels of zinc can be associated with hypogonadism, sexual dysfunction, decreased taste acuity, decreased smell, and impaired wound healing (29). If a patient has zinc deficiency, supplements may be recommended (51). However, there is conflicting evidence about the potential benefits of zinc supplementation in dialysis patients (61–64). It is recommended to continue zinc supplements only if there is a clinical response and change in serum zinc concentration levels (51).

Zinc supplements may ameliorate dysgeusia (65), improve zinc levels, and in turn increase protein catabolic rate (63). However, several studies did not show an improvement in immune function (61,62,66).

VITAMINS

Recommended daily intakes of individual vitamins are listed in Table 5.1.

Fat-Soluble Vitamins

Serum levels of vitamin A are often increased while vitamin E levels are decreased in the serum of hemodialysis patients (51). Supplementation of vitamin A or E is not recommended (51). Retinol-binding protein concentrations are elevated due to the lack of catabolic activity in the kidneys and the inability to remove both vitamin A and retinol-binding protein by dialysis (25). Hypervitaminosis A has been implicated in the development of anemia, premature atherosclerosis, retinal problems, and hypercalcemia (25). Long-term trials of vitamin E supplementation have not been conducted, but vitamin E-modified dialysis membranes suppressed hemodialysis leg cramps in combination with vitamin C (67).

Vitamin K production in the gut may be suppressed by certain antibiotics and may require vitamin K supplementation (25). However, because of vitamin K's role in promoting clot formation, supplementation is not recommended for most hemodialysis patients who receive anticoagulation therapy.

Water-Soluble Vitamins

The status of thiamin, riboflavin, and biotin is inconclusive. Serum thiamin is low to normal in hemodialysis patients (51). Biotin losses during hemodialysis are reported to be high, although normal plasma levels were found (68). Hemodialysis patients with intractable hiccups were successfully treated with 10 mg biotin daily (69).

Serum levels of folic acid are normal to high in dialysis patients (51), with some loss occurring with the use of high-flux membranes (70). High to normal folate levels can reduce homocysteine levels in dialysis patients (51), and combined with vitamins B-6 and B-12 have produced significantly decreased homocysteine levels in dialysis patients, although these levels rarely reach normalcy (71–73). Treatment for elevated levels of homocysteine in dialysis patients is not well defined. Hyperhomocysteinemia is associated with increased cardiovascular disease in both the nondialysis and dialysis populations. Analysis of epidemiological data suggests that hyperhomocysteinemia may play a protective role in the cardiovascular disease of dialysis patients in contrast to the association with adverse cardiovascular outcomes in nondialysis patients, a condition called "reverse epidemiology of cardiovascular risk factors" (74). The etiology of this association is unknown. Long-term supplementation of folic acid is not recommended unless vitamin B-12 deficiency is ruled out as "inappropriate treatment of B-12 deficiency with folic acid can precipitate severe neurologic changes, including subacute combined degeneration of the spinal cord" (51). A relationship between folic acid and iron was noted when a coexisting folate deficiency was unmasked after correcting for iron deficiency in 206 EPO-treated hemodialysis patients (75).

Pyridoxine (vitamin B-6) deficiency is present throughout the course of chronic kidney disease and may contribute to the symptoms of uremia, some of the clinical deficiency signs in adults being irritability, depression, and confusion (76). Serum pyridoxine is low to normal in hemodialysis patients with conventional dialyzers and deficient with high-flux/high-efficiency dialyzers and EPO therapy (51,77). An altered requirement for vitamin B-6 is suggested because pyridoxine supplementation response patterns are different in hemodialysis compared with predialysis patients, with hemodialysis patients more responsive to folic acid supplementation and predialysis patients more responsive to vitamin B-6 supplementation (78). Undersupplementation of vitamin B-6 may accentuate oxalate formation (79). Oversupplementation may lead to neurologic sequelae. Administration of 10 mL multivitamins (3300 IU vitamin A, 200 IU vitamin D, 3 mg thiamin, 4 mg B-6, 0.4 mg folic acid, 100 mg vitamin C, 3.6 mg riboflavin, 10 IU vitamin E, 40 mg niacin, 15 mg pantothenic acid, 60 mg biotin, and 5 μg vitamin B-12) three times per week to chronic kidney disease (CKD) patients receiving home parenteral nutrition was reported to cause elevated serum pyridoxine levels and neurologic disturbances, which resolved after discontinuation of the vitamin (21).

Serum vitamin C levels are low to normal in hemodialysis, and there is a significant loss of vitamin C with high-flux membranes (80). Supplementation of vitamin C may improve iron availability from stores (25) and successfully reduce cramps during hemodialysis when combined with vitamin E (67). Supplementation should be limited to 60 to 100 mg/day to avoid oxalate formation (51,79).

One of the current areas of research has focused on the state of decreased antioxidant defenses in uremia and hemodialysis. Antioxidant properties of vitamins E and C suppress the inflammatory response that consists of a cascade of reactions mediating cell proliferation, differentiation, and death (81). Net losses of water-soluble vitamin C during the hemodialysis process puts the hemodialysis patient in a weakened state, unable to protect against stimulation of the inflammatory response by bioincompatible membranes, and overproduction of free radicals, which oxidize proteins, lipids, DNA, and sugars, and damage biological metabolites (81). This entire process is known as oxidative stress and is suspected in many of the pathologies associated with uremia and hemodialysis, including the increased incidence of cardiovascular disease and amyloidosis. Preclinical studies have demonstrated increased red blood cell survival (82) and reduced markers of oxidative stress (83,84) when vitamin E is supplemented, and clinical studies of vitamin E-modified dialyzer membranes demonstrated increased neutrophil function (85,86). Whether supplementation would restore the pro-oxidant-antioxidant balance in hemodialysis patients is unclear at this time.

SUMMARY

The nutrient needs of the adult receiving hemodialysis are an integral part of the treatment for kidney failure. It is imperative that nutrition intervention be ongoing and developed in collaboration with the interdisciplinary health care team.

REFERENCES

1. Denker BM, Chertow Owen WF Jr. Hemodialysis. In: Brenner BM, ed. *The Kidney.* 6th ed. Philadelphia, Pa: WB Saunders Co; 2000:2373–2453.
2. Daugirdas JR, Van Stone JC. Physiologic principles and urea kinetic modeling. In: Daugirdas JT, Blake PG, Ing TS, eds. *Handbook of Dialysis*. 3rd ed. Philadelphia, Pa: Lippincott, Williams & Wilkins; 2001:15–45.
3. Daugirdas JT, Van Stone JC, Boag JT. Hemodialysis apparatus. In: Daugirdas JT, Blake PG, Ing TS, eds. *Handbook of Dialysis*. 3rd ed. Philadelphia, Pa: Lippincott, Williams & Wilkins; 2001: 46–66.
4. Kaufman AM, Levin NW. Dialyzer reuse. In: Daugirdas JT, Blake PG, Ing TS, eds. *Handbook of Dialysis*. 3rd ed. Philadelphia, Pa: Lippincott, Williams & Wilkins; 2001:169–181.
5. Kaplan AA, Halley SE, Lapkin RA, Graeber CW. Dialysate protein losses with bleach processed polysulphone dialyzers. *Kidney Int.* 1995;47: 573–578.
6. Besarab A, Raja, RM. Vascular access for hemodialysis. In: Daugirdas JD, Blake P, Ing T, eds. *Handbook of Dialysis.* 3rd ed. Philadelphia, Pa: Lippincott, Williams & Wilkins; 2001:67–101.
7. National Kidney Foundation Kidney Disease Outcomes Quality Initiative Clinical Practice Guideline for Vascular Access: Update 2000. Available at: http://www.kidney.org/professionals/doqi/guidelines/doqiupva_i.html#doqiupva3. Accessed April 25, 2003.
8. Pierratos A. Nocturnal home haemodialysis: an update on a 5-year experience. *Nephrol Dial Transplant.* 1999;14:2835.
9. Mehrota R, Kopple JD. Nutritional management of maintenance dialysis patients: why aren't we doing better? *Annu Rev Nutr.* 2001;21:343–379.
10. Mitch WE. Malnutrition: a frequent misdiagnosis for hemodialysis patients. *Am J Kidney Dis*. 2002; 40:280–290.
11. Chazot C, Laurent G, Charra B, Blanc C, VoVan C, Jean G, Vanel T, Terrat JC, Ruffet M. Malnutrition in long-term haemodialysis survivors. *Nephrol Dial Transplant.* 2001;16:61–69.
12. United States Renal Data System. The USRDS Annual Data Report (ADR) Reference Tables, 2002. Available at: http://www.usrds.org/2002/pdf/l.pdf. Accessed October 17, 2002.
13. Ikizler TA, Flakoll PJ, Parker RA, Hakim RM. Amino acid and albumin losses during hemodialysis. *Kidney Int.* 1994;46:830–837.
14. National Kidney Foundation Kidney Disease Outcomes Quality Initiative. Clinical practice guidelines for nutrition in chronic renal failure. *Am J Kidney Dis.* 2000;35(suppl):S40–S41.
15. Kelly MP, Kight MA, Migliore V. The nutritional cost of hospitalization and time needed to achieve nutritional resiliency for hemodialysis patients. *J Ren Nutr.* 1991;4:183–191.
16. Acchiardo SR, Moore LW, Burk L. Morbidity and mortality in hemodialysis patients. *ASAIO Trans.* 1990;46:M148–M151.
17. Lowrie EG, Huang WH, Lew NL. Death risk predictors among peritoneal dialysis and hemodialysis patients: a preliminary comparison. *Am J Kidney Dis.* 1995;26:220–228.
18. Wiggins K. *Guidelines for Nutrition Care of Renal Patients.* 3rd ed. Chicago, Ill: American Dietetic Association; 2002.
19. National Kidney Foundation Kidney Disease Outcomes Quality Initiative. Clinical practice guidelines for bone metabolism and disease in chronic kidney disease. *Am J Kidney Dis.* 2003;42(4 Suppl 3):S63–S68.

20. Masud T. Trace elements and vitamins in renal disease. In: Mitch WE, Klahr S, eds. *Handbook of Nutrition and the Kidney.* 4th ed. Philadelphia, Pa: Lippincott Williams & Wilkins; 2002:233–252.
21. Rocco MV, Makoff R. Appropriate vitamin therapy for renal dialysis patients. *Semin Dial.* 1997;10:272–277.
22. Institute of Medicine. *Dietary Reference Intakes for Vitamin C, Vitamin E, Selenium, and Cartenoids.* Washington, DC: National Academy Press; 2000.
23. Institute of Medicine. *Dietary Reference Intakes for Vitamin A, Vitamin K, Arsenic, Boron, Chromium, Copper, Iodine, Iron, Manganese, Molybdenum, Nickel, Silicon, Vanadium, and Zinc.* Washington, DC: National Academy Press; 2001.
24. National Kidney Foundation Kidney Disease Outcomes Quality Initiative. Clinical practice guidelines for nutrition in chronic renal failure. *Am J Kidney Dis.* 2000;35(suppl):S44–S45.
25. Kopple JD. National Kidney Foundation K/DOQI clinical practice guidelines for nutrition in chronic renal failure. *Am J Kidney Dis.* 2001; 37(suppl):S66–S70.
26. Rocco MV, Blumenkrantz MJ. Nutrition. In: Daugirdas JD, Blake P, Ing T, eds. *Handbook of Dialysis.* 3rd ed. Philadelphia, Pa: Lippincott, Williams & Wilkins; 2001:420–445.
27. National Kidney Foundation Kidney Disease Outcomes Quality Initiative. Clinical practice guidelines for nutrition in chronic renal failure. *Am J Kidney Dis.* 2000;35(suppl):S36–S37.
28. Burrowes JD, Cockram DB, Dwyer JT, Larive B, Paranandi L, Bergen C, Poole D. Cross-sectional relationship between dietary protein and energy intake, nutritional status, functional status, and comorbidity in older versus younger hemodialysis patients. *J Ren Nutr.* 2002;45:87–95.
29. Rocco MV, Paranandi L, Burrowes JD, Cockram DB, Dwyer JT, Kusek JW, Leung J, Makoff R, Maroni B, Poole D. Nutritional status in the HEMO study cohort at baseline. Hemodialysis. *Am J Kidney Dis.* 2002;39:245–256.
30. Ahmed KR, Kopple JD. Nutrition in maintenance hemodialysis patients. In: Kopple JD, Massry SG, eds. *Nutritional Management of Renal Disease.* Baltimore, Md: Williams & Wilkins; 1997:563–600.
31. Saltissi D, Morgan C, Knight B, Chang W, Rigby R, Westhuyzen J. Effect of lipid-lowering dietary recommendations on the nutritional intake and lipid profiles of chronic peritoneal dialysis and hemodialysis patients. *Am J Kidney Dis.* 2001; 37:1209–1215.
32. O'Hare AM, Tawney K, Bacchetti P, Johansen KL. Decreased survival among sedentary patients undergoing dialysis: results form the dialysis morbidity and mortality study wave 2. *Am J Kidney Dis.* 2003;41:447–454.
33. Oh-Park M, Fast A, Gopal S, Lynn R, Frei G, Drenth R, Zohman L. Exercise for the dialyzed: aerobic and strength training during hemodialysis. *Am J Phys Med Rehabil.* 2002;81:814–821.
34. Massy ZA, Keane WF. Management of lipid abnormalities in the patient with renal disease. In: Mitch WE, Klahr S, eds. *Handbook of Nutrition and the Kidney*, 4th ed. Philadelphia, Pa: Lippincott Williams & Wilkins; 2002:126–134.
35. Falkenhain M, Hartman J, Hebert L. Nutrition management of water, sodium, potassium, chloride and magnesium in renal disease and renal failure. In: Kopple JD, Massry SG, eds. *Nutritional Management of Renal Disease.* Baltimore, Md: Williams & Wilkins; 1997:371–394.
36. Schiro-Harvey K. *National Renal Diet: A Healthy Food Guide for People on Dialysis.* 2nd ed. Chicago, Ill. American Dietetic Association; 2002.
37. Daugirdas JT, Kjellstrand CM. Chronic hemodialysis prescription: a urea kinetic approach. In: Daugirdas JD, Blake P, Ing T, eds. *Handbook of Dialysis.* 3rd ed. Philadelphia, Pa: Lippincott Williams & Wilkins; 2001:121–147.
38. Vlassopoulos D, Sonikian M, Dardioti V, Pani I, Hadjilouka-Mantaka A, Hadjiconstantinou V. Insulin and mineralocorticoids influence on extrarenal potassium metabolism in chronic renal failure patients. *Renal Fail.* 2001;23:833–842.
39. De Nicola L, Bellizzi V, Minutolo R, Cioffi M, Giannattasio P, Terracciano V, Iodice C, Uccello F, Memoli B, Iorio BR, Conte G. Effect of dialysate sodium concentration on interdialytic increase of potassium. *J Am Soc Nephrol.* 2000; 11:2337–2343.
40. Martinez I, Saracho R, Montenegro J, Llach F. A deficit of calcitriol synthesis may not be the initial factor in the pathogenesis of secondary hyper-

parathyroidism. *Nephrol Dial Transplant.* 1996; 11(suppl 3):22–28.

41. Llach F, Bover J. Renal osteodystrophies. In: Brenner BM, ed. *The Kidney.* 6th ed. Philadelphia, Pa: WB Saunders Co; 2000:2013–2186.
42. Block GA, Hulbert-Shearon TE, Levin NW, Port FK. Association of serum phosphorus and calcium (phosphate product with mortality risk in chronic hemodialysis patients: a national study. *Am J Kidney Dis.* 1998;31:607–617.
43. Ahmed S, O'Neill KD, Hood AF, Evan AP, Moe SM. Calciphylaxis is associated with hyperphosphatemia and increased osteopontin expression by vascular smooth muscle cells. *Am J Kidney Dis.* 2001;37:1267–1276.
44. Block GA. Control of serum phosphorus: implications for coronary artery calcification and calcific uremic arteriolopathy (calciphylaxis). *Curr Opin Nephrol Hypertens.* 2000;10:741–747.
45. Block GA, Port FK. Re-evaluation of risks associated with hyperphosphatemia and hyperparathyroidism in dialysis patients: recommendations for change in management. *Am J Kidney Dis.* 2001;37:1331–1333.
46. Navarro-Gonzalez JF. Magnesium in dialysis patients: serum levels and clinical implications. *Clin Nephrol.* 1998;49:373–378.
47. Goldstein-Fuchs DJ. Assessment of nutritional status in renal diseases. In: Mitch WE, Klahr S, eds. *Handbook of Nutrition and the Kidney.* 4th ed. Philadelphia, Pa: Lippincott Williams & Wilkins; 2002:42–92.
48. Daugirdas JT, Ross EA, Nissenson AR. Acute hemodialysis prescription. In: Daugirdas JD, Blake P, Ing T, eds. *Handbook of Dialysis.* 3rd ed. Philadelphia, Pa: Lippincott Williams & Wilkins; 2001:102–120.
49. Navarro JF, Mora C, Jimenez A, Torres A, Macia M, Garcia J. Relationship between serum magnesium and parathyroid hormone levels in hemodialysis patients. *Am J Kidney Dis.* 1999;34: 43–48.
50. Fudin R, Jaichenko J, Shostak A, Bennett M, Gotloib L. Correction of uremic iron deficiency anemia in hemodialyzed patients: a prospective study. *Nephron.* 1998;79:299–305.
51. Fishbane S, Paganini EP. Hematologic abnormalities. In: Daugirdas JD, Blake P, Ing T, eds. *Handbook of Dialysis.* 3rd ed. Philadelphia, Pa: Lippincott Williams & Wilkins; 2001:477–494.
52. Seligman PA, Schleicher RB, Moore M. Clinical studies of HIP: an oral heme-iron product. *Nutr Res.* 2000;20:1278–1285.
53. Fairbanks VF. Iron in medicine and nutrition. In: Shils ME, Olson JA, Shike M, eds. *Modern Nutrition in Health and Disease.* 8th ed. Philadelphia, Pa: Lea & Febiger; 1994:185–213.
54. Wingard RL, Parker RA, Ismail N, Hakim RM. Efficacy of oral iron therapy in patients receiving recombinant human erythropoietin. *Am J Kidney Dis.* 1995;25:433–439.
55. Deira J, Martin M, Sanchez S, Garrido J, Nunez J, Tabernero JM. Evaluation of intestinal iron absorption by indirect methods in patients on hemodialysis receiving oral iron and recombinant human erythropoietin. *Am J Kidney Dis.* 2002;39: 594–599.
56. Magana L, Dhar SK, Smith EC, Martinez C. Iron absorption and utilization in maintenance hemodialysis patients: oral and intravenous routes. *Mt Sinai J Med.* 1984;51:180–183.
57. Eshbach J. Current concepts of anemia management in chronic renal failure: impact of NKF-K/DOQI. *Semin Nephrol.* 2000;20:320–329.
58. Infed [prescribing information]. Morristown, NJ: Watson Pharm, Inc; September 1996.
59. Venefer [prescribing information]. Shirley, NY: American Regent Laboratories, Inc; November 2000.
60. Ferrlecit [prescribing information]. Morristown, NJ: Watson Pharma, Inc; June 2001.
61. Krachler M, Scharfetter H, Wirnsberger GH. Kinetics of the metal cations magnesium, calcium, copper, zinc, strontium, barium, and lead in chronic hemodialysis patients. *Clin Nephrol.* 2000;54:35–44.
62. Erten Y, Kayatas M, Sezer S, Ozdemir FN, Ozyigit PF, Turan M, Haberal G, Guz G, Kaya S, Bilgin N. Zinc deficiency: prevalence and causes in hemodialysis patients and effect on cellular immune response. *Transplant Proc.* 1998;30:850–851.
63. Turk S, Bozfakioglu S, Ecder ST, Kahraman T, Gurel N, Erkoc R, Aysuna N, Turkmen A, Bekiroglu N, Ark E. Effects of zinc supplementation on the immune system and on antibody response to multivalent influenza vaccine in hemodialysis patients. *Int J Artif Organs.* 1998; 21:274–278.

64. Jern NA, VanBeber AD, Gorman MA, Weber CG, Liepa GU, Cochrane CC. The effects of zinc supplementation on serum zinc concentration and protein catabolic rate in hemodialysis patients. *J Ren Nutr.* 2000;10:148–153.
65. Hung KY, Ho CY, Kuo YM, Lee SH, Hseih SJ, Yang CS, Peng CJ, Wu DJ, Hung JT, Chem PY, Chen JS, Chen WY. Trace elements burden in geriatric hemodialysis patients: a prospective multicenter collaborative study. *Int J Artif Organs.* 1997;20:553–556.
66. Lew SQ, von Albertini B, Bosch JP. The digestive tract. In: Daugirdas JD, Blake P, Ing T, eds. *Handbook of Dialysis.* 3rd ed. Philadelphia, Pa: Lippincott Williams & Wilkins; 2001:601–610.
67. Kreft B, Fischer A, Kruger S, Sack K, Kirchner H, Rink L. The impaired immune response to diphtheria vaccination in elderly chronic hemodialysis patients is related to zinc deficiency. *Biogerontology.* 2000;1:61–66.
68. Khajehdehi P, Mojerlou M, Behzadi S, Rais-Jalali FA. A randomized, double-blind, placebo-controlled trial of supplementary vitamins E, C and their combination for treatment of haemodialysis cramps. *Nephrol Dial Transplant.* 2001; 16:1448–1451.
69. Jung U, Helbich-Endermann M, Bitsch R, Schneider S, Stein G. Are patients with chronic renal failure (CRF) deficient in biotin and is regular biotin supplementation required? *Z Ernahrungswiss.* 1998;37:363–367.
70. Jones WO, Nidus BD. Biotin and hiccups in chronic dialysis patients. *J Ren Nutr.* 1991;1: 80–83.
71. Lasseur C, Parrot F, Delmas Y, Level C, Ged C, Redonnet-Vernhet I, Montaudon D, Combe C, Chauveau P. Impact of high-flux/high-efficiency dialysis on folate and homocysteine metabolism. *J Nephrol.* 2001;14:32–35.
72. Henning BF, Zidek W, Riezler R, Graefe U, Tepel M. Homocysteine metabolism in hemodialysis patients treated with vitamins B6, B12 and folate. *Res Exp Med (Berl).* 2001;200:155–168.
73. Trimarchi H, Schiel A, Freixas E, Diaz M. Randomized trial of methylcobalamin and folate effects on homocysteine in hemodialysis patients. *Nephron.* 2002;91:58–63.
74. Dierkes J, Domrose U, Bosselmann KP, Neumann KH, Luley C. Homocysteine lowering effect of different multivitamin preparations in patients with end-stage renal disease. *J Ren Nutr.* 2001;11:67–72.
75. Kalantar-Zadeh K, Block G, Humphreys MH, Kopple JD. Reverse epidemiology of cardiovascular risk factors in maintenance dialysis patients. *Kidney Int.* 2003;63:793–808.
76. Polak VE, Lorch JA, Means RT Jr. Unanticipated favorable effects of correcting iron deficiency in chronic hemodialysis patients. *J Investig Med.* 2001;49:173–183.
77. Leklem JE. Vitamin B6. In: Shils ME, Olson JA, Shike M, eds. *Modern Nutrition in Health and Disease.* 8th ed. Philadelphia, Pa: Lea & Febiger; 1994:383–394.
78. Okada H, Moriwaki K, Kanno Y, Sugahara S, Nakamoto H, Yoshizawa M, Suzuki H. Vitamin B6 supplementation can improve peripheral polyneuropathy in patients with chronic renal failure on high-flux haemodialysis and human recombinant erythropoietin. *Nephrol Dial Transplant.* 2000;15:1410–1413.
79. Lindner A, Bankson DD, Stehman-Breen C, Mahuren JD, Coburn SP. Vitamin B6 metabolism and homocysteine in end-stage renal disease and chronic renal insufficiency. *Am J Kidney Dis.* 2002;39:134–145.
80. Mikalunas V, Fitzgerald K, Rubin H, McCarthy R, Craig RM. Abnormal vitamin levels in patients receiving home total parenteral nutrition. *J Clin Gastroenterol.* 2001;33:393–396.
81. Morena M, Cristol JP, Bosc JY, Tetta C, Forret G, Leger CL, Delcourt C, Papoz L, Descomps B, Canaud B. Convective and diffusive losses of vitamin C during haemodiafiltration session: a contributive factor to oxidative stress in haemodialysis patients. *Nephrol Dial Transplant.* 2002;17: 422–427.
82. Wratten ML, Tetta C, Ursini F, Sevanian A. Oxidant stress in hemodialysis: prevention and treatment strategies. *Kidney Int.* 2000;58(suppl 76):S126–S132.
83. Usberti M, Gerardi G, Bufano G, Tira P, Micheli A, Albertini A, Floridi A, Di Lorenzo D, Galli F. Effects of erythropoietin and vitamin E-modified membrane on plasma oxidative stress markers and anemia of hemodialyzed patients. *Am J Kidney Dis.* 2002;40:590–599.
84. Tsuruoka S, Kawaguchi A, Nishiki K, Hayasaka T, Fukushima C, Sugimoto K, Saito T, Fujimura A. Vitamin E-bonded hemodialyzer improves

neutrophil function and oxidative stress in patients with end-stage renal failure. *Am J Kidney Dis*. 2002;39:127–133.
85. Satoh M, Yamasaki Y, Nagake Y, Kasahara J, Hashimoto M, Nakanishi N, Makino H. Oxidative stress is reduced by the long-term use of vitamin E-coated dialysis filters. *Kidney Int*. 2001;59: 1943–1950.
86. Shimazu T, Ominato M, Toyama K, Yasuda T, Sato T, Maeba T, Owada S, Ishida M. Effects of a vitamin E-modified dialysis membrane on neutrophil superoxide anion radical production. *Kidney Int*. 2001;78(suppl):S137–S143.

Chapter 6

Nutrition Management of the Adult Peritoneal Dialysis Patient

Linda McCann, RD, CSR

Peritoneal dialysis (PD) involves the removal of body waste products and water within the peritoneal cavity, using the peritoneal membrane as a filter. Clinical application of PD was reported as early as 1923 (1), but PD did not emerge as a growing renal replacement therapy (RRT) until the mid-1970s with the advent of an "ambulatory" PD technique, called continuous ambulatory peritoneal dialysis (CAPD) (2). Although PD is thought to be underused even today, improvements in PD access, connection devices, and packaging and composition of solutions have enhanced the safety, efficacy, and acceptance of this therapy. It is simple, convenient, and relatively low in cost. In 1998 approximately 120,000 or 15% of dialysis patients worldwide were receiving PD (3). The use of PD varies among countries, depending on reimbursement, availability of hemodialysis (HD), distance from dialysis centers, and health care team biases (3).

PD is reported to have several advantages over HD, including the following (3–7):

- Freedom from the need to travel to the dialysis center two or three times per week
- Use of simple routines that are easily learned and allow the patient to travel, work, and independently manage his or her own dialysis treatment at home
- Continuous therapy that promotes steady-state chemistries and fluid balance with potentially fewer diet restrictions
- Slower decline of residual urine output
- Better blood pressure control, including reduced risk of hypotensive episodes with the avoidance of direct compromise of the vascular volume during dialysis treatment
- Elimination of the need for direct blood access

PERITONEAL PROCESSES

The process of peritoneal dialysis includes the infusion of dialysate through a catheter into the peritoneal cavity. The peritoneal membrane lines the peritoneal cavity and separates the waste-containing blood in the peritoneal capillaries from the dialysate. The peritoneal membrane is thought to have a surface area approximately equal to the individual patient's body surface area—approximately 1 to 2 m^2 in an adult. Newer research suggests that the membrane has pores of different sizes that mediate the transport of various solutes and water (4).

The dialysate typically contains electrolytes, lactate, and variable concentrations of glucose that make it hyperosmolar. The peritoneal membrane acts as a dialyzer to allow wastes and excess fluid to cross into the dialysate. Uremic solutes and potassium diffuse from the blood to the dialysate via the concentration gradient. Glucose, lactate, and potentially calcium diffuse in the opposite direction. At the same time, the hyperosmolar dialysate leads to the removal of water and associated solutes across the membrane through ultrafiltration (UF). In addition, there is a complex lymphatic system within the peritoneal cavity that facilitates the constant absorption of water and solute (4).

Infusion of peritoneal dialysate can be done manually using CAPD or automated peritoneal dialysis (APD) with a cycler machine. APD therapies include continuous cyclic peritoneal dialysis (CCPD), cyclic intermittent peritoneal dialysis (CIPD), and tidal peritoneal dialysis (TPD) (4,8).

The choice of PD modality depends primarily on the transport characteristics of the patient's peritoneal membrane, which is measured during a peritoneal equilibration test (PET) (5,8). The PET test measures solute clearance, UF, protein losses, and glucose absorption—the combined effect of diffusion and UF. Matching the dialysis prescription to the membrane type is essential for setting and achieving therapeutic goals, although patient preference is also important (3,4). Therapeutic goals include providing the dose or type of dialysis associated with the best clinical outcomes, including maintaining adequate nutritional status, achieving UF commensurate with optimal hydration status, and choosing the modality that is most convenient to the patient and his or her lifestyle (8). The PET, recommended within the first month or 6 weeks of treatment (5), classifies peritoneal transport rates (PTR) for the membrane as high, high average, low average, or low. It has been reported that the majority of patients have a high average or low average PTR (8,9).

There are significant data correlating PTR to outcomes. Those patients with high PTR are reported to have increased morbidity, mortality, malnutrition, and technique failure. The less-than-favorable prognosis for high PTR patients may be a result of their poor UF associated with chronic fluid overload and/or high peritoneal protein losses that can result in malnutrition. The cause and effect have not been absolutely established, and it is possible that the poor UF and high transport of protein may result from other processes such as low-grade chronic inflammation. The PTR can change with time on dialysis. Episodes of peritonitis can also acutely impact the PTR. The causes and consistency of PTR changes are not universal. The most common causes of PD technique failure are peritonitis and loss of UF capability. Other causes include catheter failure, patient/family fatigue, and malnutrition (3,8,10,11).

All PD patients are taught to perform CAPD even if their prescribed modality is APD. This allows them to continue with their lifesaving dialysis treatments even if the machine is unavailable for some reason. In CAPD, typically four or five "exchanges" are performed in a 24-hour period. This entails infusing a specific volume of dialysate into the peritoneum, allowing the dialysate to dwell for approximately 4 hours to filter and then drain wastes and extra fluid from the blood. The volume of dialysate instilled for each exchange varies according to the size and tolerance of the patient. Standard bags of dialysate are 1,500, 2,000, 2,500, and 3,000 mL. In CAPD, dialysate is present in the peritoneum 24 hours per day except during the 20- to 30-minute exchange when dwelling dialysate is drained and fresh dialysate is instilled. Vessels and capillaries that line the peritoneal membrane afford passive diffusion of wastes and osmotic removal of water during the time that the dialysate dwells in the peritoneum. The dextrose or other osmotic agent in the dialysate creates a gradient to facilitate the removal of fluid. Both the wastes and fluid are discarded with the drained or spent dialysate. Gravity allows the dialysate to flow into and out of the patient.

With APD, the volume of instilled dialysate is controlled by settings on the machine and can be easily adjusted to the tolerance of the patient. Generally three to five exchanges are performed during a 10-hour period. The diurnal cycle is a prolonged exchange of approximately 14 hours while the patient is disconnected from the cycler (7).

In CCPD, a greater number of exchanges are typically performed quickly with less dwell time utilizing a cycler machine to facilitate the infusion and recovery of dialysate. The blood to dialysate transfer of wastes and fluid is accomplished in the same way as CAPD. CCPD includes at least one daytime exchange.

In CIPD, the patient uses the cycler machine but has some interruption of dialysis, usually during the day when the peritoneum is "dry" or devoid of dialysate. Typically, only those patients with residual urine output are able to achieve adequate dialysis with CIPD.

Tidal peritoneal dialysis is a regimen that may decrease the time required to instill and drain dialysate. With tidal PD, a reserve volume of dialysate (usually 50% of the total volume) is always in contact with the peritoneum, and fresh dialysate cycles in on a regular basis to maintain the concentration gradient for waste and fluid removal. This method of PD has the potential of obtaining better clearances with less time (7), but the added volume of dialysate increases the cost of the treatment, which seems to limit its use.

The success of PD depends on the patient's general health, preexisting comorbid conditions, the ability to perform self-dialysis or secure an able partner, and matching the therapy to the individual needs of the patient. Psychological and metabolic needs must be considered when choosing or recommending PD as the method of RRT. The patient's modality preference should be offered as long as he or she meets the criteria and has a reasonable expectation of success with that modality. Body size, residual urine output, nutritional status, lifestyle, condition of the peritoneum, PTR, and clinical status should be considered and discussed with the patient prior to choosing the method of RRT. Many patients are transferred to PD after failure of HD and may begin PD under less than optimal conditions. Other patients may transfer from PD to HD either temporarily or permanently.

It is not uncommon for a patient with chronic kidney disease (CKD) to use several different modalities of treatment during the course of RRT. Whichever modality of RRT is used, the goals are to individualize the treatment to the specific needs of the patient, ensuring adequate dialysis to prevent uremic symptoms, maintain fluid balance, and prevent the negative impacts of CKD.

ADEQUACY OF DIALYSIS

Adequacy of dialysis is critical to the success of PD. Inadequate dialysis may result from the following:

- Large muscle mass, which increases the difficulty of providing a volume of dialysate large enough to clear wastes
- Changes in or lack of residual urine output
- Poor catheter function that prevents or prolongs fluid exchange
- Changes in PTR
- Nonadherence to prescribed PD routines

Several clinical tools are accepted as adequacy measures for PD. These include a urea kinetic modeling (UKM) Kt/V, a unitless measure of urea clearance by dialysis and urine output, and total creatinine clearance in liters per week (CrCl), a measure of creatinine removal related to patient body size. Parameters that are recommended for monitoring nutritional status and, perhaps, indirectly adequacy of dialysis, are the protein equivalent of nitrogen appearance (PNA) and edema-free, fat-free body mass. The PNA is an estimation of protein intake as calculated for the generation of urea over a 24-hour period. Edema-free, fat-free body mass is a calculation of lean tissue and can help track changes that occur over time (5).

UKM has been used to assess HD adequacy since the results of the National Cooperative Dialysis Study (NCDS) were published in 1983. The NCDS defined the level of HD, expressed as Kt/V, and protein intake, expressed as protein catabolic rate, that were associated with the most favorable patient outcomes (11). There have been two large studies to define adequacy in PD. These include the Canada-USA (CANUSA) study (12) and the Adequacy of Peritoneal Dialysis in Mexico (ADMEX) study (13). The National Kidney Foundation Kidney Disease Outcomes Quality Initiative (K/DOQI) defined PD adequacy in the Clinical Practice Guidelines for PD adequacy, published in 1998, and revised in 2001 (prior to the completion of the ADEMEX study) (5).

The K/DOQI PD adequacy workgroup explored the pertinent scientific literature and developed evidence-based guidelines for the provision of adequate PD and monitoring nutritional status. Box 6.1 provides an overview of the K/DOQI PD adequacy guidelines. A summary of K/DOQI PD adequacy targets can be found in Table 6.1 (14). Formulas for calculating Kt/V, CrCl, and PNA can be found in Figure 6.1 (14–16). Formulas for calculation of edema-free, fat-free body mass can be found in Figure 6.2 (16).

NUTRITION ASSESSMENT

Methods of nutrition assessment for PD are similar to those for HD. No single parameter can consistently and accurately assess nutritional status. Thus, several parameters are used, including biochemical, anthropometric, subjective global assessment (SGA), diet interviews, and diaries (17) (see Chapter 2).

NUTRITION RECOMMENDATIONS

Nutrient recommendations were defined in the K/DOQI Clinical Practice Guidelines for Nutrition in Chronic Renal Failure (CRF), published in 2000 (17). These recommendations, based primarily on early, landmark

Box 6.1. Summary of NKF DOQI Peritoneal Dialysis Adequacy Guidelines

1. Initiate dialysis incrementally to maintain a total Kt/V of at least 2.0 and nPNA of at least 0.8 g/kg.
2. Peritoneal dialysis (PD) adequacy testing should be performed within 1 month and at least one additional time between months 2 and 6 (depends on consistency from initial results), and then every 4 months.
3. PD targets are based on the type of PD therapy, with continuous, longer dwell time (continuous ambulatory peritoneal dialysis [CAPD]) targets lower than those for interrupted (NIPD) or shorter dwell therapies (automated peritoneal dialysis [APD]). The Kt/V and CrCl (L/week/1.73 m^2) targets are: CAPD, 2.0/60 L; NIPD, 2.2/66 L; CCPD or APD, 2.1/63 L. CrCl of 50 L/wk/1.73 m^2 may be acceptable in those patients with low or low-average transport membrane characteristics.
4. If total daily creatinine excretion differs from baseline by ≥ 15%, error analysis should be initiated (patient compliance, dialysate/urine collection procedures/accuracy, altered peritoneal transport characteristics).
5. Assess nutrition status at least every 4 months using Subjective Global Assessment (SGA) and PNA.
6. Identify and correct patient or staff errors in meeting minimum targets.
7. Regularly measure clinical outcomes (patient survival, technique survival, hospitalization rates, patient-based quality of life, albumin, Hct, nPNA, and school attendance/developmental progress in pediatric patients).
8. Indications for PD are patient preference, medical complications/no assistant for home HD. Contraindications for PD are loss of peritoneal function, inability to perform/no assistant, mechanical defects, leaks, body size, severe malnutrition, diverticular/bowel disease. Reasons to change to HD are consistent failure to achieve adequacy, unmanageable hypertriglyceridemia, recurrent peritonitis/complications, technical/mechanical problems, unmanageable severe malnutrition.

Source: Data are from reference 5.

Table 6.1. NKF K/DOQI 2000 Suggested PD Adequacy Targets

Modality	*Kt/V*	*CrCl (L/wk/ 1.73 m^2)*	*Frequency of PD Adequacy Testing*
CAPD:			Baseline:
H,*	2.0	60	• PET: within 1 month of PD initiation.
HA*	2.0	50	• Kt/V, CrCl, urine: within 1 month of PD initiation; repeat at least once within 6 months.
L/LA*	2.0	50	
			Ongoing:
			• Kt/V, CrCl, urine†: at least every 4 months or with any change in prescription or clinical status.)
NIPD	2.2	66	
CCPD	2.1	63	

Abbreviations: CAPD, continuous ambulatory peritoneal dialysis; CCPD, continuous cyclic peritoneal dialysis; CrCl, creatinine clearance; NIPD, nightly intermittent peritoneal dialysis; PD, peritoneal dialysis; PET, peritoneal equilibration test.

*Membrane transport characteristic: H = high, HA = high average, L = low, LA = low average. Low and low-average transporters have better survival and technique survival, but without residual kidney function may not be able to achieve a CrCl of 60 L/wk/1.73 m^2 even when Kt/V is adequate. Thus, the CrCl target can be set slightly lower as long as patients are observed closely for evidence of inadequate dialysis.

†Use Kt/V if discordant with CrCl. Collect urine until Kt/V_{urea} drops to < 0.1.

Source: Adapted from McCann L, ed. *Pocket Guide to Nutrition Assessment of the Patient With Chronic Kidney Disease.* 3rd ed. New York, NY: National Kidney Foundation; 2002:10–25, with permission from National Kidney Foundation.

1. **Calculate TBW* or V and BSA:**
   *TBW using Watson (15):

   Male: $V = 2.447 - (0.09516 \times Age) + (0.1074 \times Ht) + (0.3362 \times Wt)$

   Female: $V = -2.097 + (0.1069 \times Ht) + (0.2466 \times Wt)$

   Where: Age is measured in years, Height in cm, and Weight in kg.

   *TBW using Hume & Weyers (16):

   Male: $V = (0.194786 \times Ht) + (0.296785 \times Wt) - 14.012934$

   Female: $V = (0.34454 \times Ht) + (0.183809 \times Wt) - 35.270121$

   Where: Height is measured in cm and Weight in kg.

2. **Calculate residual urea clearance (mL/min):**

$$\frac{(U_U \times U_V)}{(1440 \times S_U)}$$

3. **Calculate residual (urinary) Kt/V:**

$$\frac{\text{Urea clearance} \times 1440 \times 7}{V \times 1000}$$

   Where: Urea clearance is measured in mL/min.

4. **Calculate dialysis Kt/V:**

$$\frac{D_U/S_U \times D_V \times 7}{V \times 1000}$$

5. **Calculate total Kt/V:**

   Residual Kt/V + Dialysis Kt/V

6. **Calculate residual creatinine clearance (g/d):**

$$\frac{U_{CR} \times U_V}{1440 \times S_{CR}}$$

7. **Calculate mean GFR (mL/min):**

$$\frac{\text{Residual CrCl} + \text{Residual urea clearance}}{2}$$

8. **Calculate Urinary CrCl (L/wk):**

$$\frac{\text{Mean GFR} \times 1440 \times 7}{1000}$$

9. **Calculate Dialysis CrCl (L/wk):**

$$\frac{D_{CR}/S_{CR} \times D_V \times 7}{1000}$$

10. **Calculate total CrCl (L/wk):**

    Urinary CrCl + Dialysis CrCl

11. **Normalize to patient BSA (L/wk/1.73m^2):**

$$\frac{\text{Total CrCl} \times 1.73}{\text{pt BSA}}$$

Patient Example:

	Urea, mg/dL	Creat, mg/dL	Volume, mL
Urine:	333 (U_U)	136 (U_{CR})	475 (U_V)
Serum:	60 (S_U)	6.91(S_{CR})	
Dialysate:	52 (D_U)	4.5 (D_{CR})	12485 (D_V)

1. BSA = 1.88 m^2 — TBW or V = 40.4 L
2. Residual urea clearance = (333 × 475)/(60 × 1440) = 158175/86400 = **1.83 mL/min**
3. Residual Kt/V = (1.83 × 1440 × 7)/(40.4 × 1000) = 18446.4/40400 = **0.46/wk**
4. Dialysate Kt/V = (52/60 × 12485 × 7)/(40.4 × 1000) = 75742.32/40400 = **1.87**
5. Total Kt/V = 0.46 + 1.87 = **2.33**
6. Residual CrCl = (135 × 475)/(1440 × 6.91) = 64600/9950 = **6.49 g/d**
7. Mean GFR = (2.33 + 1.83)/2 = **2.08 mL/min**
8. Urinary CrCl = (2.08 × 1440 × 7)/1000 = 20966.4/1000 = **21 L/wk**
9. Dialysis CrCl = [(4.5/6.91) × 12485 × 7]/1000 = (0.651 × 12485 × 7)/1000 = 56894.2 /1000 = **56.9 L/wk**
10. Total CrCl = 21 + 56.9 = **77.9 L/wk**
11. Normalized CrCl = (77.9 × 1.73)/1.88 = **71.7 L/wk/ 1.73 m^2**

KEY: BSA = body surface area (m^2); D_{CR} = dialysate creatinine (mg/dL); D_{PRO} = protein in dialysate (mg/dL); D_U = dialysate urea (mg/dL); D_V = dialysate volume (mL); nPNA = normalized protein equivalent of total nitrogen (g/kg/d); PCR = protein catabolic rate; PNA = protein equivalent of total nitrogen appearance (g/d); S_{CR} = serum creatinine (mg/dL); S_U = serum urea (mg/dL); TBW = total body water (L); U_{CR} = urine creatinine (mg/dL); UNA = urinary nitrogen apearance (g/d); U_{PRO}= protein in urine (mg/dL); U_U = urine urea (mg/dL); U_V = urine volume (mL); V = volume (L).

Figure 6.1. Peritoneal dialysis (PD) adequacy formulas. Adapted from McCann L, ed. *Pocket Guide to Nutrition Assessment of the Patient With Chronic Kidney Disease.* 3rd ed. New York, NY: National Kidney Foundation; 2002:10–23,10–24, with permission from National Kidney Foundation.

PNA Formulas

1. **Calculate UNA:**

$$\frac{(D_U/100 \times D_V) + (U_U/100 \times U_V)}{1000}$$

2. **Determine whether the patient has protein losses > 15 g/d.**
   Potential: Nephrotic patients, those with high transport membranes and those whose clinical picture doesn't correspond with chemistries (well nourished, eating well, but low protein parameters).
   Obtain 24–hr protein levels for dialysate and urine. Convert to g/d.

$$\frac{D_{PRO} \times (D_V/100) + U_{PRO} \times (U_V/100)}{1000}$$

3. **Calculate PNA (if protein losses > 15 g/d)**

$$PCR = (6.49 \times UNA) + (0.294 \times V)$$

$$PNA = PCR + \text{protein losses}$$

4. **Calculate PD PNA (if protein losses < 15 g/d)**
   (Incorporates average PD protein loss of 7.3 g/d)

$$10.76 \times (0.69 \times UNA + 1.46)$$

5. **Calculate nPNA**

$$nPNA = \frac{PNA}{(V/0.58)}$$

Patient Example:

	Urea, mg/dL	Creat, mg/dL	Volume, mL
Urine:	333 (U_U)	136 (U_{CR})	475 (U_V)
Serum:	60 (S_U)	6.91(S_{CR})	
Dialysate:	52 (D_U)	4.5 (D_{CR})	12485 (D_V)

1. UNA = [(52/100 × 12485) + (333/100 × 475)]/1000
   = (6492.2 + 1581.75)/1000
   = 8.07 g/d
2. Obtain 24–hour protein levels from urine and dialysate. Sample patient has D_{PRO} = 117 mg/dL and U_{PRO} = 107 mg/dL.
   Protein loss = [117 × (12485/100) + 107 × (475/100)]/1000
   = [(117 × 124.9) + (107 × 4.75)]/1000
   = (14613.3 + 508.25)/1000
   Total protein loss = **15.1 g/d**
3. PNA = (6.49 × 8.07) + (0.294 × 40.4)
   + 24–hr protein loss
   = 52.4 + 11.8 + 15.1
   = 64.2 + 15.1
   = 79.3 g/d
4. PNA = 10.76 × (0.69 × 8.07 + 1.46)
   = 10.69 × 7.028
   = 75.1 g/d
5. nPNA = 75.1/(40.4/0.58)
   = 75.1/69.7
   = 1.08 g/kg/d

Figure 6.1. (Continued).

scientific evidence, are similar to those that have been used since the early days of PD. The need for nutrient recommendations is underscored by the incidence of protein-energy malnutrition in the CKD population. Recommendations for PD patients differ slightly from those for HD patients. A summary of nutrient requirements can be found in Table 6.2 (18–19).

ENERGY

Energy levels should be prescribed to maintain a reasonable body weight and are based on age, activity levels, and standard (SBW) or adjusted body weight (17). Although the goal of the K/DOQI SBW guideline was to facilitate standardization of the weight used to calculate nutrient requirements, clinicians may still use other references or clinical judgment to determine the most appropriate weight for an individual patient. Thirty-five kcal/kg per day are recommended for individuals younger than 60 years of age. For those 60 and older, 30 kcal/kg are recommended. Calories are reduced in older individuals due to lower activity levels and decreases in lean body mass (17). Research has indicated that 35 kcal/kg is necessary to maintain both nitrogen balance and stable body composition (18). Calories provided from the dialysate should be included in the total allowance for PD patients. The most accurate method of determining the caloric load from peritoneal dialysate is to measure the grams of glucose in the effluent and compare that to the grams of glucose that were infused. Several other formulas have been published and can be found in Table 6.3 (14). PD patients can absorb as much as one third of their daily energy from the dialysate depending on the modality. Fewer calories are typically absorbed with APD because of more rapid exchanges of fluid and shorter dwell time. With APD, a shorter dura-

The creatinine (Cr) index is defined as the creatinine synthesis or production rate and is used to assess skeletal muscle mass. It is determined by the size of the skeletal muscle mass and the intake of creatine and creatinine. Creatinine production is approximately proportional to skeletal muscle mass in metabolically stable adults who have consistent protein intake. In maintenance dialysis patients creatinine is synthesized and serum levels rise at a rate that is approximately proportional to somatic protein mass and dietary protein intake. The creatinine index is measured as the sum of creatinine removed from the body (urine, dialysate, ultrafiltrate), any increase in the body creatinine pool, and the creatinine degradation rate.

Creatinine Index* mg/24 hr = dialysate (ultrafiltrate) Cr mg/24 hr + urine Cr mg/24 hr + change in Cr body pool mg/24 hr + Cr degradation mg/24 hr.

Change in body creatinine pool mg/24 hr = (Final serum Cr mg/L – initial serum Cr) × (24 hour/time interval between creatinine measurements) × (BW kg × 0.5 L/kg)

If body weight is variable:

Change in body creatinine pool mg/24 hr = [final serum Cr mg/L × (final BW kg × 0.5 L/kg)] – [initial serum Cr mg/L × (initial BW kg × 0.5 L/kg)] × (24 hr/time interval between creatinine measurements)

Creatinine Degradation (gut) mg/24 hr = 0.038 dL/kg/24 hr × serum Cr mg/dL × BW kg
Edema-free lean body mass kg = 0.029 kg/mg/24 hr × Cr index mg/24 hr + 7.38 kg

SAMPLE CALCULATION OF EDEMA-FREE LEAN BODY MASS

PD patient:
Urine volume = 475 mL
Effluent volume = 12,485 mL
Serum Cr = 6.91
Body weight (BW) = 70.6 kg

Urine creatinine = 136 mg/mL
Effluent creatinine = 4.5 mg/mL

Cr degradation (gut)

$= 0.038 \times (S_{CR} \times Wt_{kg})$
$=0.038 \times 6.91 \times 70.6$
$= 18.5$ mg/d

Cr production

$= D_{CR} (D_V /100) + U_{CR} \times (U_V /100)/1000$
$= 4.5 \times (12{,}845/100) + 136 \times (475/100)$
$= 562 + 646$
$= 1208$ mg/d

Creatinine Index (Total creatinine production) = 1208 +18.5 or *1226.5 mg/d*

Edema Free LBM = 0.029 × 1226.5 + 7.38 or *42.95 kg*
Edema Free LBM = 61% of total weight is LBM

*Creatinine Index or Total creatinine production = Creatinine excretion + Creatinine degradation

Figure 6.2. Creatinine index (for estimating edema-free lean body mass. Reprinted from McCann L, ed. *Pocket Guide to Nutrition Assessment of the Patient With Chronic Kidney Disease.* 3rd ed. New York, NY: National Kidney Foundation; 2002:1–23, with permission from National Kidney Foundation.

Table 6.2. Peritoneal Dialysis Nutrient Recommendations

Nutrient	*Recommended Daily Level*	*Comment*
Protein	1.2 to 1.3 g/kg SBW or adjusted BW; > 50% HBV protein	Consider increased levels with peritonitis, malnutrition, or other metabolic stress.
Energy	35 kcal/kg SBW or adjusted BW if <60 yrs old. 30–35 kcal/kg if 60 and older.	Includes kilocalories from dialysate and should be individualized to achieve or maintain desirable body weight.
Sodium	2–4 g	Some patients may require no restriction at all, whereas others may need to limit sodium to minimize the use of hypertonic exchange.
Potassium	2–4 g (considered to be consistent with unrestricted diet)	Individualized to maintain serum potassium within the desired range. Some patients require supplementation.
Calcium	≤ 2000 mg total elemental calcium including diet and binders	Low-calcium dialysate is most commonly used and does not add a calcium load unless the patient has a very low serum level.
Phosphorus	800–1000 mg or 10–15 mg phosphorus/g protein	Minimize phosphorus load while allowing adequate protein intake.
Fluids	1–3 L per day	Individualized to patient tolerance with minimal use of hypertonic solutions to maintain fluid balance.
Vitamins and minerals	Renal formulation with 800 µg-5 mg folic acid. Individualized vitamin D, E, zinc, and iron	Replace dialysis losses of B complex plus vitamin C.
Cholesterol and triglycerides	Advise patient of ways to limit simple sugars and saturated fats while maintaining intake of other essential nutrients.	Should not be restricted to the point of compromising essential nutrients.

Abbreviations: BW, body weight; HBV, high biological value; SBW, standard body weight.

Source: Data are from references 18(pp3-3,3-4) and 19.

tion of contact between blood and dialysate allows the removal of excess fluid with less dextrose absorption. In addition, Icodextrin (Extraneal, Baxter Healthcare Renal Division, Deerfield, IL 60025-4625), a high molecular weight, starch-derived glucose polymer can be used in place of sugar-based hypertonic solutions to reduce the calorie load, although its use may be limited by the cost.

PROTEIN

Protein recommendations are formulated to meet protein needs and replace the protein that is lost to dialysate during PD treatment. Between 5 and 15 g of protein are lost each day, primarily as albumin (17,20). Blumenkrantz and associates showed that CAPD patients with daily protein intake less than 1.1 g/kg body weight were at high risk for negative nitrogen balance (20). A positive nitrogen balance could be achieved by some patients with a lower protein intake; however, it is impossible to predict which patients might be able to do this. In addition, that level of protein would not provide any measure of safety for acute problems or stresses. Thus, it is recommended that individuals on PD be encouraged to eat 1.2 to 1.3 g of protein per kg SBW or adjusted body weight (17).

In countries other than the United States, commercial amino acid-containing dialysate, Nutrineal (Baxter Healthcare Renal Division, Deerfield, IL 60025-4625), is available for use in PD. This solution uses amino acids as the osmotic agent rather than glucose or dextrose. Amino acid solutions have the potential to replace protein that is normally lost to the dialysate, as well as decrease the calorie load from sugar-based hypertonic exchanges. Without Food and Drug Administration approval of Nutrineal, intraperitoneal protein replacement or supplementation in the United States can only be done on a limited, individual-patient basis with variable reimbursement by private insurance providers and no reimbursement by Medicare.

Table 6.3. Estimates of Calories Absorbed From Peritoneal Dialysate

The most accurate method of determining the caloric load from peritoneal dialysate is to measure the grams of glucose in the effluent and compare that with the grams of glucose that were infused. The following table compares several other formulas.

Reference	*Formula*	*Example*	*Comment*
Grodstein GP, Blumenkrantz MJ, Kopple JD, Moran JK, Coburn JW. Glucose absorption during continuous ambulatory peritoneal dialysis. *Kidney Int.* 1981;19: 564–567.	Glucose absorbed (kcal) = (11.3X – 10.9) × L inflow × 3.4 Where: X = average glucose concentration infused.	4 L of 1.5% (1.36) + 4 L of 4.25% (3.8) solution = average 2.6%. [(11.3 × 2.6) – 10.9] × 8 L = (29.4 – 10.9) × 8 L = 18.5 × 8 L 18.5 × 8 L = 148 g glucose 148 × 3.4 = 503 kcal	Developed before differences in membranes were recognized but gives a rough glucose absorption/kcal estimate.
Bodnar DM, Busch S, Fuchs J, Piedmonte M, Schreiber M. Estimating glucose absorption in peritoneal dialysis using peritoneal equilibration tests. *Adv Perit Dial.* 1993;9:114–118.	Glucose absorbed (kcal) = $(1 - D/D_o)x_i$ Where: D/D_o is the fraction of glucose remaining and the x_i is the initial glucose.	Infused = 4 L of 38 g/L + 4 L of 13.6 g/L = 152 + 54.4 = 206 g = x_i Measured remaining glucose = 1200 mg/dL in 10 L effluent = 1200 × (10000 mL/100000) = 1200 × 0.1 = 120 g D/D_o = 120/206 = 0.58 (1 – 0.58) × 206 = 86.5 g 86.5 × 3.4 = 294 kcal	This considers dialysis modality and membrane transport characteristics.
Podel J, Hodelin-Wetzel R, Saha DC, Burns G. Glucose absorption in acute peritoneal dialysis. *J Ren Nutr.* 2000;10:93–97.	With acute peritoneal dialysis (APD) in the critical care setting, the mean total glucose absorbed was 43% ± 15%. This finding suggests that the Grodstein formula overestimates glucose absorption with 4.25% APD exchanges and underestimates glucose absorption with 1.5% APD exchanges.		
Simple estimate	Glucose absorbed (kcal) = Glucose infused (mL) × 40% (APD) or Glucose infused (mL) × 60% absorption (CAPD) 1 L: 1.5% = 15 g × 3.4 = 51 × 60% = 31 kcal/L 2.5% = 25 g × 3.4 = 85 × 60% = 51 kcal/L 4.25% = 42.5 g × 3.4 = 144.5 × 60% = 86.7 kcal/L	4 L, 1.5% = 124 kcal 4 L, 4.25% = 346 kcal Total kcal = 470	Does not consider membrane transport characteristics or PD modality.

Abbreviations: APD, automated peritoneal dialysis; CAPD, continuous ambulatory peritoneal dialysis; PD, peritoneal dialysis.

Intraperitoneal nutrition (IPN) in the United States is typically compounded and provided by home care companies such as those that provide home total parenteral nutrition.

SODIUM

Sodium is easily cleared on PD, making a severe sodium restriction unnecessary. Older studies in CAPD showed sodium clearances of up to 5.7 g/day (21), and some patients tolerate as much as 6 to 8 g per day (22). However, extra sodium can create thirst, which in turn causes fluid weight gain. If the individual on PD gains too much fluid weight, they must use higher dextrose (hypertonic) exchanges to remove that fluid. Frequent use of high-dextrose exchanges may cause alterations and even loss of UF capability within the peritoneal membrane. In addition, constant use of hypertonic exchanges can aggravate diabetes, hypertriglyceridemia, and insulin resistance. Thus, the dietary sodium prescription should be tailored to the individual needs of the patient, usually between 2 and 4 g per day. A more limited sodium intake may be necessary if the patient is unable to maintain fluid balance without the constant use of hypertonic solutions. Icodextrin, a high-molecular weight, starch-derived glucose polymer, can be used in place of hypertonic solutions, but it is significantly more expensive. Icodextrin is capable of sustaining UF during prolonged PD dwells (12 to 16 hours) without the negative effects of traditional sugar-based hypertonic solutions (19).

POTASSIUM

Potassium is easily cleared by PD. Most individuals on PD will not need a potassium restriction, and some may need potassium supplementation. Monthly biochemical monitoring provides guidance for adjustment in dietary intake or supplementation based on the serum potassium levels. Most patients tolerate at least 3 g of potassium daily, similar to what might be found in a general diet without excessive dairy products, fruits, and vegetables (14).

CALCIUM

The amount of dietary calcium in PD meal plans is minimal. Most of the calcium comes from calcium-based phosphate binders. Current recommendations are to limit the total elemental calcium to 2,000 mg per day, with no more than 1,500 mg from calcium-based phosphate binders (23). This recommendation is based on the discovery of increased soft-tissue calcification in patients with CKD, which may contribute to the higher incidence of cardiovascular disease in this population. It is recommended that serum calcium (adjusted for low visceral protein stores) be maintained in the low-normal range for the laboratory being used, about 8.4 to 9.5 mg/dL (23).

PHOSPHORUS

The K/DOQI clinical practice guidelines for bone and mineral metabolism suggest that dietary phosphorus be restricted to 800 to 1,000 mg per day and to maintain serum phosphorus levels between 3.5 and 5.5 mg/dL (23). This level of dietary phosphorus is difficult to accomplish with the increased protein levels needed with PD. High-protein foods are also high in phosphorus. Thus, to ensure the palatability of the diet, additional phosphorus may need to be allowed in the diet. In addition to dietary phosphorus limits, phosphorus control is also maintained with the help of phosphate binders. Those patients who have consistently high serum calcium levels or signs of soft-tissue calcification should use non-calcium binders or a combination of binders to control serum phosphorus (23). (See Chapter 16 for further information.)

FLUIDS

Fluid balance in PD is maintained by varying the dextrose concentrations of the dialysate. PD patients are taught how to determine which concentration of dialysate to use based on the fluctuations in their weight. As with sodium, fluids may need to be limited if the patient is unable to maintain fluid balance without frequent use of hypertonic exchanges. Fluid allowance is typically approximately 2 L per day (14).

CHOLESTEROL AND TRIGLYCERIDES

Strict hyperlipidemia guidelines are not usually followed for PD patients. Studies have shown that dietary modification in PD patients have minimal effect on lipid profiles and may compromise the intake of calories and protein (24,25). However, patients should be taught ways to minimize added sugars, saturated fats, and cholesterol. Priority should be given to protein requirements, with guidance on how minimize saturated fat. Often the protein-rich foods that are higher in cholesterol or saturated fats, such as eggs and cheese, are most acceptable to patients.

VITAMINS AND MINERALS

Vitamins and mineral recommendations for PD are similar to those of HD. Water-soluble vitamins are lost to the peritoneal dialysate and must be replaced. Vitamin D is prescribed based on the needs of the patient and in response to the serum levels of calcium, phosphorus, and parathyroid hormone (see Chapter 16). Other vitamin and mineral recommendations can be found in Table 6.2 (14).

PROBLEMS AND SOLUTIONS

PD is an effective form of RRT, but there are some unique issues and problems with this therapy, including significant protein loss, malnutrition, energy absorption, potassium depletion, and physical aberrations (abdominal fullness, slow gastrointestinal transit time, reflux, loss of UF capabilities). Table 6.4 lists some potential problems and interventions for issues that are common to PD.

CONCLUSION

Currently, therapy outcomes on PD and HD are similar in risk factor-adjusted studies, yet PD, for the reasons outlined in this chapter, is not as widely used as HD. While opinions vary and change, neither modality has emerged as the absolute best choice for all patients. PD may become more popular as new, improved techniques and solutions are developed. Current adequacy targets preclude PD for some patients with large muscle mass and little or no urine output. Newer research, such as the ADEMEX (13), may elicit adequacy targets that expand the pool of patients for whom PD is appropriate. In addition, PD, home HD, and self-care therapies will need to expand to accommodate the predicted increase in people requiring renal replacement therapy over the next decade (26).

REFERENCES

1. Ganter G. Ueber die Beseitigung giftiger Stoffe aus dem Blute durch Dialyse. *Munch Med Wochenshcr*. 1923;70:1478–1480.

Table 6.4. Common Side Effects Associated With Peritoneal Dialysis and Potential Interventions

Issues	*Interventions*
Weight gain, hypertriglyceridemia, hyperglycemia	1. Increase exercise as allowed by MD. 2. Limit sodium and fluid to minimize hypertonic exchanges. 3. Use solutions with alternate osmotic agents such as Icodextrin.* 4. Modify energy intake to facilitate weight loss. 5. Modify intake of sugars and fats, especially saturated fats.
Protein losses, malnutrition	1. Education/continual follow-up with the patient regarding protein goals and ways to meet those goals. 2. Advise the patient to eat protein foods first and to limit fluids at mealtime. 3. Advise the patient to eat frequent smaller portions of protein and easy to eat proteins such as egg white, cottage cheese, etc. 4. Education and follow-up on sterile technique to avoid peritonitis. 5. Use Nutrineal,* if available, or refer for intraperitoneal nutrition if the patient is unable to sustain adequate intake with conventional foods. (See Chapter 14). 6. Encourage the patient to build up their intake slowly.
Fullness, abnormal GI function	1. Advise frequent, smaller meals. 2. Limit fluid intake with meals. 3. Advise the patient to eat while draining. 4. Advise an increased fiber diet.
Hypokalemia, potassium depletion	1. Advise the patient to increase intake of higher potassium fruits and vegetables. 2. Supplement potassium if serum levels are significantly low and/or the patient is unable to adequately increase dietary intake.
Ultrafiltration loss	1. Preventive intervention includes avoiding peritonitis and the constant use of hypertonic exchanges. 2. Modify intake of sodium and water. 3. Use alternate solutions such as Icodextrin.†

*Nutrineal (Baxter Healthcare Renal Division, Deerfield, IL 60025-4625)

†Icodextrin (Extraneal, Baxter Healthcare Renal Division, Deerfield, IL 60025-4625)

2. Popovich RP, Moncrief JW, Decherd JF, Bomar JB, Pyle WK. The definition of a novel portable/wearable equilibrium peritoneal dialysis technique (abstract). *ASAIO Trans.* 1976;5:64.
3. Thodis E, Passadeakis P, Vargemezis V, Oreopoulos DG. Peritoneal dialysis: better than, equal to, or worse than hemodialysis? Data worth knowing before choosing a dialysis modality. *Perit Dial Int.* 2001;21:25–35.
4. Daugirdas JT, Blake PG, Ing TS. *Handbook of Dialysis*. 3rd ed. Philadelphia, Pa: Lippincott Williams & Wilkins; 2001.
5. NKF DOQI 2000 update: clinical practice guidelines for peritoneal dialysis adequacy. *Am J Kidney Dis.* 2001;37(Suppl 1):S1–S236.
6. Dimkovic N, Oeopoulos DG. Chronic peritoneal dialysis in the elderly. *Semin Dial.* 2002;15: 94–97.
7. Diaz-Buxo JA. Automated peritoneal dialysis therapies: patient selection and dialysis prescription. *Adv Perit Dial.* 1989;5:207–211.
8. Mujais S, Nolph K, Gokal R, Blake P, Burkhart J, Coles G, Kawaguchi Y, Kawanishi H, Korbet S, Krediet R, Lindholm B, Oreopolis D, Rippe B, Selgas R. Evaluation and management of ultrafiltration problems in peritoneal dialysis. *Perit Dial Int.* 2000;20(Suppl 4):S5–S21.
9. Churchill DN, Thorpe KE, Nolph KD, Keshaviah PR, Oreopoulos DG, Page D. Increased peritoneal membrane transport is associated with decreased patient and technique survival for continuous peritoneal dialysis patients. *J Am Soc Nephrol.* 1998;9:1285–1292.
10. Diaz-Buxo JA. Peritoneal dialysis: matching the prescription to the membrane. *Adv Perit Dial.* 1999;15:96–100.
11. Gotch FA, Sargent JA. A mechanistic analysis of the National Cooperative Dialysis Study. *Kidney Int.* 1985;28:526–534.
12. Churchill DN. Implications of the Canada-USA (CANUSA) study of adequacy of dialysis on peritoneal dialysis schedule. *Nephrol Dial Transplant.* 1998;13(Suppl 6):158–163.
13. Paniagua R, Amato D, Vonesh E, Correa-Rotter R, Ramos A, Moran J, Mujais S, Mexican Nephrology Collaborative Study Group. Effects of increased peritoneal clearances on mortality ratesin peritoneal dialysis; ADEMEX, a prospective, randomized, controlled trial. *J Am Soc Nephrol.* 2002;13:1307–1320.
14. McCann L, ed. *Pocket Guide to Nutrition Assessment of the CKD Patient*. 3rd ed. New York, NY: National Kidney Foundation; 2002.
15. Watson PE, Watson ID, Batt RD. Total body water volumes for adult males and females estimated from simple anthropometric measurements. *Am J Clin Nutr.* 1980;33:27–39.
16. Hume R, Weyers E. Relationship between total body water and surface area in normal and obese subjects. *J Clin Pathol.* 1971;24:234–238.
17. National Kidney Foundation. NKF K/DOQI clinical practice guidelines for nutrition in chronic renal failure. *Am J Kidney Dis.* 2000;35(6 Suppl 2):S1–S140.
18. Bergstrom J, Furst P, Alvestrand A, Lindholm B. Protein and energy intake, nitrogen balance, and nitrogen losses in patients treated with continuous ambulatory peritoneal dialysis. *Kidney Int.* 1993; 44:1048–1057.
19. Baxter Web site. Available at: http://www.baxter.com. Accessed April 5, 2004.
20. Blumenkrantz MJ, Kopple JD, Moran JK, Coburn JW. Metabolic balance studies and dietary protein requirements in patients undergoing continuous ambulatory peritoneal dialysis. *Kidney Int.* 1982; 21:849–861.
21. Moncrief JW. Continuous ambulatory peritoneal dialysis. *Dial Transplant.* 1979;8:1077.
22. Nolph KD, Sorkin MI, Moore H. Autoregulation of sodium and potassium removal during continuous ambulatory peritoneal dialysis. *Trans Am Soc Artif Internal Organs.* 1980;26:334–338.
23. National Kidney Foundation. K/DOQI Clinical Practice Guidelines on Bone Metabolism and Disease in Chronic Kidney Disease. *Am J Kidney Dis.* 2003;42(Suppl 3): S1–S202.
24. Saltissa D, Morgan C, Knight B, Chang W, Rigby R, Westhuyzen J. Effect of lipid-lowering recommendations on the nutritional intake and lipid profiles in chronic peritoneal dialysis and hemodialysis patients. *Am J Kidney Dis.* 2001;37: 1209–1215.
25. Fried L, Hutchisonh A, Stegmayr B, Prichard S, Bargman J. ISPD guidelines/recommendations: recommendations for the treatment of lipid disorders in patients on peritoneal dialysis. *Perit Dial Int.* 1999;19:7–16.
26. United States Renal Data System. *USRDS 2003 Annual Data Report: Atlas of End-Stage Renal Disease in the United States.* Bethesda, Md: Na-

tional Institutes of Health, National Institute of Diabetes and Digestive and Kidney Diseases; 2003. Available at: http://www.usrds.org/adr.htm. Accessed April 8, 2004.

ADDITIONAL RESOURCES

Kopple JD, Massry SG, eds. *Nutritional Management of Renal Disease.* 2nd ed. Lippincott Williams and Wilkins, Philadelphia Pa; 2004 (in press).

Mitch WE, Klahr S, eds. *Handbook of Nutrition and the Kidney*. 3rd ed. Philadelphia, Pa: Lippincott-Raven; 1998.

Wiggins K. *Guidelines for Nutrition Care of Renal Patients.* 3rd ed. Chicago, Ill: American Dietetic Association; 2002.

Chapter 7

Nutrition Management of the Adult Renal Transplant Patient

Carolyn C. Cochran, MS, RD, CDE,
and Pamela S. Kent, MS, RD, CSR

Renal transplantation is the preferred method of treatment for many end-stage renal disease (ESRD) patients and is the most common solid organ transplant. Kidney transplantation is economically advantageous, costing less than long-term dialysis, which is an important factor in today's health care economy. In 2002, 14,775 kidney transplants were performed, with the waiting list increasing to more than 58,000 candidates as of September 2003 (1). Insufficient organ donation accounts for the discrepancy between the number of recipients and candidates. Although the number of cadaveric organs has not been increasing in recent years, there has been an increase in living related and nonrelated donations. Living donation affords the option, in some recipient cases, to bypass the need for dialysis before transplant.

Nutrition care of the renal transplant recipient is a dynamic process. It involves integrating knowledge of the patient's complex medical condition related to chronic renal disease and the impact of ongoing therapeutic interventions on the patient's nutritional status. Continual reassessment of the nutrition goals and efficacy of therapy allow for the adjustment of nutrition priorities during different phases of care.

Three phases of care have been identified for organ transplant recipients: pretransplantation, the acute posttransplantation phase, and the chronic posttransplantation phase (2). In the pretransplantation period, the goal is to meet current education and nutrition needs, optimize the patient's nutritional status, and assist the patient in meeting body weight criteria for transplantation (as per transplant facility guidelines). In the acute posttransplantation period (up to 8 weeks after transplantation), the goal is to support the increased metabolic demands of surgery and high-dose immunosuppressive therapy. A plan for nutritional rehabilitation is formulated and initiated. During the chronic posttransplantation period, nutritional rehabilitation can be realized. Of concern is the nutrition management of complications related to long-term immunosuppressive therapy, especially in individuals genetically predisposed to diabetes and cardiovascular disease (3,4).

THE PRETRANSPLANTATION PERIOD

A complete evaluation of the patient's nutritional status before transplantation is imperative to identify deficits and, when possible, to correct these before surgery. Dietitians must keep in mind that the transplant candidate has been subjected to the deleterious effects of a chronic disease with organ failure and that not all deficiencies identified can be corrected without organ replacement. The baseline data gathered during initial assessment are used to develop a plan of care for that candidate. Assessment of the patient with ESRD and chronic kidney disease (CKD) is discussed in Chapter 2.

The pretransplantation evaluation should include a medical history, dietary history, anthropometric data, biochemical indices of nutritional status, evaluation of gastrointestinal (GI) abnormalities, nutrition supplement and vitamin and mineral use, herbal/botanical product use, and information about current renal replacement therapy, if any. The dietitian can then assess nutritional needs and formulate recommendations. For the severely malnourished patient, specialized nutrition support before surgery may be warranted.

Although the clinical relevance of specific nutritional indices in the ESRD population related to posttransplantation complications has not been extensively investigated, obesity is one index that has been studied. In 2002, Meier-Kriesche et al (5) retrospectively analyzed the impact of body mass index (BMI) on transplant outcomes in 51,927 adult renal transplant patients registered in the United States Renal Data System (USRDS). Their findings suggest that underweight and obese patients have a higher mortality and reduced allograft (graft) survival. These patients experienced a higher incidence of perioperative complications resulting in delayed graft function, early graft loss, and increased length of hospital stay.

Due to the limited availability of organs, the selection of transplant candidates who are likely to have a positive outcome remains an important issue. Both cadaveric and living-related or living-unrelated transplant recipients should meet specific weight criteria prior to transplantation. These criteria vary by medical facility, but the scientific literature indicates that the patient should have a BMI greater than 22 but less than 30 (5,6). Aggressive attempts at pretransplantation weight reduction should be made for the obese candidate. Only by treating the complex behavioral, nutritional, and medical aspects of obesity together can successful weight loss be achieved. Future studies should investigate whether weight adjustment can favorably impact posttransplant outcomes in underweight and obese patients, and if pharmacologic agents or surgical treatment for obesity are feasible options for the pretransplant population.

THE ACUTE POSTTRANSPLANTATION PERIOD

Immunosuppressive Therapy

Pharmacologic immunosuppression is used to prevent acute rejection and maintain long-term graft survival. In multidrug therapy, each drug mediates the immunocompetence cascade at a different point. The goal of immunosuppression is to inhibit the adaptive immune response while allowing nonspecific immune functions to remain intact (7). Unfortunately, this therapy has yet to be perfected. Immunosuppressive agents also have nonimmunologic side effects. The common use of multitherapy regimens is an attempt to use lower doses of individual agents to minimize associated side effects. Some of the currently used agents are listed in Table 7.1 (7–18).

Cyclosporine A (Sandimmune/Neoral)

Cyclosporine A (CsA; Sandimmune/Neoral, Novartis Pharmaceuticals, St. Louis, MO 63166–6556) revolutionized solid organ transplantation in the 1980s and was considered the gold standard for maintenance immunosuppression (8). CsA and its successors are cyclic polypeptides extracted from the fungus *Tolypocladium inflatum gams.* CsA is lipophilic, with the intravenous preparation stabilized in castor oil and the oral preparation stabilized in olive or corn oil. CsA selectively inhibits adaptive immune responses but also has some nonimmunologic side effects, which may include gingival hyperplasia, GI disturbances, hyperglycemia, hyperkalemia, hypophosphatemia, hypomagnesemia, hepatotoxicity, and nephrotoxicity. This drug is absorbed in the upper small intestine and can be affected by food, drug-drug interactions, bile flow, and the patient's lipoprotein and hematocrit status (9). Due to the nephrotoxic side effects, CsA peak and/or trough levels and renal function are closely monitored. Neoral is a microemulsion preparation of CsA and has better absorption because it is not dependent on bile. There are usually fewer side effects with Neoral.

Tacrolimus (Prograf/FK506)

Tacrolimus (Prograf/FK506, Fujisawa Healthcare, Inc, Chantilly, VA 20153–1644) was approved as an immunosuppressive agent in kidney transplantation in 1997. It is 10 to 100 times more potent than CsA (10). Whereas both tacrolimus and CsA inhibit interleukin-2 (IL-2) synthesis and release, each reacts differently at the cellular level. The ingestion of food with tacrolimus affects the rate and extent of the absorption of the drug. Side effects include insulin resistance, hyperkalemia or hypokalemia, hypophosphatemia, and hypomagnesemia, as well as GI distress

Table 7.1. Potential Adverse Effects of Immunosuppressants With Nutritional Implications

Agent	*Adverse Effects*	*Interventions*
Cyclosporine A (Sandimmune, Neoral)*	• Hyperkalemia • Hyperglycemia • Gingival hyperplasia • Hypertension • Hypomagnesemia • Gastrointestinal distress • Hyperlipidemia	• Restrict potassium intake • Address carbohydrate load • Good oral hygiene • Restrict sodium intake • Supplement magnesium • Provide clear liquids, oral nutritional supplements • Therapeutic lifestyle changes
Azathioprine (Imuran)†	• Infection • Mouth ulcers • Folate deficiency • Gastrointestinal distress	• Increased nutrient demands • Diet texture medications • Folate supplementation • Provide clear liquids, oral nutritional supplements
Corticosteroids (prednisone,‡ prednisolone,‡ Solumedrol)§	• Cushingoid appearance • Sodium retention • Enhanced appetite • Hyperlipidemia • Hyperglycemia • Protein catabolism • Gastrointestinal ulceration	• Address carbohydrate load and increase protein intake • Restrict sodium intake • Low-calorie snacks • Therapeutic lifestyle changes • Address carbohydrate load • Increase protein provision • Limit/restrict caffeine if sensitive
Tacrolimus (Prograf, FK506)‖	• Hypertension • Hyperglycemia • Hyperkalemia • Hypomagnesemia • Gastrointestinal distress	• Restrict sodium intake • Restrict simple carbohydrate intake/address carbohydrate distribution • Restrict potassium intake • Supplement magnesium • Provide clear liquids, oral nutritional supplements
Mycophenolate mofetil (CellCept, RS-61443)¶ Antithymocyte Globulin (ATG)# Muromonab CD3 (Orthoclone OKT3)** Daclizumab (Zenepax)¶ Basiliximab (Simulect)*	• Gastrointestinal distress	• Provide clear liquids during acute gastrointestinal distress, oral nutritional supplements
Sirolimus (Rapamune)††	• Hyperlipidemia • Delayed wound healing • Hypokalemia	• Therapeutic lifestyle changes • Vitamin supplementation, increased protein • Potassium supplementation

*Novartis Pharmaceuticals, St. Louis, MO 63166-6556

†Faro Pharmaceuticals, San Diego, CA 92121

‡Watson Laboratories, Inc., Corona, CA 92880

§Pharmacia and Upjohn, Peapack, NJ 07977

‖Fujisawa Healthcare, Inc. Chantilly, VA 20153-1644

¶Roche, Centreville,VA 20120

#Upjohn Co., Kalamazoo, MI 49001

**Otho Biotech, Bridgewater, NJ 08807-0914

††Wyeth Pharmaceuticals, Philadelphia, PA 19101

Source: Data are from references 7–18.

including anorexia, nausea, vomiting, and diarrhea or constipation.

Mycophenolate Mofetil (CellCept/RS-61443)

Mycophenolate mofetil (MMF; CellCept/RS-61443, Roche, Centerville, VA 20120) became available for use in kidney transplantation in 1995. It is mainly used as an adjunctive agent in multitherapy protocols with CsA, corticosteroids, or tacrolimus. Its primary effect on the immune system is to inhibit T-cell proliferation (7). There are several side effects of this drug, but the most common involves GI distress with diarrhea, nausea, or vomiting. Distribution of dosages throughout the day has been shown to be helpful.

Sirolimus (Rapamycin/Rapamune)

Sirolimus (Rapamune, Wyeth Pharmaceuticals, Philadelphia, PA 19101) was approved for use in transplantation in 1999 (11). Sirolimus is a macrolide antibiotic that is structurally similar to tacrolimus and inhibits the proliferation of immune cells. Potential side effects include dyslipidemias (hypertriglyceridemia and hypercholesterolemia), increased liver enzymes, delayed wound healing, and hypokalemia. When sirolimus is used in combination therapy with CsA and corticosteroids, the dyslipidemias can be further exacerbated (12).

Azathioprine (Imuran)

Azathioprine (Imuran, Faro Pharmaceuticals, San Diego, CA 92121) was initially used as standard immunosuppressive therapy in the 1960s. Azathioprine is thought to be a nonspecific immunosuppressant whose mode of action is to inhibit the proliferation of immunocompetent cells. It is typically used in multidrug therapy and may be administered intravenously or orally. Common GI side effects include diarrhea and cholestasis (13).

Corticosteroids (Prednisone, Prednisolone, Solumedrol)

Corticosteroids became available in the 1960s to reverse rejection in kidney transplantation (14). The most commonly prescribed corticosteroids used in transplant programs include prednisone and methylprednisolone. Corticosteroids have anti-inflammatory properties and inhibit the production of lymphokines. This class of immunosuppressants can be administered either in high oral or parenteral doses for acute rejection or as oral pulse doses, which are then tapered to maintenance levels or in some cases discontinued (15). Associated side effects are believed to be dose-dependent and may include impaired wound healing, avascular necrosis of long bones, upper GI ulceration, protein catabolism, hypertension, steroid-induced diabetes mellitus, cataract formation, and stimulation of appetite with resultant weight gain, among others (16).

Other Agents

Monoclonal antibodies (muromonab-CD3; Orthoclone OKT3, Ortho Biotech, Bridgewater, NJ 08807–0914) and antithymocyte globulin (ATG; Upjohn Co, Kalamazoo, MI 49001) are examples of immunosuppressants used either perioperatively for induction therapy or for acute rejection episodes. These agents may cause GI distress and flu-like symptoms, and appropriate adjustments in nutritional therapy should be made (7). Daclizumab (Zenapax, Roche, Centerville, VA 20120) is a genetically engineered monoclonal antibody that is an IL-2 receptor antagonist. This drug can be combined with traditional immunosuppressive therapy. It is an intravenous preparation administered in 1 to 5 doses within the first 8 weeks postoperatively. There are no known side effects (17). Another IL-2 antagonist without side effects is Basiliximab (Simulect, Roche, Centerville, VA 20120). It is used in combination therapy usually with CyA and corticosteroids. This medication is administered preoperatively and then given on the fourth postoperative day (18).

There are several immunosuppressive agents currently being investigated in clinical trials. Dietitians are challenged to stay informed about the various nutrition-related side effects of each agent and to assist patients in appropriate management.

Nutritional Requirements

Currently accepted practice approaches on nutrition recommendations for adult kidney transplantation are shown in Table 7.2 (16,19). Nutrient requirements are increased during the acute posttransplantation phase, which lasts up to 8 weeks.

Table 7.2. Daily Nutrient Recommendations for Adult Kidney Transplantation

Nutrient	*Acute Period*	*Chronic Period*
Protein	1.3–2.0 g/kg*	0.8–1.0 g/kg; limit with chronic graft dysfunction.
Calories	30–35 kcal/kg* or BEE × 1.3; May increase with postoperative complications.	Maintain desirable body weight.
Carbohydrate	Limit simple carbohydrate intake if intolerance is apparent.	Emphasize complex carbohydrate intake and distribution.
Fat	Remainder of calories; emphasize PUFA and MUFA.	Emphasize PUFA and MUFA.
Sodium	2–4 g	2–4 g with hypertension.
Potassium	2–4 g if hyperkalemic.	Unrestricted unless hyperkalemic.
Calcium	1200–1500 mg	1200–1500 mg
Phosphorus	DRI; may need supplementation to normalize serum levels.	DRI†
Other vitamins	DRI†	DRI†
Other minerals	DRI†	DRI†
Trace elements	DRI†	DRI†
Fluid	Limited only by graft function.	Limited only by graft function; generally unrestricted.

Abbreviations: BEE, basal energy expenditure; DRI, dietary reference intake; MUFA, monounsaturated fatty acids; PUFA, polyunsaturated fatty acids.

*Based on standard or adjusted body weight.

†Due to lack of research, no specific recommendations are available for this population. Currently the DRI is used as the guideline.

Source: Data are from references 16 and 19.

Protein

The acceleration of the transplant recipient's protein catabolic rate (PCR) is related to the administration of large doses of corticosteroids as well as postoperative stress (20). This increase in PCR seems to persist at least through the third postoperative week and increases during rejection therapy. Maintenance of protein balance during this period is a formidable task, and negative protein balance will ensue if the intake of protein does not equal the PCR. The present recommendation for initial protein intake is 1.3 to 2.0 g/kg of standard body weight or adjusted body weight (21). Advances in immunosuppression have lessened the need for corticosteroids. There are currently no studies available that address nitrogen balance with the latest immunosuppression regimens.

Energy

Energy requirements are increased in the acute posttransplantation phase and can be estimated by calculating 30 to 35 kcal/kg standard body weight or adjusted body weight (22). This recommendation seems adequate for maintaining or achieving neutral nitrogen balance. Energy needs may further increase in the presence of fever, infection, surgical stress, and high-dose corticosteroid therapy. Estimation of energy needs can also be calculated using the Harris-Benedict equation to determine basal energy requirements multiplied by a stress factor of 1.3 to 1.5 (23).

Carbohydrate

Glucose intolerance postoperatively can result from immunosuppression, surgical stress, genetic predisposition, obesity, increased age, and infection (24). Hyperglycemia may be short lived during this acute postoperative period and can be managed with sliding scale insulin or oral hypoglycemic agents, as well as a carbohydrate-controlled diet. Complex carbohydrates may provide up to 70% of the estimated calorie requirements (23).

Transplant recipients are encouraged to have a liberal fluid intake to maintain adequate hydration. Some patients think that fruit juice is a healthful beverage choice, but overconsumption results in significant carbohydrate and calorie intake. Alternative low-carbohydrate fluid choices should be encouraged.

Fat

During the acute postoperative period, fat is used to supply the remainder of the total energy after calculating the amount provided by protein and carbohydrate. The amount of fat is only limited by the appropriate energy level and often provides up to 30% of the total energy, with intake of saturated fat limited to 10% of calories (23). Dyslipidemia is usually addressed during the chronic posttransplantation period. Nutrition education in the acute period should introduce the importance of a "heart-healthy" lifestyle.

Sodium

Sodium intake should only be restricted in the acute postoperative period in the presence of poor allograft function or posttransplant hypertension. Some immunosuppressive medication can cause hypertension and fluid retention, which may necessitate sodium restriction of 4 gram per day. Blood pressure, fluid status, and electrolyte levels should be closely monitored to determine whether sodium restriction is warranted (25).

Potassium

A moderate dietary potassium restriction is indicated if serum potassium levels are elevated. Poor graft function as well as impaired potassium excretion associated with cyclosporine immunosuppression and potassium-sparing diuretics may contribute to hyperkalemia (26). Hypokalemia has also been reported in kidney transplant recipients due to potassium-wasting diuretics.

Vitamins and Minerals

Little research has been done regarding the vitamin and mineral needs of the renal transplant recipient in the acute postoperative period. A diagnostic approach is helpful to identify vitamin and mineral deficiencies when determining requirements. Additional vitamin and mineral requirements during the chronic posttransplantation phase will be discussed later in this chapter. Information about the effect of renal transplantation on trace element nutriture is scarce, with the exception of the effects on zinc and magnesium. Because uremic patients have abnormal zinc metabolism, zinc is one of the trace elements most likely to become deficient in patients with ESRD (27,28). Candidates presenting for renal transplantation may therefore be zinc deficient. In a study by Mahajan and colleagues (27), patients with subnormal plasma and hair zinc levels as well as abnormal taste detection and recognition thresholds during the pretransplantation period did not show normalization of these parameters until 1 year after transplantation. These patients showed a persistence of zinc depletion, despite correction of uremia. The suboptimal zinc nutriture seems to be related to increased urinary zinc losses. The mechanism underlying hyperzincuria and the clinical significance of zinc depletion after renal transplantation may be immune-mediated because zinc metabolism is affected by inflammation (27). When faced with wound complications, zinc status should be considered, with supplementation if dietary zinc intake is insufficient.

Hypomagnesemia has been reported in kidney transplant recipients treated with CsA. Thirty-one hypertensive postrenal transplant patients receiving multidrug immunosuppression (CsA, azathioprine, and Prednisolone) and not receiving magnesium supplementation were prospectively studied (29). Conclusions were that high serum CsA levels are associated with hypomagnesemia and that serum magnesium should be monitored regularly and supplemented if indicated.

Herbals/Botanicals

Herbal products and botanicals have an enormous presence in the US health care system (30). The Dietary Supplement Health and Education Act , which became a law in 1994, established a formal definition of dietary supplement (31). No proof of efficacy, safety, nor quality control standards is required, thus increasing the risks of adverse effects from these products. Some herbal preparations are advertised to enhance the immune system (such as ginseng and echinacea), which theoretically may increase the risk of organ rejection. Others, like St. John's wort, can cause drug-drug interactions, requiring higher doses of immunosuppression to maintain trough levels (32). The use of herbals and botanicals in the transplant population is currently contraindicated.

Common Postsurgical Problems

Hyperglycemia

Insulin resistance is a common response to corticosteroids and is also a documented side effect of tacrolimus and cyclosporine (13). Prior personal or family history of diabetes mellitus and obesity predisposes a patient to hyperglycemia, especially during the period of high-dose corticosteroids used during the initial postoperative days or during treatment for acute rejection. Oral hypoglycemic agents or insulin therapy combined with nutrition counseling may be necessary for glycemic control.

Gastrointestinal Issues

The majority of immunosuppressive agents are associated with a wide range of GI symptoms, including diarrhea, nausea, and vomiting. There is an increased incidence of GI complications due to infections, mucosal injury, and ulceration, which can manifest anywhere in the GI tract from the mouth to the anus in the kidney transplant recipient (33).

Viral infections such as cytomegalovirus (CMV) are common in the immunocompromised patient. CMV can affect any portion of the GI tract and may mimic ischemic colitis, intestinal pseudo-obstruction, and toxic megacolon (34). Symptoms may include dysphagia, odynophagia, nausea, vomiting, abdominal pain, diarrhea, GI bleeding, or gut perforation. It is imperative to minimize any delay in diagnosis because CMV can quickly spread to critical organs. Herpes simplex virus (HSV) is another common viral infection that can affect any region of the GI tract but most often infects the oral cavity and esophagus. One report of 221 kidney transplant patients found HSV esophagitis in only five patients, an incidence of 2.2%, over an 8–year period (35).

Fungal infections are also common in the early posttransplantation phase and usually present as candida esophagitis with or without thrush (33). Transplant programs typically prescribe prophylactic antifungal agents to prevent fungal infections.

Bacterial infections of the gut are also frequently diagnosed in the transplant recipient and include *clostridium difficile* colitis. Symptoms include diarrhea and abdominal tenderness and usually respond to appropriate medical treatment (33).

Several factors can be responsible for posttransplantation ulcer formation, including the administration of corticosteroids and a prior history of peptic ulcer disease. One study showed that the prevalence of *Helicobacter pylori* was 70% in renal transplant recipients and that gastritis was present in 65% of the transplant recipients (36). Transplant candidates need to be evaluated for *H. pylori* if there is no other obvious indication for peptic ulcer disease. Most transplant programs initially prescribe prophylactic histamine-2 receptor blockers.

Although the incidence is low, the stress of surgery, nonsteroidal anti-inflammatory drugs, corticosteroids, or immunosuppression may impact the formation of ulcers after renal transplantation (37). Prophylaxis for posttransplantation ulceration may complicate immunosuppression (33). CsA drug levels may be affected by administration of cimetidine (Tagamet, GlaxoSmithKline, Phoenix, AR 85038–9038) or ranitidine (Zantac, GlaxoSmithKline, Phoenix, AR 85038–9038). Cimetidine may cause serum creatinine to be falsely elevated by inhibiting the tubular secretion of creatinine. CsA levels may also be altered by concomitant administration of proton-pump inhibitors. Due to the decrease in gastric secretions, the GI flora may be altered, increasing overgrowth of undesirable organisms and resulting in an infection.

Hypophosphatemia

Abnormalities of renal phosphate handling occur even with stable, functioning allografts. Hypophosphatemia is common when glomerular filtration rate normalizes in transplant recipients with preexisting hyperparathyroidism (38). Other factors that may contribute to the development of hypophosphatemia in the acute postoperative period include the use of phosphate binders, intracellular phosphorus shifts associated with high levels of dextrose provision and aggressive refeeding, use of calcium supplements with meals, and inadequate phosphorus intake. Low intake may be seen with lactose-intolerant patients, or those who inadvertently continue a phosphorus-restricted diet. In the acute setting, it may be necessary to use IV phosphorus to normalize serum levels in addition to oral supplementation for maintenance (refer to Table 7.3) (39). Some phosphorus supplements contain significant amounts of potassium and require close monitoring of

Table 7.3. Phosphorus Supplements

Product	*Phosphorus, mg (mmol)*	*Potassium, mEq*	*Usage*
Neutraphos*	250 (8)	7	Use if potassium is within normal limits
K-Phos Neutral†	250 (8)	1	Use if potassium level is high
Neutraphos-K*	250 (8)	14	Use if potassium level is low

*Ortho-McNeil Pharmaceutical, San Bruno, CA 94066

†Beach Pharmaceuticals, Tampa, FL 33611

Source: Data are from reference 39.

serum potassium levels. With persistent hyperkalemia, a change to a sodium phosphate preparation for phosphorus supplementation may be suggested. Doses should be less than that which would affect a laxative response. Sodium phosphate preparations in a flavored liquid may be more palatable. Patients should also be counseled about high-phosphorus food choices.

Hyperkalemia

Postsurgical hyperkalemia is associated with poor graft function, cyclosporine therapy, and cell lysis related to the catabolic effect of both surgery and corticosteroids. Interventions include restriction of potassium intake (dietary and supplements) and the provision of adequate calories and protein to minimize catabolism of endogenous tissue (40). If hyperkalemia persists, a binding resin may be used. Patients may find this situation confusing because they may have been told there would be no more dietary potassium control after transplantation. A high dietary phosphorus intake may have been encouraged by the medical staff to treat hypophosphatemia, which then contributes to the dietary potassium load, thus complicating the situation. Selection of a phosphorus supplement should include comparison of potassium content as well.

Inadequate Intake

Successful renal transplantation corrects the abnormalities of taste suppression and anorexia typically observed in the ESRD patient. Despite an increased appetite after transplant, there are those patients whose postsurgical experience is more complicated. Some recipients may experience temporary loss or a slow return of appetite. In these cases, nutritional supplementation to facilitate surgical recovery is the priority. After several months, the patient may have an increased appetite and need behavior modification to avoid unwanted weight gain.

General Considerations

Interactions

Grapefruit juice and grapefruit products can cause changes in absorption of certain medications, including calcium channel blockers, and some immunosuppressants, antilipidemics, and estrogen products, and should not be consumed by patients taking these drugs. It is thought that grapefruit inhibits the cytochrome P450 isoenzyme CYP3A4 in the gut wall. More than 20 drugs have been identified as having this potential effect. The pharmacokinetics of cyclosporine showed intraindividual variability when this drug was administered with grapefruit in a study by Hollander et al (41). Bailey and colleagues published research showing that the duration of the effect of grapefruit juice can last 24 hours, and that repeated intake can have a cumulative effect (42).

Food Safety

Foodborne infections are a common and sometimes life-threatening problem for millions of individuals in the United States and around the world (43). There are currently 250 known foodborne diseases, but there is limited information reported on the risk of infection from food sources in the immunosuppressed patient (43–46). Individuals infected with foodborne microorganisms exhibit symptoms ranging from mild intestinal distress to severe dehydration, which can jeopardize adequate immunosuppression and renal perfusion. Given the increased prevalence of foodborne outbreaks, it is prudent to reinforce food safety guidelines.

Specialized Nutrition Support Considerations

Kidney transplant recipients are most often able to meet their nutrition needs with an oral diet. Liquid nutrition supplements may be used to assist patients experiencing difficulty with adequate intake. Problems that may benefit from enteral supplementation range from dental work or short-term gastric irritation to gastroenteropathy.

Tube feeding is not commonly needed after kidney transplantation. If a patient is unable to meet metabolic demands orally and has a functional GI tract, standard high-nitrogen tube feedings should be initiated. Nutrient-dense enteral formulas may be indicated in the event of poor allograft function with volume overload. (See Chapter 13 for additional information.)

Parenteral nutrition (PN) is rarely indicated after kidney transplantation. If PN is required, consider allograft function, urine output, electrolytes, and whether renal replacement therapy is used. (See Chapter 14 for additional information.)

THE CHRONIC POSTTRANSPLANTATION PERIOD

Nutritional rehabilitation of patients with ESRD can be realized after successful renal transplantation. During the chronic posttransplant phase, overnutrition may lead to transplant complications, including obesity, dyslipidemias, diabetes mellitus, and hypertension. The nutrition goals of the chronic posttransplantation phase are to provide adequate nutrition, prevent infection, and manage long-term nutritional complications. Since the passage of the Beneficiary Improvement and Protection Act of 2000, transplant recipients in the United States are eligible for medical nutrition therapy (MNT) for 3 years after transplant (47). The ICD-9 diagnosis code for renal transplant is V42.0 and must be accompanied by a physician's order for MNT. (See Appendix A.)

Nutritional Requirements

Once maintenance levels of immunosuppressive agents have been reached, renal transplant recipients without complicating factors can enjoy a dietary regimen consistent with guidelines for the healthy population, addressing specific issues as needed. In general, the diet is moderate in sodium and fat. It is prudent to have a protein intake of 0.8 to 1.0 g/kg of standard or adjusted body weight. Calorie requirements can be estimated using the Harris-Benedict equation to determine basal energy requirements, multiplied by a stress factor of 1.3 (16). Adjustment can be made based on weight gain trends. (Refer to Table 7.2.)

Calcium

Osteoporosis, secondary to preexisting hyperparathyroidism, abnormalities in vitamin D metabolism, and corticosteroid use, is a major complication after transplantation (48). One year posttransplant, hyperparathyroidism is present in 43% of long-term renal transplant patients with normal serum creatinine (49).

To evaluate vitamin D metabolism, 61 renal transplant recipients were studied for 2 years after transplantation. Immunosuppressive therapy consisted of CsA and a corticosteroid (prednisone). At time of transplantation, 1,25–dihydroxy vitamin D levels were low in all candidates and remained abnormal for at least 6 months in nearly half of the participants. Bone mineral density subsequently decreased during the first 6 months posttransplant but remained stable for the duration of the study (50).

Long-term corticosteroid therapy with resultant inhibition of bone formation and the stimulation of bone resorption can also lead to osteoporosis (48). Corticosteroids also decrease the intestinal absorption of elemental calcium to approximately 42% of that ingested, compared with 61% for individuals not being treated with corticosteroids. The amount of calcium excreted in the urine is also increased with corticosteroid therapy (19). For these reasons, it has been suggested that the renal transplant recipient requires a higher level of calcium intake to absorb the amount equal to that expected to be provided by the dietary reference intake (DRI), and calcium supplementation may be indicated. Some centers recommend calcium with vitamin D to maintain good bone health.

Vitamins and Trace Minerals

Typically, vitamin supplementation is not usually required after kidney transplantation, although many programs recommend a general multivitamin product. Vitamin A levels are elevated in patients with ESRD and can remain elevated for 2 years posttransplant (51). Iron supplementation may be clinically indicated in some patients.

Long-Term Care Challenges

Exercise

In addition to playing a significant role in the management of body weight and obesity, exercise offers significant health benefits, including the reduction of cardiovascular risk factors improvement in diabetes management and bone health. The patient's physical condition prior to dialysis and transplant may be predictive in forecasting exercise capacity. Patients are typically cleared to resume exercise 6 weeks after surgery if complications are not present.

Few studies have evaluated the impact of exercise after kidney transplantation, but one study concluded that exercise training is beneficial in kidney transplant recipients (52).

Cardiovascular Disease

Cardiovascular disease is the leading cause of mortality in kidney transplantation. The cardiovascular risk factors that accompany postrenal transplantation include an atherogenic lipid profile, hypertension, diabetes mellitus, chronic prothrombotic state, and obesity (53,54).

The occurrence of dyslipidemias in kidney transplantation has been recognized for nearly 30 years. Approximately 70% of kidney recipients will experience serum lipid abnormalities sometime during the posttransplant course (48,55). Contributing factors for dyslipidemias after transplant include immunosuppressive therapy (CsA, corticosteroids, tacrolimus, sirolimus, etc), graft dysfunction, obesity, diuretic and/or antihypertensive drug therapy, age, gender, diabetes mellitus, and proteinuria.

Although most risk factors cannot be modified, diet and obesity are two factors that may be manipulated. Therapeutic lifestyle changes should be considered as a first step in treatment of obesity and lipid disorders. These involve reducing intake of saturated fat and cholesterol, increasing physical activity, and maintaining a healthy weight (56). Lipid profiles can improve with MNT, but renal transplant recipients often still require lipid-lowering agents to reach target lipid levels as suggested by the Adult Treatment Panel guidelines. The HMG-CoA reductase inhibitors have emerged as the agents of first choice in the treatment of posttransplant hyperlipidemia in combination with therapeutic lifestyle changes (57).

The Food and Drug Administration has approved plant stanol esters as a food ingredient that can reduce low-density lipoprotein (LDL) cholesterol. Plant stanols are combined with canola oil to form stanol esters. The plant stanols inhibit the absorption of cholesterol from the small intestine. More than 20 clinical studies in the general population have demonstrated the safety and effectiveness of 2 to 3 g of plant stanol esters per day with a subsequent reduction of LDL ranging from 6% to 15% (56). There is currently no documented literature regarding the safety of these products in the transplantation population.

The management of cardiovascular disease has become an increasingly important problem in renal transplantation. Hyperhomocysteinemia has been reported in kidney transplant recipients (58–63). The mechanism for elevated homocysteine levels in transplant recipients is unknown, but factors such as inadequate folate status or renal dysfunction have been identified. It has also been reported that CsA can interfere with the folate-assisted remethylation of homocysteine (64). The effect of folate therapy on plasma homocysteine levels in renal transplant recipients was evaluated, and a 21.6% reduction in fasting serum homocysteine level after 5 mg/day of folate therapy was reported. Folate supplementation can be an effective intervention in reducing the homocysteine levels in renal transplant recipients (63).

Obesity

The negative impact of obesity on the outcomes of kidney transplant recipients is well known. The majority of studies have investigated the effects of pretransplant obesity on posttransplant outcomes. Transplant recipients often experience a significant increase in body weight after transplantation, which adversely affects posttransplant comorbid complications (65). The cause of posttransplantation obesity is multifactorial and includes hyperphagia from steroid administration, elimination of the cachectic effects of dialysis, lack of physical activity, genetic predisposition, age, gender, and race (66,67). Clunk et al (67) conducted a retrospective review of 977 renal transplant recipients to identify variables affecting weight gain in this population. The primary influences on weight gain were female sex, low median household income, and age. The mean weight gain was 10.3 kg within 1 year posttransplant.

Obesity management is a difficult challenge. Lifestyle changes involving diet, behavior modification, and physical activity are the cornerstone of successful weight control. In one study, the effect of early intensive dietary intervention on recently transplanted kidney patients showed reduced weight gain (68). Future studies should investigate whether posttransplant weight reduction can favorably impact outcomes.

Diabetes Mellitus, New Onset

The development of posttransplantation diabetes mellitus (PTDM) is a recognized long-term complication of renal transplantation and is an independent predictor of reduced survival in kidney transplant recipients (69,70). The incidence of PTDM ranges from 10% to 46% according to several reports (71). The etiology of PTDM is multifactorial and includes genetic predisposition; diabetogenic effects of CsA, tacrolimus, and corticosteroids; age; posttransplant weight gain; and ethnicity (particularly prevalent in African Americans, Hispanics, and Native Americans) (71).

Transplant recipients with glucose intolerance should be treated aggressively. Management of PTDM typically includes a carbohydrate-controlled diet, exercise, and weight management. Use of oral hypoglycemic agents (thiazolidinediones, sulfonylureas) individually or in combination may be needed. In some cases insulin will be needed. If so, various types of insulin regimens should be investigated to determine the system best suited to meet the patient's personal and physiological needs.

Hypertension

Hypertension is the most common posttransplant complication and occurs in 90% of renal allograft recipients (72,73). The etiology of hypertension is multifactorial and includes impaired renal function, use of calcineurin immunosuppressants, uncontrolled renin secretion from the native organ, stenosing lesions of the transplant artery, genetic predisposition, and obesity (73). Mild hypertension can accelerate the loss of allograft function and impact the survival of the transplant recipient (73). Antihypertensive treatment may include sodium modification, weight management, diuretics, and calcium channel blockers.

Cancer

The development of malignancies posttransplant is a long-term complication of immunosuppression. Tremblay and colleagues reported a 12.2% cancer incidence in patients who were treated with CsA (74). There is a higher incidence of skin and genitourinary cancers in immunosuppressed populations as compared with the general population. Aggressive nutrition support during chemotherapy or radiation is warranted.

Pregnancy

Along with the restoration of kidney function after successful renal transplantation comes the return of fertility. For many patients, the possibility of pregnancy becomes a reality (75,76). There have been more frequent reports of successful pregnancy outcomes after transplantation. To improve positive outcomes, general guidelines have been suggested for the transplant recipient wanting to conceive. The patient should be in good general health and have adequate kidney function for approximately 2 years after transplantation and minimal or no hypertension or proteinuria (77). Once confirmed, the patient should be monitored as a high-risk pregnancy. Despite the high-risk status assigned to these patients, there is little or no mention of maternal nutritional status, weight gain, or differences in nutritional requirements in comparison with pregnancies in women without renal transplants.

Immunosuppressive agents are secreted in breast milk, and no definitive data exist regarding their effects on the infant. Therefore, breastfeeding is presently discouraged (77).

CONCLUSION

The nutrition interventions associated with kidney transplantation vary according to phase of care as well as nutritional status of the transplant recipient. During the acute posttransplantation phase, the goals are to maintain protein stores, promote wound healing, prevent infection associated with surgery and immunosuppression, and normalize electrolyte imbalances. The goals for the chronic posttransplantation phase are to achieve and maintain good overall nutritional status, manage the nutrition-related preexisting medical concerns, and prevent or minimize the side effects of immunosuppressive therapy, including hyperlipidemia, obesity, hypertension, glucose intolerance, and bone disease. The registered dietitian is a valued member of the health care team, providing timely MNT to enhance the transplant recipient's ability to prevent or minimize the nutrition-related complications.

REFERENCES

1. Organ Procurement and Transplantation Network. View data reports. Available at: http://www.optn.org. Accessed September 13, 2003.
2. Kumar MR, Coulston AM. Nutritional management of the cardiac transplant patient. *J Am Diet Assoc*. 1983;83:463–465.
3. Aguilar-Salinas CA, Diaz-Polanco A, Quintana E, Macias N, Arellano A, Ramirez E, Ordonez ML, Velasquez-Alva C, Gomez Perez FJ, Alberu J, Correa-Rotter R. Genetic factors in the pathogenesis of hyperlipidemia posttransplantation. *Am J Kidney Dis*. 2002;40:169–177.
4. Nampoory MR, Johny KV, Costandi JN, Gupta RK, Nair MP, Samhan M, Al-Muzairai IA, Al-Mousawi M. Inferior long-term outcomes of renal transplantation in patients with diabetes mellitus. *Med Princ Pract*. 2002;11:29–34.
5. Meier-Kriesche HU, Arndorfer JA, Kaplan B. The impact of body mass index on renal transplant outcomes: a significant independent risk factor for graft failure and patient death. *Transplantation.* 2002;73:70–74.
6. Halme L, Eklund B, Kyllonen L, Salmela K. Is obesity still a risk factor in renal transplantation? *Transpl Int*. 1997;10:284–288.
7. Fisher JS, Woodle ES, Thistlethwaite JR. Kidney transplantation: graft monitoring and immunosuppression. *World J Surg*. 2002;26:185–193.
8. Morris PJ. Cyclosporine. In: Morris PJ, ed. *Kidney Transplantation: Principles and Practice*. Philadelphia, Pa: WB Saunders Co; 1994:179–201.
9. Bennett W, Burdmann E, Andoh T, Houghton D, Lindsley J, Elzinga L. Nephrotoxicity of immunosuppressive drugs. *Nephrol Dial Transplant*. 1994;9:141–145.
10. Kahan B. Cyclosporine. *N Engl J Med*. 1989; 321:1725–1738.
11. Gelone DK, Lake KD. Transplantation pharmacotherapy. In: Cupples SA, Ohler L, eds. *Solid Organ Transplantation: A Handbook for Primary Health Care Providers*. New York, NY: Springer Publishing; 2002:114–116.
12. Gonzalez-Posada JM, Rodriquez AP, Tamajon P, Hdez-Marrero D, Maceira B. Immunosuppression with sirolimus, cyclosporine and prednisone in renal transplantation. *Transplant Proc*. 2002; 34:99.
13. DiCecco SR, Francisco-Ziller N, Moore D. Overview and immunosuppression. In: Hasse JM, Blue LS, eds. *Comprehensive Guide to Transplant Nutrition*. Chicago, Ill: American Dietetic Association; 2002:1–30.
14. Starzl T, Marchiono T, Waddell W. The reversal of rejection in human renal homografts with subsequent development of homograft tolerance. *Surg Gynecol Obstet*. 1963;117:385–395.
15. Gelone DK, Lake KD. Transplantation pharmacotherapy. In: Cupples SA, Ohler L, eds. *Solid Organ Transplantation: A Handbook for Primary Health Care Providers*. New York, NY: Springer Publishing; 2002:120–121.
16. McCann L. *Pocket Guide to Nutrition Assessment of the Patient With Chronic Kidney Disease.* 3rd ed. Redwood City, Calif: Satellite Healthcare; 2002.
17. Vincenti F, Nashan B, Light S. Double Therapy and the Triple Therapy Study Groups. Daclizumab: outcome of phase III trials and mechanisms of action. *Transplant Proc*. 1998;30:2155–2158.
18. Kahan B, Rajagopalan P, Hall M. Reduction of the occurrence of acute cellular rejection among renal allografts recipients treated with basiliximab, a chimeric anti-interleukin-2 receptor monoclonal antibody. *Transplantation*. 1999;67:276–284.
19. Hahn TJ, Halstead LR, Baran DT. Effects of short-term glucosteroid administration on intestinal calcium absorption and circulating vitamin D metabolite concentrations. *J Clin Endocrinol Metab*. 1981;2:111.
20. Seagraves A, Moore EE, Moore FA, Weil R 3rd. Net protein catabolic rate after kidney transplantation: impact of corticosteroid immunosuppression. *JPEN J Parenter Enteral Nutr*. 1986;10: 453–455.
21. Jequler E. Energy, obesity and body weight standards. *Am J Clin Nutr*. 1987;45:1035.
22. Glynn C, Greene G, Winkler M, Albina J. Predictive versus measured energy expenditure using limits-of-agreement analysis in hospitalized, obese patients. *JPEN J Parenter Enteral Nutr*. 1999;23:147–154.

23. Hasse JM, Weseman RA. Solid organ transplantation: In: Gottschlich MM, Fuhrman MP, Hammond KA, Holcombe BJ, Seidner DL, eds. *Nutrition Support Dietetics Core Curriculum*. Dubuque, Iowa: ASPEN; 2001:605.
24. Blue LS. Nutrition considerations in kidney transplantation. *Top Clin Nutr*. 1992;7:7–23.
25. Blue LS. Adult kidney transplantation. In: Hasse JM, Blue LS, eds. *Comprehensive Guide to Transplant Nutrition*. Chicago, Ill: American Dietetic Association; 2002:49.
26. Rosenberg ME. Nutrition and transplantation. *Kidney*. 1986;18:19.
27. Mahajan SK, Prasad AS, Rabbani P, Briggs WA, McDonald FD. Zinc deficiency: a reversible complication of uremia. *Am J Clin Nutr*. 1982;36: 1177–1183.
28. Sandstead HH. Trace elements in uremia and hemodialysis. *Am J Clin Nutr*. 1980;33:1501–1508.
29. Thakur V, Kumar R, Dhawan IK. Correlation between serum magnesium and blood cyclosporine A concentrations in renal transplant recipients. *Ann Clin Biochem*. 2002;39:70–72.
30. Bell. AD. Herbal medicine and the transplant patient. *Nephrol Nurs J*. 2002;29:269–274.
31. Dietary Supplement Health and Education Act of 1994. US Food and Drug Administration, Center for Food Safety and Applied Nutrition. Available at: http://vm.cfsan.fda.gov/~dms/dietsupp.html. Accessed November 17, 2003.
32. Ruschitzka F, Meier PJ, Turina M. Acute heart transplant rejection due to St. John's wort. *Lancet*. 2000;355:548–549.
33. Helderman JH, Goral S. Gastrointestinal complications of transplant immunosuppression. *J Am Soc Nephrol*. 2002;13:277–287.
34. Bardaxoglou E, Maddern G, Ruso L, Siriser F, Campion JP, Le Pogamp P, Catheline JM, Launois B. GI surgical emergencies following kidney transplantation. *Transpl Int*. 1993;6:148–152.
35. Mosimann F, Cuenoud PF, Steinhauslin F, Wauters JP. Herpes simplex esophagitis after renal transplantation. *Transpl Int*. 1994;7:79–82.
36. Ozgur O, Boyacioglu S, Ozdogan M, Gur G, Telatar H, Haberal M. Helicobacter pylori infection in haemodialysis patients and renal transplant recipients. *Nephrol Dial Transplant*. 1997; 12:289–291.
37. Troppman C, Papalois BE, Chiou A, Benedetti E, Dunn DL, Matas AJ, Najarian JS, Gruessner RW. Incidence, complications, treatment, and outcome of ulcers of the upper GI tract after renal transplantation during the CsA era. *J Am Coll Surg*. 1995;80:433–443.
38. Torres A, Lorenzo V, Salido E. Calcium metabolism and skeletal problems after transplantation. *J Am Soc Nephrol*. 2002;13:551–558.
39. *Drug Facts and Comparisons*. St Louis, Mo: Wolters Kluwer; 2000.
40. Beto J, Bansal VK. Hyperkalemia: evaluating dietary and nondietary etiology. *J Ren Nutr.* 1992;1: 28–29.
41. Hollander A, van Rooij J, Lentjes E, Arbouw F, van Bree J, Schoemaker R, van Es L, van der Woude F, Cohen A. The effect of grapefruit juice on cyclosporine and prednisone metabolism in transplant patients. *Clin Pharm Ther.* 1995;57: 318–324.
42. Bailey DG, Malcolm J, Arnold O, Spence JD. The effect of grapefruit juice on CsA and prednisone metabolism in transplant patients. *Br J Clin Pharm*. 1998;46:101–110.
43. National Institute of Allergy and Infectious Diseases. National Institutes of Health. Fact Sheet: Foodborne Diseases. April 2002. Available at: http://www.niaid.nih.gov/factsheets/foodbornedis.htm. Accessed November 12, 2002.
44. Daniels N, Shafie A. A review of pathogenic vibrio infections for clinicians. *J Infect Med.* 2000;17:665–685.
45. US Food and Drug Administration, Center for Food Safety and Applied Nutrition. Foodborne Pathogenic Microorganisms and Natural Toxins Handbook, Bag Bug Book. (2000). Available at: http://www.cfsan.fda.gov/~mow/intro.html. Accessed March 21, 2004.
46. US Environmental Protection Agency. Safe drinking water—guidance for people with severely weakened immune systems. June 1999. Available at: http://www.epa.gov/OGWDW/crypto.html. Accessed November 12, 2002.
47. Beneficiary Improvement and Protection Act of 2000. *Federal Register*. November 2001;66. Available at: http://www.eatright.org/member/files/federal-register-8.2.01.doc. Accessed March 21, 2004.
48. Torres, A, Lorenzo, V, Salido, E. Calcium metabolism and skeletal problems after transplantation. *J Am Soc Nephrol.* 2002;13:551–558.
49. Messa P, Sindici C, Cannella G, Miotti V, Risaliti A, Gropuzzo M, Di Loreto PL, Bresadola F,

Mioni G. Persistent secondary hyperparathyroidism after renal transplantation. *Kidney Int.* 1998;54:1704–1713.

50. De Sevaux RG, Hoitsma AJ, Van Hoof HJ, Corstens FJ, Wetzels JF. Abnormal vitamin D metabolism and loss of bone mass after renal transplantation. *Nephrol Clin Pract.* 2004 (in press).
51. Yatzidis H, Digenis P, Koutsicos D. Hypervitaminosis A in chronic renal failure after transplantation. *Br Med J.* 1976;1076:1675.
52. Painter PL, Hector L, Ray K, Lynes L, Dibble S, Paul SM, Tomlanovich SL, Ascher NL. A randomized trial of exercise training after renal transplantation. *Transplantation.* 2002;74:42–48.
53. Hricik DE. Hyperlipidemia in renal transplant recipients. *Graft.* 2000;4:11–19.
54. Tonstad S, Holdaas C, Gorbitz C, Ose L. Is dietary intervention effective in post-transplant hyperlipidaemia? *Nephrol Dial Transplant.* 1995; 10:82–85.
55. Andany MA, Kasiske BL. Dyslipidemia and its management after renal transplantation. *J Nephrol.* 2001;14(suppl):S81–S88.
56. Expert Panel on Detection, Evaluation, and Treatment of High Blood Cholesterol in Adults. Executive summary of the Third Report of the National Cholesterol Education Program (NCEP) Expert Panel on Detection, Evaluation, and Treatment of High Blood Cholesterol in Adults (Adult Treatment Panel III). *JAMA.* 2001;285:2486–2497.
57. Martinez-Castelao, A, Grinyo JM, Gil-Vernet S, Seron D, Castineiras MJ, Ramos R, Alsina J. Lipid-lowering long-term effects of six different statins in hypercholesterolemic renal transplant patients under cyclosporine immunosuppression. *Transplant Proc.* 2002;34:398–400.
58. Savaj S, Ghorbani G, Ghoda AJ. Hyperhomocysteinemia in renal transplant recipients. *Transplant Proc.* 2002;33:2701.
59. Mor E, Helfmann L, Lustig S, Bar-Nathan N, Yussim A, Sela BA. Homocysteine levels among transplant recipients: effect of immunosuppressive protocols. *Transplant Proc.* 2001;33:2945–2946.
60. Zantvoort FA, Waldeman J, Colic D, Lison AE. Incidence and treatment of hyperhomocysteinemia after renal transplantation. *Transplant Proc.* 2001;33:3679–3680.
61. Merouani A, Rozen R, Clermont MJ, Genest J. Renal function, homocysteine and other plasma thiol concentrations during the postrenal transplant period. *Transplant Proc.* 2002;34:1159–1160.
62. Friedman AN, Rosenberg IH, Selhub J, Levey AS, Bostom AG. Hyperhomocysteinemia in renal transplant recipients. *Am J Transplant.* 2002;2: 308–313.
63. Savaj S, Rezakhani S, Porooshani F, Ghods AJ. Effect of folic acid therapy on serum homocysteine level in renal transplant recipients. *Transplant Proc.* 2002;34:2419.
64. Arnadottir M, Hultberg B, Vladov V, Nilsson-Ehle P, Thysell H. Hyperhomocysteinemia in cyclosporine-treated renal transplant recipients. *Transplantation.* 1996;61:509–512.
65. Hricik DE. Weight gain after kidney transplantation. *Am J Kidney Dis.* 2001;38:409–410.
66. Hasse JM. Nutritional issues in adult transplantation. In: Cupples SA, Ohler L, eds. *Solid Organ Transplantation: A Handbook of Primary Health Care Providers.* New York, NY: Springer Publishing; 2002:64–87.
67. Clunk J, Lin C, Curtis J. Variables affecting weight gain in renal transplant recipients. *Am J Kidney Dis.* 2001;73:53–55.
68. Patel MG. The effect of dietary intervention on weight gains after renal transplantation. *J Ren Nutr.* 1998;8:137–141.
69. Cosio FG, Pesavento TE, Kim S, Osei K, Henry M, Ferguson RM. Patient survival after renal transplantation: IV. Impact of post-transplant diabetes. *Kidney Int.* 2002;62:1440–1446.
70. Markell MS. Post-transplant diabetes: incidence, relationship to choice of immunosuppressive drugs, and treatment protocol. *Adv Ren Replace Ther.* 2001;8:64–69.
71. Bartucci MR, Hricik DE. Kidney transplantation. In: Cupples SA, Ohler L, eds. *Solid Organ Transplantation: A Handbook of Primary Health Care Providers.* New York, NY: Springer Publishing; 2002:189–239.
72. Schwenger V, Zeier M, Ritz E. Hypertension after renal transplantation. *Ann Transplant.* 2001;6: 25–30.
73. Zeier M, Dikow R, Ritz E. Blood pressure after renal transplantation. *Ann Transplant.* 2001;6: 21–24.

74. Tremblay F, Fernandes M, Habbab F, Edwardes MD, Loertscher R, Meterissian S. Malignancy after renal transplantation: incidence and role of immunosuppression. *Ann Surg Oncol*. 2002;8: 785–788.
75. Armenti VT, Moritz MJ, Cardonick EH, Davison JM. Immunosuppression in pregnancy: choices for infant and maternal health. *Drugs*. 2002;62: 2361–2375.
76. Fernando O. Pregnancy in transplantation. *Transplant Proc*. 2002;34:2403.
77. Armenti VT, Radomski JS, Moritz MJ, Gaughan WJ, Philips LZ, McGrory CH, Coscia LA, and the National Transplantation Pregnancy Registry. Report from the National Transplantation Pregnancy Registry (NTPR): outcomes of pregnancy after transplantation. *Clin Transplant*. 2002;10: 121–130.

Chapter 8

Nutrition Management of HIV/AIDS in Chronic Kidney Disease

D. Jordi Goldstein-Fuchs, DSc, RD

EPIDEMIOLOGY

The human immunodeficiency virus (HIV) and acquired immunodeficiency syndrome (AIDS) have affected more than 60 million people around the world since first appearing 20 years ago. As of December 2002, the Centers for Disease Control and Prevention (CDC) estimated the number of diagnoses of AIDS in the United States to be 886,575 (1,2). More than 40,000 new cases are reported in the United States annually. Approximately 90% of people infected with HIV do not realize that they carry the virus (1,2). Three states have a cumulative total of 45% of AIDS cases diagnosed in the United States: New York, California, and Florida. The Joint United Nations Programme on HIV/AIDS reports that during 2002, AIDS was responsible for the death of 3.1 million people, including 1.2 million women and 610,000 children younger than 15 years of age (3).

DEFINITIONS OF HIV AND AIDS

HIV is a chronic disease that can develop into AIDS. The acute phase of HIV is characterized by fever, malaise, lymphadenopathy, pharyngitis, headache, myalgia, and sometimes rash (1–4). AIDS is defined as HIV infection accompanied by a CD4 cell count of 200 or less; or dementia, wasting syndrome, or malignant diseases such as Kaposi's sarcoma or non-Hodgkin's lymphoma; or one of 26 opportunistic infections (1–4). AIDS was initially described by the CDC in 1981, when young adults were presenting with unusual opportunistic infections (*Pneumocystis carinii* pneumonia, cytomegalovirus) or Kaposi's sarcoma (a rare skin cancer), accompanied by severe depression of cellular immunity (5).

Key terms associated with clinical management are viral load testing and CD4 lymphocyte counts (T cells). Viral load testing measures free virus circulating in the blood and is expressed as HIV-RNA copies per milliliter of blood plasma. The goal of treatment is to obtain undetectable levels (4). The pathophysiology of the HIV virus is due in large part to a decrease in the number of T cells that express the CD4 receptor (6). Depletion of CD4 T cells is correlated with severe HIV disease and an unfavorable prognosis (6). HIV infects the CD4 cells by becoming part of the cell such that when the CD4 cell multiplies to fight infection, it also replicates copies of the HIV virus. The normal range of CD4 cell counts vary by laboratory, but is usually between 500 and 1,600 cells/mm^3 of blood (1,3,6). The goal of treatment is to maintain CD4 levels more than 200; generally the higher the better.

RENAL DISEASES ASSOCIATED WITH HIV/AIDS

Renal disease associated with HIV was first reported in 1984 (7). The most common renal lesion observed among HIV-infected patients is HIV-associated focal segmental glomerulosclerosis and related mesangiopathies, collectively referred to as HIV-associated nephropathy (HIVAN) (7–10). Other lesions observed in this patient population include thrombotic microangiopathies and immune-complex glomerulonephritis (see Box 8.1) (7–11). The rate of patients with HIV that develop end-stage kidney disease has steadily increased (10). HIVAN was the third leading cause of end-stage renal disease among black men aged 20 to 64 years in 1999 (10).

Most people with HIVAN are young black men (there is a male to female ratio of 10:1), and about 50% of these men use intravenous drugs (10,12). The other subset of patients are gay or bisexual men, heterosexual contacts of infected persons, or children born to HIV-infected mothers (9). The mortality rate among individuals with HIVAN is significant: 30% to 50% at 1 year after initiating dialysis (10). These statistics do not include the number of people infected with HIV who have early renal insufficiency. As the prevalence of HIV increases due to new cases and increased survival, there will be an increased number of patients with complications of HIV, including renal disease (10).

Renal disease in HIV-positive patients may be a primary effect from the infection, a side effect of drug therapy, a secondary effect from drug therapy or a result of comorbid illnesses accompanying or complicating the HIV, or a coincident finding (7,11). HIVAN typically presents as a nephrotic syndrome with more than 3.5 g of proteinuria, hypoalbuminemia, and edema with or without hematuria (9,10). There is progressive loss of renal function and an increased risk of mortality (8,9). The usual progression is loss of kidney function to end-stage within 8 to 16.6 months from the time of diagnosis (13,14). Despite these observations, there is only a limited understanding of the epidemiology and clinical course of HIVAN. This is in part because of the lack of large population studies. In addition, many studies to date had selection bias that impedes applicability of the results to the HIVAN population (10).

Box 8.1. Types of Nephropathies Observed in Patients With HIV

Acute renal failure

- Prerenal azotemia
- Obstructive uropathy
- Acute tubular necrosis
- Hemolytic uremic syndrome (HUS)

Chronic Renal Failure

- HIVAN
- Immune complex glomerulonephritis
- Thrombotic microangiopathies
- HUS
- Glomerulonephritis (membranoproliferative, membranous nephropathy, postinfectious glomerulonephritis)
- IgA nephropathy

Source: Data are from references 7,11.

MEDICAL MANAGEMENT GUIDELINES

Clinical practice guidelines for HIVAN do not currently exist, but recommendations have been reported. (2,7–12). Early intervention is extremely important. HIV-positive individuals should be screened for proteinuria with annual follow-up of high-risk patients. In the presence of proteinuria, further evaluation with a 24–hour urine collection and serologic studies to assess the presence of chronic infection with hepatitis B or C or syphilis should also be completed with renal biopsy to guide therapy (7–12). Box 8.2 summarizes a recommended clinical approach to treatment (7,9).

Available Treatment Options

Treatment options for HIV nephropathies include immunosuppression with cyclosporine and glucocorticoids, highly active antiretroviral therapy (HAART), and angiotensin converting enzyme inhibitors (7–12). The effectiveness observed with the latter class of agents is thought to be due to their hemodynamic effects of lowering intraglomerular pressure, reducing proteinuria, and modulating cytokine-mediated renal injury (8,9). Both hemodialysis and peritoneal dialysis are available for HIV-positive patients with end-stage kidney failure. Transplantation requires meeting strict criteria, which include absence of AIDS-related opportunistic infections, CD4 counts more than 200 for 6

Box 8.2. Clinical Recommendations for Diagnosing and Treating Kidney Disease in HIV-Positive Individuals

Diagnosis

- *Blood tests:* blood urea nitrogen, serum creatinine, electrolytes, calcium, phosphate, albumin, full blood count.
- *Urinalysis:* dip testing for blood and protein; microscopy for red and white blood cells, eosinophils, and casts; 24-hour urine collection for protein and creatinine clearance.
- *Renal imaging:* ultrasound to assess renal size, echogenicity, and cortical thickness; plain abdominal film if nephrocalcinosis suspected; intravenous urogram if obstruction/stones; etc.

Treatment

- Eliminate or reduce viral load to stop continued infection of renal cells.
- Block or minimize cytokine-mediated renal injury.
- Eliminate cells infiltrating the interstitium to reduce further renal damage.
- Stop or minimize protein loss (marker of nephropathy and risk factor for renal deterioration).

Source: Data are from references 7,9.

months, and adequate weight for height as evaluated by body mass index (2).

Nutrition Guidelines for Patients With Kidney Disease and HIV/AIDS

Similar to medical management, clinical guidelines for the nutrition care of the patient with HIV and kidney disease have not been formally established. However, there is substantial literature describing nutrition problems and interventions for this patient population (15–20). At the current time, the best nutrition intervention for the HIV/AIDS patient with kidney disease is individualized assessment, integrating the specific nutrition challenges of HIV/AIDS with appropriate guidelines for patients with chronic kidney disease and for those receiving renal replacement therapy. The second part of this chapter will summarize the nutrition problems associated with HIV/AIDS and discuss how to apply interventions appropriately for the patient with kidney disease.

Nutrition concerns for the patient with HIV are related to the AIDS wasting syndrome, side effects of medications, impact of complicating opportunistic infections, malabsorption, endocrine problems, psychosocial issues, neurologic impairments, and immunosuppression. Newer complications arising as a side effect of HAART and longer survival include lipodystrophy (often referred to as fat redistribution), lipid abnormalities, insulin resistance, bone disease, and lactic acidosis (21–23). A less recognized but very important issue is food safety (24). Early nutrition intervention is important because weight loss, hypoalbuminemia, low CD4 lymphocyte counts, and low body cell mass are associated with increased morbidity (15,19,20).

Nutrition challenges specific to the patient with HIV can be addressed by first categorizing the factors contributing to the development of nutrition problems (Box 8.3) and then identifying specific problems that the dietitian may need to address for both nutrition screening and developing an individualized intervention (Box 8.4) (19). All of these factors need to be considered when providing nutrition care to the kidney patient with HIV.

Wasting Syndrome

The HIV/AIDS wasting syndrome is similar to the wasting observed in renal failure in that it is compli-

Box 8.3. Identification of Factors Contributing to Nutritional Challenges in the Patient With HIV/AIDS

- Wasting syndrome
- Lipodystrophy syndrome
- Anorexia
- Diarrhea
- Nausea
- Vomiting
- Malabsorption
- Hormonal imbalances
- Metabolic abnormalities
- Side effects of drug therapies

Box 8.4. Factors Associated With Significant Nutritional Risk

Diabetes
HTN
> 10% intentional weight loss over 4 to 6 months
> 5% unintentional weight loss within 4 weeks
Oral (or esophageal) thrush
Dental problems
Dysphagia
Chronic nausea or vomiting
Chronic and/or severe diarrhea
CNS disease
Intercurrent or active opportunistic infection
Enteral or parenteral feedings
Medical comorbidities
Dialysis
Complicated food-drug-nutrient interactions
Severely dysfunctional psychosocial situation
Obesity
Evidence for lipodystrophy
Dyslipidemia (cholesterol > 200mg/dL or < 100 mg/dL; or triglycerides > 250 mg/dL)
Evidence of excessive use of vitamins, minerals, or other nutritional supplements or products
Inappropriate use of over-the-counter medications
Substance abuse
Food allergies and intolerances
Chronic pain
Sedentary life style or excessive exercise

Source: Data are from reference 19.

cated, multifaceted, and poorly understood. Anorexia/inadequate intake, malabsorption due to intestinal dysfunction, diarrhea, excessive cytokine production, HIV itself, hypogonadism, and metabolic alterations are thought to be the major contributors to the development of HIV-associated wasting (15,17,20). The CDC case definition of AIDS wasting requires a net weight loss of 10% (20). Loss of both fat and lean muscle mass has been observed, and weight loss has been associated with an increase in risk of death in this patient population (18,20). Patients with kidney disease and HIV with active weight loss should be evaluated for gastrointestinal disease, malignancy, opportunistic infections, hypogonadism, and adrenal insufficiency. Early intervention of the comorbid condition is important as an effort to improve oral intake. Similar to the intervention for kidney disease, therapeutic interventions used for AIDS wasting include nutrition supplements, appetite stimulants, and growth hormones (5,18–20). It is unclear whether cytokine suppression, anabolic agents (testosterone and oxandrolone), and progressive resistance exercise training, which have been used in patients with HIV/AIDS, would be helpful for those with kidney disease. Because it can be difficult to differentiate underlying causes of wasting in the HIV/AIDS patient who also has kidney disease, the more recent interventions being used in patients with HIV/AIDS need to be evaluated in the HIV/AIDS patient with kidney disease.

Lipodystrophy

Lipodystrophy is a new syndrome, also referred to as "fat redistribution syndrome" and peripheral lipodystrophy (15,24). The constellation of symptoms associated with lipodystrophy includes elevated blood lipids, insulin resistance, and an enlarged truncal girth due to the deposition of adipose tissue in the visceral area (15,20,23). Body habitus changes may be due in part to the use of certain protease inhibitors (PI), nucleoside reverse transcriptase inhibitors (NRTIs), or combination therapy (24). One study completed in patients taking HAART showed that 88% of individuals taking PIs reported the incidence of lipodystrophy to be 5% at 6 months, 9% at 12 months, and 26% at 24 months (24). Interventions that have been initiated for this syndrome include diet (low-saturated fat, high-fiber, low-glycemic index carbohydrates) and exercise programs (5,22,24). Other interventions include human growth hormone, insulin-sensitizing agents, androgens, and modification of HAART regimen (15,24). However, effectiveness of these interventions has not been demonstrated, and research is needed in this area. It is unknown whether patients with kidney disease and HIV/AIDS develop body habitus changes of lipodystrophy with similar distribution. The exact pathogenesis of lipodystrophy remains unclear and is an area of continued research.

Hyperlipidemia

Hyperlipidemia can be a separate problem from lipodystrophy that occurs in HIV (22). Progression of HIV is associated with elevated triglycerides and decreased total and high-density lipoprotein. The use of PI therapy increases serum total cholesterol and low-density lipoprotein cholesterol on average 23% and 27%, respectively (22). Elevations in triglycerides can be extreme. Volunteers without HIV who took PIs had a 137% increase in serum triglycerides. The concern is the potential increase in cardiovascular disease in the HIV patient population. How the combination of both HIV and the dyslipidemia of renal disease interact is unclear. Currently, recommendations for the hyperlipidemia of HIV and renal disease are the same: therapeutic lifestyle interventions that utilize the National Cholesterol Education Program guidelines (22,25). (Refer to Chapter 10 for specific guidelines for dyslipidemia management in chronic kidney disease.)

Bone Disease

The development of bone problems, specifically osteopenia and osteoporosis, is increasing in prevalence (26). This seems to be associated with HIV itself and is more pronounced in those patients receiving HAART therapy (26). Risk factors for bone density loss in individuals with HIV include past steroid use, hormonal deficiencies, HIV-related immune system activation, immune reconstitution, and wasting or poor nutrition (26). Intervention currently recommended includes daily: 1,500 mg calcium, 400 to 1,000 IU vitamin D, and moderate physical activity. Hormone replacement therapy, including biphosphates, calcitonin, or raloxifene, is reserved for advanced cases. Due to the increased propensity of bone disease in the individual with renal disease (as described in Chapter 16), treatment guidelines for renal disease should be prioritized, while closely monitoring the patient with the additional diagnosis of HIV.

Protein and Energy

Data from studies measuring resting energy expenditure in patients with HIV suggest a 10% to 25% increase due to the progression of the disease, or the disease itself (15). Therefore, it is prudent to add 10% to 15% to energy expenditure calculations when approximating energy needs. Patients with active weight loss may be best served by adding 15% to 25% to the resting energy expenditure. Current recommendations for energy intake for patients with chronic kidney disease not requiring renal replacement therapy and for those receiving dialysis as recommended by the National Kidney Foundation Dialysis Outcome Quality Initiative is 35 kcal/kg/day for those who are younger than 60 years and 30 to 35 kcal/kg/day for individuals who are 60 years of age or older (27).

Similar to energy, there is not much data available about the protein requirements of patients with HIV/AIDS. General recommendations are to provide 100 to 150 g/day for men and 80 to 100 g/day for women, or 1.2 to 2.0 g of protein per kilogram of body weight per day (15). This recommendation is within the range of the guideline for kidney patients receiving renal replacement therapy (28). For the patient with chronic kidney disease, prioritizing adequacy of nutritional status and prevention of malnutrition may take precedence over the possible benefit of protein restriction on progression of the disease.

SUMMARY

Nutrition guidelines specific for the kidney patient with HIV/AIDS are not currently available. Therefore, the nutrition professional should be aware of potential nutrition problems specific to HIV/AIDS (see Boxes 8.3 and 8.4) that need to be addressed in conjunction with the specifics for kidney disease. Side effects from the specialized medications present additional challenges. The type of kidney disease can also indicate the type of nutrition interventions that might be required, such as electrolyte balance in patients with glomerulonephritis or the nephrotic syndrome symptoms found to accompany HIVAN. Lipodystrophy and hyperlipidemia are newer consequences observed in patients living with HIV/AIDS on HAART. Effective therapies for these conditions will require clinical trials. Research is also needed to identify optimal nutrition interventions for wasting and maintenance of an adequate nutritional status.

REFERENCES

1. Centers for Disease Control and Prevention, Division of HIV/AIDS Prevention Web site. Available at: http://www.cdc.gov/hiv.stats.htm. Accessed November 19, 2003.
2. Burns J, Longton S, Robinson FP, Wolfe G. HIV/AIDS and HIV nephropathy. *Nephrol Nurs J.* 2003;30:64–69,73.
3. Joint United Nations Programme on HIV/AIDS Web site. Available at: http://www.UNAIDS.org. Accessed July 18, 2003.

4. Fenton M, Silverman E. Medical nutrition therapy for human immunodeficiency virus (HIV) infection and acquired immunodeficiency syndrome (AIDS). In: *Krause's Food, Nutrition, and Diet Therapy.* 10th ed. Philadelphia, Pa: WB Saunders Co; 2000:889–911.
5. Roubenoff R. Acquired immunodeficiency syndrome wasting, functional performance, and quality of life. *Am J Manag Care.* 2000;6:1003–1016.
6. Mandy F, Nicholson J, Autran B, Janossy G. T-cell subset counting and the fight against AIDS: reflections over a 20–year struggle. *Cytometry.* 2002;50:39–45.
7. Dellow EL, Unwin RJ, Miller RF. Presentation, diagnosis, and management of renal failure in patients with HIV infection. *AIDS Patient Care STDs.* 2000;14:71–77.
8. Hedayati SS, Reddan DN, Szczech LA. HIV-associated nephropathy: a review of the epidemiology and clinical course in the HAART era. *AIDS Patient Care STDs.* 2003;17:57–63.
9. Rao TK. Human immunodeficiency virus infection and renal failure. *Infect Dis Clin North Am.* 2001;15:833–850.
10. Szczech LA. Renal diseases associated with human immunodeficiency virus infection: epidemiology clinical course, and management. *Clin Infect Dis.* 2001;33:115–122.
11. Kimmel PL. The nephropathies of HIV infection: pathogenesis and treatment. *Curr Opin Nephrol Hypertens.* 2000;9:117–122.
12. Winston JA, Burns GC, Klotman PE. Treatment of HIV-associated nepthropathy. *Semin Nephrol.* 2000;20:293–298.
13. Szczech LA, Edwards LJ, Sanders LL, van der Horst C, Bartlett JA, Heald AE, Svetkey LP. Protease inhibitors are associated with a slowed progression of HIV-associated renal diseases. *Clin Nephrol.* 1991;35:110–118.
14. Laradi A, Mallet A, Beaufils H, Allouache M, Martinez F. HIV-associated nephropathy: outcome and prognosis factors. *J Am Soc Nephrol.* 1998;9:2327–2335.
15. Gerrior J, Wanke C. Nutrition and immunodeficiency syndromes. In: Coulston AM, Rock CL, Monsen ER, eds. *Nutrition in the Prevention and Treatment of Disease.* San Diego, Calif: Academic Press; 2001:741–748.
16. Karlsson A, Nordstrom G. Nutritional status, symptoms experienced and general state of health in HIV-infected patients. *J Clin Nurs.* 2001;10: 609–617.
17. Knox TA, Zafonte-Sanders M, Fields-Gardner C, Moen K, Johansen D, Paton N. Assessment of nutritional status, body composition, and human immunodeficiency virus-associated morphologic changes. *Clin Infect Dis.* 2003;36(Suppl 2):S63–S68.
18. Mulligan K, Schambelan M. Anabolic treatment with GH, IGF-I, or anabolic steroids in patients with HIV-associated wasting. *Int J Cardiol.* 2002; 85:151–159.
19. Nerad J, Romeyn M, Silverman E, Allen-Reid J, Dietrich D, Merchant J, Pelletier VA, Tinnerello D, Fenton M. General nutrition management in patients infected with human immunodeficiency virus. *Clin Infect Dis.* 2003:36(Suppl 2):S52–S62.
20. Grinspoon S, Mulligan K. Weight loss and wasting in patients infected with human immunodeficiency virus. *Clin Infect Dis.* 2003;36(Suppl 2): S69–S78.
21. Bartlett JG. Introduction: integrating nutrition therapy into medical management of human immunodeficiency virus. *Clin Infect Dis.* 2003; 36(Suppl 2):S51.
22. Dube M, Fenton M. Lipid abnormalities. *Clin Infect Dis.* 2003;36(Suppl 2):S79–S83.
23. Gelato MC. Insulin and carbohydrate dysregulation. *Clin Infect Dis.* 2003;36(Suppl 2):S91–S95.
24. Sattler F. Body habitus changes related to lipodystrophy. *Clin Infect Dis.* 2003;36(Suppl 2): S84–S90.
25. National Kidney Foundation. K/DOQI clinical practice guidelines for managing dyslipidemias in chronic kidney disease. *Am J Kidney Dis.* 2003; 41(Suppl 3):S43.
26. Mondy K, Tebas P. Emerging bone problems in patients infected with human immunodeficiency virus. *Clin Infect Dis.* 2003;36(Suppl 2):S101–S105.
27. National Kidney Foundation. K/DOQI clinical practice guidelines for chronic kidney disease: evaluation, classification, and stratification. *Am J Kidney Dis.* 2002;39(Suppl 1):S128.
28. National Kidney Foundation. K/DOQI clinical practice guidelines for nutrition in chronic renal failure. *Am J Kidney Dis.* 2000;35(Suppl 2): S128.

Chapter 9

Nutrition Management of Diabetes in Chronic Kidney Disease

Joni J. Pagenkemper, MS, MA, RD

OVERVIEW OF DIABETES CLASSIFICATIONS

Diabetes mellitus is characterized by hyperglycemia resulting from defects in insulin secretion, insulin action, or both (1). Table 9.1 contrasts the characteristics of type 1 and type 2 diabetes (2). Type 1 diabetes is usually an autoimmune destruction of the beta cells of the pancreas leading to absolute insulin deficiency. These individuals present with markedly elevated blood glucose levels and acute symptoms of diabetes. Box 9.1 outlines the diagnostic criteria for diabetes mellitus (1).

Type 2 diabetes ranges from predominantly insulin resistance with relative insulin deficiency to a predominantly insulin secretory defect with insulin resistance (1). Type 2 diabetes frequently goes undiagnosed for many years because the hyperglycemia develops gradually and the classic symptoms are not severe enough for the patient to notice. Consequently, type 2 diabetes often is not diagnosed until complications appear. As Table 9.1 indicates, the risk of developing this form of diabetes increases with age, obesity, and lack of physical activity (2). Certain ethnic groups, especially Native Americans, Mexican Americans, and African Americans, are at higher risk for type 2 diabetes (1).

The categories of impaired glucose tolerance (IGT) or impaired fasting glucose (IFG) are associated with the insulin resistance syndrome (also known as syndrome X or the metabolic syndrome), which consists of insulin resistance, compensatory hyperinsulinemia to maintain glucose homeostasis, abdominal obesity, hypertension, and dyslipidemia including high triglycerides and low high-density lipoprotein cholesterol (1). The insulin resistance syndrome contains many features that increase cardiovascular risk, making diagnosis and intervention crucial for this intermediate group. Table 9.2 outlines the criteria for glycemic classifications (1).

Like chronic kidney disease, diabetes, particularly type 2, needs to be viewed as a progressive disease with clinical practice guidelines that provide a basis for the continuum of care, as illustrated in Figure 9.1 (1). The early stage of diabetes is characterized by mild fasting hyperglycemia. If diabetes is identified early prior to intractable insulin resistance, medical nutrition therapy (MNT), lifestyle interventions, and physical activity can be effective in maintaining euglycemia. As the disease progresses and blood glucose becomes more difficult to control, MNT and physical activity are an ongoing part of therapy, but now pharmacologic management with a single agent may be needed. Eventually, the need for medication will increase, requiring a combination of oral diabetes medications and/or insulin to achieve euglycemia (3). With such a diverse and heterogeneous diabetes population, dietitians need to be familiar with the variety of medical treatments

Table 9.1. Comparison of Type 1 and Type 2 Diabetes

Type 1	*Type 2*
Characteristics	
• Insulin dependent	• Non-insulin dependent
• Autoimmune destruction of pancreatic beta cells causing absolute insulin deficiency	• Insulin resistance or defect in insulin secretion; decreased tissue glucose uptake
• 5%–10% of all diabetes cases	• 90%–95% of all diabetes cases
• Most cases diagnosed in youth < 30 y	• Generally diagnosed at older age > 40 y
• Prone to diabetes ketoacidosis (DKA)	• Not DKA-prone
• Usually lean	• 80% are obese at diagnosis
• Rapid onset of symptoms	• Gradual onset of symptoms
• 15%–20% inherited	• Family history of diabetes
	• Race or ethnicity
	• Lack of physical activity
Acute Symptoms at Diagnosis	
• Marked elevation in blood glucose level	• Elevated blood glucose level
• Frequent urination (polyuria)*	• Blurred vision*
• Abnormal thirst (polydipsia)*	• Tingling in feet*
• Unusual hunger (polyphagia)	• Slow wound healing*
• Rapid weight loss	• Excess weight
• Fatigue and weakness	• Easily fatigued*
• Dehydration	• Skin infections*
• Irritability	• Drowsiness*
• Nausea and vomiting	• Itching

*These particular symptoms, while common to both types, are more likely to be evident in the particular type of diabetes noted in the column.

Source: Adapted from McCann L, ed. *Pocket Guide to the Nutrition Assessment of the Patient With Chronic Kidney Disease (CKD).* 3rd ed. New York, NY: National Kidney Foundation; 2002, with permission from the National Kidney Foundation:4–2.

Box 9.1. Diagnostic Criteria for Diabetes Mellitus

Symptoms* of diabetes with a casual† plasma glucose level ≥ 200 mg/dL (11.1 mmol/L) *confirmed on a subsequent day* by a

1. Fasting‡ plasma glucose (FPG) levels of ≥ 126 mg/dL (7.0 mmol/L)
   or
2. Symptoms of diabetes plus a casual† plasma glucose level ≥ 200 mg/dL (11.1 mmol/L)
   or
3. A 2–hour plasma glucose level ≥ 200 mg/dL (11.1 mmol/L) during an oral glucose tolerance test (OGTT)§

*The classic symptoms of diabetes include polyuria, polydipsia, and unexplained weight loss.
†*Casual* is defined as any time of day without regard to time since last meal.
‡*Fasting* is defined as no caloric intake for at least 8 hours.
§OGTT is not recommended for routine clinical use.

Source: Adapted from American Diabetes Association. Clinical practice recommendations 2002. *Diabetes Care.* 2002;25(Suppl 1):S22, with permission from the American Diabetes Association.

Table 9.2. Criteria for Glycemic Classifications

Normoglycemia	*IFG or IGT*	*Diabetes*
FPG < 110 mg/dL 2-h PG* < 140 mg/dL	FPG ≥ 110 and < 126 mg/dL (IFG) 2-h PG* ≥ 140 and < 200 mg/dL (IGT)	FPG ≥ 126 mg/dL 2-h PG* ≥ 200 mg/dL Symptoms of diabetes and casual plasma glucose ≥ 200 mg/dL

Abbreviations: FPG, fasting plasma glucose; IFG, impaired fasting glucose; IGT, impaired glucose tolerance; PG, postload glucose.

*This 2-hour postload glucose test requires the use of a glucose load containing the equivalent of 75 g anhydrous glucose dissolved in water. Conversions: 110 mg/dL (6.1 mmol/L); 140 mg/dL (8.7 mmol/L); 126 mg/dL (7.0 mmol/L); 200 mg/dL (11.1 mmol/L).

Source: Adapted from American Diabetes Association. Clinical practice recommendations 2002. *Diabetes Care.* 2002;25(Suppl 1):S22, with permission from American Diabetes Association.

that are available and determine where the patient is along the continuum of care to individualize education and meal plans accordingly. Figure 9.1 describes the continuum of glycemia by type and stages.

Diabetes continues to be the most common cause of end-stage renal disease (ESRD) in the United States, accounting for more than 40% of new cases of ESRD annually (1,4). Approximately 20% to 30% of patients with type 1 or type 2 diabetes develop evidence of nephropathy, but a much smaller fraction of those with type 2 diabetes progress to ESRD. However, because there is a much greater prevalence of type 2 diabetes, these patients constitute more than half of the diabetic population starting dialysis. Recent studies have demonstrated that both the onset and course of diabetic nephropathy can be delayed if several interventions are implemented early in the course of the disease process (1,5,6).

CHRONIC KIDNEY DISEASE/PREDIALYSIS

The earliest clinical evidence of "incipient nephropathy" is microalbuminuria (≥ 30 mg/day). At this point, without specific interventions, approximately 80% of people with type 1 diabetes will progress over a period of 10 to 15 years to overt nephropathy or clinical albuminuria (> 300 mg/day) with hypertension. The glomerular filtration rate (GFR) will gradually decline over a period of years, with ESRD developing in 50% of individuals with type 1 diabetes within 10 years and in more than 75% of these patients by 20 years. In contrast, without specific interventions, 20% to 40% of pa-

Stages / Type	Normoglycemia	Hyperglycemia			
	Normal glucose regulation	Impaired glucose tolerance or Impaired fasting glucose	Diabetes mellitus: Not insulin requiring	Insulin requiring for control	Insulin required for survival
Type 1*					
Type 2					

*Even after presenting in ketoacidosis, these patients can briefly return to normoglycemia without requiring continuous therapy (ie, "honeymoon" remission).

Figure 9.1. Continuum of glycemia by type and stages. Adapted from American Diabetes Association. Clinical practice recommendations 2002. *Diabetes Care.* 2002;25(Suppl 1):S8, with permission from the American Diabetes Association.

tients with type 2 diabetes and microalbuminuria progress to overt nephropathy, but by 20 years after this point, only 20% will have progressed to ESRD (7). Box 9.2 outlines the stages of diabetic nephropathy with some of their defining characteristics (2,8).

Yearly urine testing for microalbuminuria is essential to detect kidney disease at its earliest and most treatable stages (5–7). People with type 1 diabetes should be screened for microalbuminuria yearly starting 5 years after the diagnosis of diabetes. People with type 2 diabetes should be screened every year from the time of diagnosis because they often go undiagnosed for years (6,7). Albuminuria is a marker of greatly increased cardiovascular morbidity and mortality for patients with either type 1 or type 2 diabetes (9). (Refer to Chapter 10 for more detail on dyslipidemias in kidney disease.) The clinical course of the diabetic nephropathy can be modified by the following possible early interventions (5,7,10–13).

Box 9.2. Stages of Diabetic Nephropathy

Stage 1: Hyperglycemia leads to increased kidney filtration due to osmotic load and toxic effects of high blood glucose. There is increased GFR with enlarged kidneys.

Stage 2: Clinically silent phase, but continued kidney hyperfiltration and hypertrophy. Mild decrease in GFR to 60–89 mL/min/1.73 m^2.

Stage 3: Microalbuminuria (defined as 30 to 300 mg/day); loss of albumin in urine.
Within 5 years, 20% of patients develop nephropathy on standard care; 50% do not progress.
Microalbuminuria is a better predictor of progression in type 1 than type 2.
Microalbuminuria is a predictor of increased cardiovascular disease.
Microalbuminuria is associated with higher HbA_{1c} levels (> 8.1%).
Moderate decrease in GFR to 30 to 59 mL/min/1.73 m^2.

Stage 4: Overt nephropathy.
Almost always with hypertension, > 300 mg/day albumin in urine, about 10% have nephrotic range proteinuria, GFR decreased to 15 to 29 mL/min/1.73 m^2.

Stage 5: CKD needing renal replacement therapy with GFR < 15 mL/min/1.73 m^2.
Older than 30 years, > 24% of patients with type 1 progress to this stage.
Older than 25 years, about 8% of patients with type 2 progress to this stage.

Source: Adapted from McCann L, ed. *Pocket Guide to the Nutrition Assessment of the Patient With Chronic Kidney Disease (CKD)*. 3rd ed. New York, NY: National Kidney Foundation; 2002:4–3, with permission from the National Kidney Foundation.

Optimize Glycemic Control

The landmark Diabetes Control and Complications Trial (DCCT) proved that tight blood glucose control (ie, mean blood glucose of 155 mg/dL and mean hemoglobin A1c [HbA_{1c}] of 7.2%) reduced the risk of microalbuminuria by one third (34%) in patients with type 1 diabetes. In people with microalbuminuria, the risk of progressing to proteinuria was reduced by about half (56%) in people with tight control (1,14). The United Kingdom Prospective Diabetes Study (UKPDS) in type 2 diabetic patients demonstrated a 25% reduction in nephropathy with intensive diabetes therapy and that for every percentage point decrease in HbA_{1c}, there was a 35% reduction in the risk of complications (1,15,16).

It is now recommended that intensive diabetes management with the goal of achieving euglycemia be implemented as early as possible in as many patients with diabetes as is safely possible using a collaborative and integrated health care team approach (17). Because diet is the most complex aspect of intensive diabetes therapy, it is important to simplify and streamline nutrition priorities for the chronic kidney disease patient.

Research on the DCCT patients who received intensive diabetes therapy showed that adherence to the following dietary behaviors were associated with lower HbA_{1c} levels: a) adherence to the prescribed meal plan, b) adjusting food and/or insulin in response to hyperglycemia, c) adjusting insulin dose for changes in food intake, and d) consistency in consumption of a bedtime snack. In contrast, overtreatment of hypoglycemia and consumption of extra nighttime snacks beyond the meal plan were associated with higher HbA_{1c} levels (17,18).

Careful attention to the relationship between diet, insulin, and activity is necessary to achieve HbA_{1c} goals without undesired hypoglycemia and weight gain. Food variations often explain erratic blood glucose results and episodes of hypoglycemia and hyperglycemia (18). However, fluctuations in blood glucose can also occur due to alterations in insulin metabolism with changing kidney function. Because insulin is broken down in the kidneys, patients with chronic kidney disease often begin to require less exogenous insulin and need to be alert to the signs and symptoms of hypoglycemia and how to treat it (19).

Use of ACE inhibitors or ARBs

Large, prospective randomized studies in patients with type 1 and type 2 diabetes have demonstrated that angiotensin-converting enzyme (ACE) inhibitors and angiotensin receptor blockers (ARBs) are the drugs of choice instead of other antihypertensive agents to delay the clinical progression of microalbuminuria and slow the decline in GFR (20–23). Use of ACE inhibitors or ARBs may exacerbate hyperkalemia in patients with advanced renal insufficiency, so serum potassium should be monitored routinely. It is likely a patient will also be on a diuretic for blood pressure and/or fluid control, which may cause potassium wasting.

Maintain Tight Blood Pressure Control at Less Than 130/80 mmHg

For years, aggressive management of hypertension has been the first and most important intervention known to greatly slow the decrease of GFR (10). In type 2 diabetes, hypertension is often present as part of the metabolic syndrome. Hypertension substantially increases the risk of both macrovascular and microvascular complications, including stroke, peripheral vascular disease, coronary artery disease, retinopathy, and nephropathy. Initial treatment should focus on lifestyle modifications, such as weight loss, reducing sodium and alcohol intake, and exercise (24). Severe calorie restriction is not recommended, particularly if weight-loss efforts hinder glycemic control. Because the hypertension associated with diabetes is usually related to volume expansion, a daily sodium restriction of approximately 100 mEq (2,400 mg) is recommended. If hyponatremia develops, a fluid restriction may also be required (4,24).

Recommend a Diet With Adequate Energy

A meta-analysis of several small studies has shown that protein restriction may be of benefit in some patients whose nephropathy seems to be progressing despite optimal glucose and blood pressure control (25). With the onset of overt nephropathy, initiate a protein restriction of no more than 0.8 g/kg/day (approximately 10% of daily calories), which is the current adult Dietary Reference Intake (DRI) for protein. Further protein restriction (0.6 g/kg/day) may be useful in slowing the decline in selected patients who are stable and closely monitored (26,27). This needs to be balanced with the possibility of undernutrition on low-protein diets in diabetic patients because insulin deficiency stimulates gluconeogenesis and increases protein degradation. Metabolic acidosis also needs to be corrected to maintain positive nitrogen balance. The National Kidney Foundation Kidney Disease Outcomes Quality Initiative (K/DOQI) nutrition guidelines recommend 35 kcal/kg/day as necessary to maintain positive nitrogen balance on a low-protein diet (28). When lower protein intakes are indicated, protein restriction should not be at the expense of glycemic control.

Additional Recommendations

To reduce cardiovascular morbidity, individuals should reduce low-density lipoprotein cholesterol, stop smoking, and increase exercise. Because more than 80% of patients with diabetes die of cardiovascular disease, aggressive management of other cardiovascular risk factors (smoking, blood pressure, lipids, and weight management) are at least as important as diabetes management (3). (Refer to Chapter 10 for more detail on clinical practice recommendations related to cardiovascular disease.)

HEMODIALYSIS

It is generally recommended that for diabetic patients, dialysis should be initiated at a higher GFR, usually at 15 mL/min/1.73 m^2, because renal function deteriorates more rapidly compared with nondiabetic patients (4). Hypertension also becomes more difficult to control. At initiation of dialysis, patients with diabetes have more comorbid conditions, a higher incidence of complications, and are less well nourished in comparison with patients with other types of kidney disease. Thus, they require more time from health care professionals and demonstrate less rehabilitation potential than those without diabetes. Survival, although greatly improved from the past, remains significantly lower in patients with diabetes than in other types of patients treated with hemodialysis (HD) (4).

Fluctuations in blood glucose often occur due to changes in eating patterns with dialysis scheduling and disruption of nutrient absorption with gastropathy (29). HD solutions always contain about 200 mg/dL of glucose to keep blood glucose stable. Because of the absence of glycosuria, these patients are prone to rapid increases and wide fluctuations in blood sugar. High blood glucose levels often lead to excess thirst, which complicates fluid control. Serum potassium levels may also fluctuate due to extremely high blood glucose levels and cellular shifts of potassium or due to gastropathy and the erratic absorption of food (4).

Gastroparesis

Gastroparesis (delayed emptying of the stomach), caused by autonomic neuropathy, is common among patients on dialysis and may occur in more than 50% of patients with type 1 and type 2 diabetes (30,31). Associated with alternating bouts of constipation and diarrhea, symptoms may vary in severity and range from early satiety and epigastric pain, to nausea and vomiting, which, if prolonged, may result in dehydration.

Retained food in the stomach is termed a bezoar and indicates delayed gastric emptying. Food, especially high-fat food, stays in the stomach longer, causing unpredictable glucose levels and late insulin reactions. Patients with gastroparesis should have small, frequent meals of low-fat, low-fiber foods with liquids. Patients should chew food thoroughly and maintain an upright posture for at least 30 minutes after each meal (30–32). Parrish (32) provides a useful appendix on food-related tips for gastroparesis.

More frequent monitoring of blood glucose levels will help determine insulin requirements and adjustments. Changing insulin types and/or the timing of injections to improve blood glucose control is often necessary (19). The antiemetic, prokinetic gastrointestinal motility drug, metoclopramide (Reglan, AH Robins Co., Richmond, VA 23220) can be given in small starting dosages (5 mg twice daily), and increased in small increments until results are seen (4). Other prokinetic medications include domperidone (given 10 to 20 mg before meals and at bedtime) and erythromycin (125 to 250 mg up to four times daily) (2,31). Cisapride, which has been removed from the US market, should not be used in the renal population because it is associated with potentially fatal dysrhythmias (4). Some patients with prolonged problems may require postpyloric tube feedings or parenteral nutrition to maintain nutritional status (19,32). (Refer to Chapters 13 and 14 for more specific recommendations.)

Patients with diabetes are more likely to be hospitalized with infections or for surgery. The stress of illness frequently aggravates glycemic control and requires more frequent monitoring of blood glucose and urine or blood ketones. The patient treated with oral glucose-lowering agents or MNT alone may temporarily require insulin. Adequate fluid, protein, and energy intake must be assured during these periods of increased need (1). Diabetic enteropathy with resulting diarrhea can complicate nutritional status, causing poor food intake and hypoglycemia. Severe cases can be treated with broad-spectrum antibiotics. Use of loperamide hydrochloride (Imodium, McNeil Consumer Healthcare, Fort Washington, PA 19034) can be helpful to decrease bowel motility (4). Also effective in the management of diarrhea is diphenoxylate hydrochloride, atropine sulfate (Lomotil, GD Searle and Co., Chicago, IL 60680).

PERITONEAL DIALYSIS

Continuous ambulatory peritoneal dialysis (CAPD) results in more steady-state serum chemistries and fluid balance that provides better control of blood pressure than does hemodialysis. In addition, residual renal function is better preserved, allowing a more liberal diet and fluid regimen. Despite glucose absorption from the dialysate, good blood sugar control can be achieved with intraperitoneal regular insulin added to the dialysate, allowing for ongoing delivery of insulin to the portal circulation (4). There will be some loss of insulin activity due to delayed absorption as a consequence of the dilution in the dialysate fluid and the adsorption to the plastic surface of the dialysate delivery system (33). If necessary, supplemental subcutaneous insulin injections can be given as indicated by blood glucose monitoring (4). The effectiveness of peritoneal dialysis is not affected by intraperitoneal insulin administration. The frequency of peritonitis during intraperitoneal insulin administration increases slightly only in CAPD, but not with intermittent peritoneal dialysis (33). The incidence and severity of hypoglycemic episodes is reduced in CAPD compared with HD due to the constant presence of glucose in the abdomen (4).

For stable maintenance chronic peritoneal dialysis patients, the K/DOQI nutrition guidelines recommend a daily calorie intake of 30 to 35 kcal/kg, which needs to include the glucose absorbed from the peritoneal dialysate (28). The absorption of glucose from the dialysate can be significant, accounting for 15% to 30% of daily energy (4). A patient who maintains optimal sodium and fluid intake is less likely to require frequent use of the higher dextrose concentrations and therefore may have fewer problems with hyperglycemia, hyperlipidemia, and excess weight gain.

In general, the diets advocated for hemodialysis and peritoneal dialysis patients without diabetes also apply to patients with diabetes. Please refer to Chapters 5 and 6 for more detail.

TRANSPLANTATION

Diabetes is the most common cause of ESRD, and kidney transplantation, alone or combined with pancreas transplantation for type 1 patients, is the treatment of choice for these patients. Diabetes may become more difficult to manage after transplantation, and patients with type 2 diabetes may require insulin for adequate blood sugar control. Approximately 20% of transplant recipients with no prior evidence of diabetes develop hyperglycemia after transplantation, and 5% to 10% require treatment with oral hypoglycemic agents or insulin (34,35). Older patients, obese patients, African Americans, and patients with a strong family history of diabetes are at higher risk of developing posttransplant diabetes. Corticosteroids, cyclosporine, and tacrolimus all contribute to glucose intolerance. Diabetes is also the most important risk factor for posttransplant cardiovascular disease. The presence of posttransplant diabetes is associated with decreased graft survival and increased risk for infection (34,35).

In the preoperative period, patients with severe gastroparesis may need a nasogastric tube placed. Poor gastrointestinal function may compromise the absorption of immunosuppressive medications, thus requiring intravenous solutions to be used. Bowel function may be slow to return following transplantation, and with a prolonged ileus nutrition support may be indicated. Preoperatively, when the patient is receiving nothing by mouth, half the normal dose of insulin should be given. Blood glucose levels should be monitored every 4 hours and a sliding scale used for regular insulin dosing (34).

High-dose corticosteroids given postoperatively necessitate frequent blood glucose monitoring and a probable insulin drip initially, with sliding scale regular insulin to control episodes of hyperglycemia. In patients with poor blood sugar control, hypovolemia can cause elevations in blood urea nitrogen and creatinine levels that mimic a rejection episode. Careful assessment of volume status and blood glucose records can diagnose and correct the problem (34). Hyperlipidemia should be aggressively treated. (See Chapter 10.)

Nutrition guidelines for the well-functioning simultaneous pancreas-kidney (SPK) transplant are essentially the same as for solitary kidney transplants (refer to Chapter 7). The only exception would be for pancreas transplantation with bladder drainage, which requires supplemental sodium and bicarbonate intake and increased fluids. This is due to the significant urinary losses of sodium chloride and sodium bicarbonate that may result in metabolic acidosis and extracellular fluid volume contraction in these patients. Enteric drainage of the exocrine pancreas secretions is increasingly being used and helps prevent these metabolic complications (34–36).

Current United Network for Organ Sharing data from 1994 to 1998 show an overall 1-year pancreas graft survival of 83%, kidney graft survival of 90%, and patient survival of 94% (37). A successful SPK transplant offers better long-term quality of life with freedom from insulin therapy and dietary constraints, as well as greater potential for stabilization or reduction of diabetic complications (38).

MEDICAL NUTRITION THERAPY

MNT is an integral component of diabetes management and should emphasize patient involvement in problem solving as much as possible, using a variety of education strategies and techniques. General goals include the following (1,19):

- Maintenance of near-normal blood glucose levels by balancing food intake, exercise, and available insulin with kidney function and/or dialysis
- Achievement of optimal serum lipids and blood pressure to reduce the risk of cardiovascular disease
- Adequate energy intake to attain or maintain reasonable weight
- Achievement of acceptable biochemical parameters and fluid status
- Prevention and treatment of acute and long-term complications of diabetes
- Improvement in overall health through appropriate food choices and physical activity

- Consideration of lifestyle, personal and cultural preferences, and financial situation while respecting the individual's willingness to make changes

Monitoring glucose, HbA_{1c}, lipids, blood pressure, and renal status is essential to evaluate nutrition-related outcomes. If goals are not met, changes must be made in the overall management plan. The role of the dietitian is to help patients learn a problem-solving approach that evaluates diet as one of many factors that impact these goals.

Dietary Strategies for Carbohydrate Management

Careful management of carbohydrate (CHO) intake is integral to any diabetes meal planning approach, with emphasis on knowing how much and when CHO should be consumed. Many strategies are used to achieve dietary consistency, and the dietitian is best qualified to match the appropriate meal planning strategy to each patient's lifestyle and capabilities.

A "constant carbohydrate" meal plan is suited for patients who use diet alone to control their blood sugars, for those on fixed doses of insulin, or for patients with low literacy. Emphasis is placed on keeping the amount of CHO relatively constant for each meal and eating meals at the same times every day. Insulin should be adjusted around usual CHO intake as much as possible rather than CHO adjusted to meet insulin regimens. Some modifications in food choices may be needed to accommodate sodium, potassium, and phosphorus restrictions (19).

The "carbohydrate counting" method provides the most flexibility and is the preferred meal-planning approach for adjusting insulin around usual dietary intake. The patient simply counts the grams of total CHO to be eaten and then matches it with the proper amount of insulin. This method does require motivation and a higher literacy level. Careful record keeping is essential until an accurate ratio of insulin to grams of CHO is established. Insulin dosage must also take into account exercise and current blood glucose levels. It is highly recommended that blood glucose be checked 2 hours after a meal (19). To avoid excess energy intake and undesired weight gain at the expense of blood sugar control, protein and fat intake should be relatively constant and carbohydrate consumption should not vary widely.

The "exchange list" meal plan is the one most familiar to many people with diabetes. Foods are grouped into six food groups with similar amounts of carbohydrate, protein, fat, and calories. Foods within each group can be traded, depending on the amounts consumed (19). Although the exchange lists can provide structure and a higher degree of metabolic control, they also require a higher level of literacy due to their complexity.

Protein, Fat, Sugar, and Fiber Guidelines

Dietary guidelines for diabetes are often liberalized on the renal diet to provide adequate calories from increased amounts of fats and simple carbohydrates, especially for those on low-protein diets. The American Diabetes Association recommends that protein provide 10% to 20% of calories, with the remaining 60% to 70% of energy intake divided between carbohydrate and fat (emphasizing monounsaturated fats and reducing saturated fats). The metabolic profile and need for weight loss should be considered when determining the fat content of the diet (39,40).

Scientific evidence has concluded that sucrose does not cause a greater increase in blood glucose levels than an equivalent amount of starch (39,40), so sugars and sucrose-containing foods may be included as part of the total carbohydrate in the meal plan. For best results, sugars should be distributed throughout the day, in conjunction with other foods, and intake should be consistent. Regarding glycemic index, the position of the American Diabetes Association 2002 evidence-based nutrition principles and recommendations is that the total amount of carbohydrate in meals and snacks is more important than the source or the type. "Although it is clear that carbohydrates do have differing glycemic responses, the data reveal no clear trend in outcome benefits" (39,40). In particular, no improvements have been seen in HbA_{1c} levels. The report goes on to state: "Although the use of low glycemic index foods may reduce postprandial hyperglycemia, there is not sufficient evidence of long-term benefit to recommend use of low glycemic index diets as a primary strategy in food/meal planning" (39,40). Fiber should be encouraged within the constraints of the renal diet, but "it appears that ingestion of very large amounts of fiber are necessary to confer metabolic benefits on glycemic control, hyperinsulinemia, and plasma lipids" (39,40).

Treating Hypoglycemia

The 15/15 rule should be used to treat hypoglycemia. Namely, take 15 g of CHO, wait 15 minutes, and retest the blood sugar or evaluate relief of symptoms. If necessary, repeat with another 15 g of CHO and continue the process until the blood sugar improves (41). The usual methods of treating hypoglycemia (for example, with orange juice) may result in fluid overload and/or hyperkalemia in the oliguric diabetic patient. Better choices that will provide 15 g of carbohydrate are 10 jelly beans, 6 hard candies (eg, Lifesavers), or 4 commercial glucose tablets. Once the glucose returns to normal, and if the next regular meal will be delayed for more than 1 hour, the patient should eat a snack that contains both protein and carbohydrate to stabilize the glucose (19).

Table 9.3 provides a useful summary of the dietary modifications recommended for each stage of diabetic nephropathy (1,2,19,28).

Table 9.3. Recommended Dietary Modifications at Various Stages of Diabetic Nephropathy

Nutrient	*Pre-Clinical Nephropathy Stages 1-2-3*	*Progressive Nephropathy Stage 4*	*Hemodialysis*	*Peritoneal Dialysis*	*Transplantation*
Energy (kcal/kg/d)	30–35; adequate to achieve and maintain DBW	30–35; adequate to achieve and maintain DBW	30–35; adequate to achieve and maintain DBW	30–35; allow for dialysate calories	30–35; adequate to achieve and maintain DBW
Protein	12%–15% of calories 0.8–1.0 g/kg/day	10% of calories; 50% HBV 0.6–1.0 g/kg/day*	12%–20% of calories; 50% HBV 1.2 g/kg/day*	12%–20% of calories; 50% HBV 1.2–1.3 g/kg/day*	1.3–2.0 g/kg after surgery 0.8–1.0 g/kg in stable patients
Carbohydrate	50%–60% of calories; ↑ fiber to 20–30 g	50%–60% of calories ↑ fiber to 20–30 g	50%–60% of calories ↑ fiber to 20–30 g	50% of calories (35% oral and 15% dialysate) ↑ fiber to 20–30 g	50%-60% of calories ↑ fiber to 20–30 g
Fat	25%–35% calories as fat < 7% saturated fat Emphasis on MUFA < 200 mg cholesterol/d	25%–35% calories as fat < 7% saturated fat Emphasis on MUFA < 200 mg cholesterol/d	25%–35% calories as fat < 7% saturated fat Emphasis on MUFA < 200 mg cholesterol/d	25%–35% calories as fat < 7% saturated fat Emphasis on MUFA < 200 mg cholesterol/d	25%–35% calories as fat < 7% saturated fat Emphasis on MUFA < 200 mg cholesterol/d
Sodium (mg/d)	No HTN: ≤ 3000 HTN: ≤ 2400	No HTN: ≤ 3000 HTN: ≤ 2400 mg/d	2000–2400	No HTN: ≤ 2000–4000 Monitor fluid balance	No HTN: ≤ 3000 HTN: ≤ 2400
Potassium (g/d)	No restriction	Monitor labs; 2 if hyperkalemic	2–3; adjust to serum levels	Unrestricted if serum levels normal	Unrestricted unless hyperkalemic
Phosphorus	Maintain serum value WNL; 800–1000 mg/d; adjust for protein	10–12 mg/g protein or 10 mg/kg/d; 800–1000 mg/d	10–12 mg/g protein or 800–1000 mg/d; adjust for protein	10–12 mg/g protein or 800–1000 mg/d; adjust for protein	RDA; supplement as needed
Calcium (g/d)	Maintain serum value WNL 1.0–1.5	1.0–1.5; daily limit including binder load: < 2.0	Daily limit including binder load: < 2.0	Daily limit including binder load: < 2.0	0.8–1.5
Fluid	No restriction	Output plus 1000 mL	Output plus 1000 mL	Maintain balance	Unrestricted unless overloaded

Abbreviations: DBW, desired body weight; HBV, high biological value protein; HTN, hypertension; MUFA, monounsaturated fatty acids; RDA, Recommended Dietary Allowance; SFA, saturated fatty acids; WNL, within normal limits.

*1.2–1.5 g/kg/d during catabolic stress.

Source: Data are from references 1,2,19,28.

GOALS OF THERAPY

The American Diabetes Association's evidence-based clinical practice recommendations state that a fasting plasma glucose (FPG) less than 120 mg/dL (6.7 mmol/L) and HbA_{1c} levels less than 7% are the glycemic goals for monitoring the effective treatment of diabetes and determining when to make changes in therapy (1). Daily glucose goals are 70 to 120 mg/dL before meals and 150 to 180 mg/dL 2 hours after meals. The guidelines acknowledge that "less stringent treatment goals may be appropriate for patients with limited life expectancies, in the very young or older adults, and in individuals with comorbid conditions" (1). Reasonable goals for glycemic control in dialysis patients are a fasting serum glucose less than 140 mg/dL, a postprandial value of less than 200 mg/dL, HbA_{1c} levels less than 7%, and avoidance of hypoglycemia (4). Table 9.4 outlines the clinical goals of therapy for people with diabetes and chronic kidney disease or who are being treated with hemodialysis or peritoneal dialysis (1,2,4).

An accurate picture of the patient's daily and long-term blood glucose values is necessary to evaluate diabetes control. The HbA_{1c} test indicates the mean blood glucose value over the previous 2 to 3 months and should be done routinely to assess treatment efficacy. New standards recommend HbA_{1c} testing twice a year for patients with stable glycemic control and quarterly for patients not meeting glycemic goals or who have a change in management, such as a change in medication type and/or dosage (1). Randomized controlled clinical trials have documented relative risk reductions of 15% to 30% for each 1% absolute reduction in HbA_{1c} (1,14–16,42,43).

Table 9.4. Goals of Therapy for Diabetic Nephropathy

	Chronic Kidney Disease	*Hemodialysis*	*Peritoneal Dialysis*
FPG (mg/dL)	< 120	< 140	"fasting" PG*: < 160
HbA_{1c} (%)	< 7	< 7	< 7
Blood pressure (mm Hg)	< 130/80	< 130/80	< 130/80
LDL-C (mg/dL)	< 100	< 100	< 100
2-h PPG (mg/dL)	150–180	< 200	< 200
Blood glucose (mg/dL)	Avoid hypoglycemia < 70	Avoid hypoglycemia < 70	Avoid hypoglycemia < 70

Abbreviations: FPG, fasting plasma glucose; HbA_{1c}, hemoglobin A1c; LDL-C, low-density lipoprotein cholesterol; 2-h PPG, postprandial glucose 2 hours after meals.

*PD patients are never truly "fasting" because they always have 2 to 3 L of glucose dialysate exchanges dwelling in their peritoneal cavity.

Source: Data are from references 1, 2, and 4.

The oral glucose tolerance test cannot be used to diagnose diabetes in dialysis patients because of uremia-induced insulin resistance (which will result in greater and more prolonged glucose levels). However, FPG can be used for diagnosis (4). In CAPD patients, a true fasting state is never achieved due to constant absorption of glucose from the dialysis solution. The "fasting" serum glucose value rarely exceeds 160 mg/dL, even when using a 4.25% dextrose solution. Higher levels would suggest that the patient has diabetes (4). Additionally, when renal function is absent, the "safety valve" effect of glucosuria may result in the development of severe hyperglycemia (>1,000 mg/dL). The severe hyperosmolality can cause thirst, weight gain, and hyperkalemia, but not the polyuria or usual alteration in mental status because of the absence of water loss induced by osmotic diuresis (4).

MEDICAL MANAGEMENT AND SELF-MONITORING OF BLOOD GLUCOSE

Until 1995, insulin and sulfonylureas were the only classes of drugs available in the United States for the treatment of diabetes. Since then, new insulin analogues and four new classes of oral medications have been approved for improved diabetes management (1, 3,4,41,44–48). (Refer to Chapter 15 for more detail on medications.)

Dialysis patients should be encouraged to continue or resume self-monitoring of blood glucose (SMBG) because many stop testing once they go on dialysis. Monthly and random blood glucose testing done at the time of dialysis treatments is not a substitute for home testing (49). For persons diagnosed with diabetes who require insulin, SMBG is recommended three or more times daily to detect variations in blood glucose levels that may require insulin adjustments (1). Intensive insulin therapy for tight control may require checking blood glucose up to eight times per day (fasting, prior to and 2 hours after each meal, at bedtime or during the night). The American Diabetes Association acknowledges that the benefits of tight control may not be indicated for patients with ESRD or advanced complications. The optimal frequency and timing of SMBG for patients with type 2 diabetes is not known, but testing frequency should be sufficient to reach glucose goals (1). A reasonable goal would be to monitor fasting blood sugars and then vary a second blood check by rotating different days and times to see if a pattern emerges prior to certain meals, 2 hours postprandial, or at bedtime.

It is important for health care providers to evaluate each person's monitoring technique for accuracy, both initially and at regular intervals thereafter. Because laboratory methods measure plasma glucose, it is crucial that people with diabetes know whether their monitor and strips provide whole blood or plasma results, since plasma glucose values are 10% to 15% higher than whole blood values (1). Patients should be taught how to use the SMBG data to adjust food intake, exercise, or pharmacologic management to achieve specific glycemic goals.

CONCLUSION

The incidence of both diabetes and chronic kidney disease is on the rise. Living with either diabetes or chronic kidney disease is challenging for anyone. Managing diabetes in the presence of chronic kidney disease requires additional effort on the part of patients and the health care team to improve outcomes and decrease the morbidity and mortality in this population. The nutrition needs of patients with diabetes and chronic kidney disease change as the progression and treatment of the disease changes. Understanding the treatment goals of each stage is crucial to maximize the nutritional status of patients throughout the course of their disease and to individualize their education and meal plans accordingly.

REFERENCES

1. American Diabetes Association. Clinical practice recommendations 2004. *Diabetes Care*. 2004; 27(Suppl 1):S-3–S143.
2. McCann L, ed. *Pocket Guide to the Nutrition Assessment of the Patient With Chronic Kidney Disease (CKD)*. 3rd ed. New York, NY: National Kidney Foundation; 2002.
3. Kulkarni K. Intensive therapy in type 2 diabetes: finding the right combination. *On the Cutting Edge: Diabetes Care and Education*. 2000;21: 8–11.
4. Tzamaloukas AH, Friedman EA. Diabetes. In: Daugirdas JT, Blake PG, Ing TS, eds. *Handbook of Dialysis*. 3rd ed. Philadelphia, Pa: Lippincott Williams & Wilkins; 2001.
5. Bakris GL, Williams M, Dworkin L, Elliott WJ, Epstein M, Toto R, Tuttle K, Douglas J, Hsueh W, Sowers J. Preserving renal function in adults with hypertension and diabetes: a consensus approach. *Am J Kidney Dis*. 2000;36:646–661.
6. Bennett PH, Haffner S, Kasiske BL, Keane WF, Mogensen CE, Parving HH, Steffes MW, Striker GE. Diabetic renal disease recommendations: screening and management of microalbuminuria in patients with diabetes mellitus: recommendations to the scientific advisory board of the National Kidney Foundation from an ad hoc committee of the council on diabetes mellitus of the National Kidney Foundation. *Am J Kidney Dis*. 1995;25:107–112.
7. American Diabetes Association. Diabetic nephropathy (position statement). *Diabetes Care*. 2002;25(Suppl 1):S85–S89.
8. National Kidney Foundation. K/DOQI clinical practice guidelines for chronic kidney disease: evaluation, classification, and stratification. *Am J Kidney Dis*. 2002;39(Suppl 1):S1–S266.
9. Levey AS, Beto JA, Coronado BE, Eknoyan G, Foley RN, Kasiske BL, Klag MJ, Mailloux LU, Manske CL, Meyer KB, Parfrey PS, Pfeffer MA, Wenger NK, Wilson PWF, Wright JT. Controlling the epidemic of cardiovascular disease in chronic renal disease: what do we know? What do we need to learn? Where do we go from here? National Kidney Foundation Task Force on Cardiovascular Disease. *Am J Kidney Dis*. 1998;32:853–906.
10. Edelman SV. Prevention, early detection, and aggressive management of diabetic kidney disease. *Clin Diabetes*. 1998;16:77–80.
11. O'Connell BS. Early renal disease in diabetes: a brief review. *Newsflash: Diabetes Care and Education*. 2001;22:7–11.
12. Molitch ME. Management of early diabetic nephropathy. *Am J Med*. 1997;102:392–398.
13. Ritz E, Orth SR. Nephropathy in patients with type 2 diabetes mellitus. *N Engl J Med*. 1999;341: 1127–1133.

14. Diabetes Control and Complications Trial Research Group. The effect of intensive treatment of diabetes on the development and progression of long-term complications in insulin-dependent diabetes mellitus. *N Engl J Med.* 1993;329:977–986.
15. UK Prospective Diabetes Study Group. Intensive blood-glucose control with sulphonylureas or insulin compared with conventional treatment and risk of complications in patients with type 2 diabetes (UKPDS 33). *Lancet.* 1998;352:837–853.
16. UK Prospective Diabetes Study Group. Effect of intensive blood-glucose control with metformin on complications in overweight patients with type 2 diabetes (UKPDS 34). *Lancet.* 1998;352:854–865.
17. Delahanty LM. Implications of the Diabetes Control and Complications Trial for renal outcomes and medical nutrition therapy. *J Ren Nutr.* 1998; 8:59–63.
18. Delahanty LM, Halford BN. The role of diet behaviors in achieving improved glycemic control in intensively treated patients in the Diabetes Control and Complications Trial. *Diabetes Care.* 1993;16:1453–1458.
19. *National Renal Diet Professional Guide.* 2nd ed. Chicago, Ill: Renal Practice Group of the American Dietetic Association; 2002.
20. Lewis EJ, Hunsicker LG, Bain RP, Rohde RD for the Collaborative Study Group. The effect of angiotensin-converting enzyme inhibition on diabetic nephropathy. *N Engl J Med.* 1993;329: 1456–1462.
21. Lewis EJ, Hunsicker LG, Clarke WR, Berl T, Pohl MA, Lewis JB, Ritz E, Atkins RC, Rohde R, Raz I. Renoprotective effect of the angiotensin-receptor antagonist irbasartin in patients with nephropathy due type 2 diabetes. *N Engl J Med.* 2001;345:851–860.
22. Brenner BM, Cooper ME, de Zeeuw D, Keane WF, Mitch WE, Parving HH, Remuzzi G, Snapinn SM, Zhang Z, Shahinfar S. Effects of losartan on renal and cardiovascular outcomes in patients with type 2 diabetes and nephropathy. *N Engl J Med.* 2001;345:861–869.
23. Anderson S, Tarnow L, Rossing P, Hansen BV, Parving HH. Renoprotective effects of angiotensin II receptor blockade in type 1 diabetic patients with diabetic nephropathy. *Kidney Int.* 2000;57:601–606.
24. American Diabetes Association. Treatment of hypertension in adults with diabetes (position statement). *Diabetes Care.* 2002;25(Suppl 1):S71–S73.
25. Pedrini MT, Levey AS, Lau J, Chalmers TC, Wang PH. The effect of dietary protein restriction on the progression of diabetic and nondiabetic renal disease: a meta-analysis. *Ann Intern Med.* 1996;124:627–632.
26. Kasiske BL, Lakatua JD, Ma JZ, Louis TA. A meta-analysis of the effects of dietary protein restriction on the rate of decline in renal function. *Am J Kidney Dis.* 1998;31:954–961.
27. Levey AS, Greene T, Beck GJ, Caggiula AW, Kusek JW, Hunsicker LG, Klahr S, for the MDRD Study Group. Dietary protein restriction and the progression of chronic renal disease: what have all of the results of the MDRD study shown? *J Am Soc Nephrol.* 1999;10:2426–2439.
28. National Kidney Foundation. K/DOQI clinical practice guidelines for nutrition in chronic renal failure. *Am J Kidney Dis.* 2000;35(suppl):S40–S45,S58–S61.
29. Kleinbeck C. Challenges of diabetes and dialysis. *Diabetes Spectrum.* 1997;10:135–141.
30. Valentine V, Barone JA, Hill JVC. Gastropathy in patients with diabetes: current concepts and treatment recommendations. *Diabetes Spectrum.* 1998;11:248–253.
31. Koch KL. Diabetic gastropathy: gastric neuromuscular dysfunction in diabetes mellitus: a review of symptoms, pathophysiology, and treatment. *Dig Dis Sci.* 1999;44:1061–1075.
32. Parrish CR. Nutritional care of the patient with gastroparesis. *On the Cutting Edge: Diabetes Care and Education.* 1999;20(4):8–13.
33. Quellhorst E. Insulin therapy during peritoneal dialysis: pros and cons of various forms of administration. *J Am Soc Nephrol.* 2002;13(Suppl 1):S92–S96.
34. Pirsch JD, Sollinger HW. Kidney and kidney-pancreas transplantation in diabetic patients. In: Danovitch GM, ed. *Handbook of Kidney Transplantation.* 3rd ed. Philadelphia, Pa: Lippincott Williams & Wilkins; 2001:313–331.
35. Robertson RP, Davis C, Larsen J, Stratta R, Sutherland DER. Pancreas and islet transplantation for patients with diabetes mellitus (Technical Review). *Diabetes Care.* 2000;23:112–116.

36. Elkhammas EA, Henry ML, Yilmaz S, Bumgardner GL, Ferguson RM. The kidney/pancreas transplant: an alternative for type 1 diabetics. *Nephrol News Issues*. 1997;11:41–44.
37. Gruessner AC, Sutherland DER. Analysis of United States (US) and non-US pancreas transplants as reported to the International Pancreas Transplant Registry (IPTR) and to the United Network for Organ Sharing (UNOS). In: Cecka JM, Terasaki PI, eds. *Clinical Transplants 1998*. Los Angeles, Calif; 1999:53–71.
38. Gross CR, Limwattananon C, Matthees BJ. Quality of life after pancreas transplantation: a review. *Clin Transplant*. 1998;12:351–361.
39. American Diabetes Association. Evidence-based nutrition principles and recommendations for the treatment and prevention of diabetes and related complications (position statement). *Diabetes Care*. 2002;25(Suppl 1):S50–S60.
40. Franz MJ, Bantle JP, Beebe CA, Brunzell JD, Chiasson JL, Garg A, Holzmeister L, Hoogwerf BJ, Mayer-Davis E, Mooradian AD, Purnell JQ, Wheeler M. Evidence-based nutrition principles and recommendations for the treatment and prevention of diabetes and related complications (technical review). *Diabetes Care*. 2002;25:148–198.
41. Stanley K. American Diabetes Association resource guide 2002. *Diabetes Forecast*. 2002;55:42–99.
42. Lawson ML, Gerstein HC, Tsui E, Zinman B. Effect of intensive therapy on early macrovascular disease in young individuals with type 1 diabetes. *Diabetes Care*. 1999;22(Suppl 1):B35–B39.
43. Stratton IM, Adler AI, Neil HA, Matthews DR, Manley SE, Cull CA, Hadden D, Turner RC, Holman RR. Association of glycaemia with macrovascular and microvascular complications of type 2 diabetes (UKPDS 35): prospective observation study. *BMJ*. 2000;321:405–412.
44. Edelman SV. Prescribing oral antidiabetic agents: general considerations. *Clin Diabetes*. 1998;16:37–40.
45. White JR. The pharmacological reduction of blood glucose in patients with type 2 diabetes mellitus. *Clin Diabetes*. 1998;16:58–67.
46. Clark CM. Oral therapy in type 2 diabetes: Pharmacological properties and clinical use of currently available agents. *Diabetes Spectrum*. 1998;11:211–221.
47. Buse JB. Progressive use of medical therapies in type 2 diabetes. *Diabetes Spectrum*. 2000;13:211–220.
48. McCarren M. Class action: type 2 drugs. *Diabetes Forecast*. 2002;55:62–66.
49. McDougall K, Borman D, Mitchell EK. Diabetes care in the dialysis setting. *RenaLink/National Kidney Foundation*. 2001;2(2):1,4–6.

Chapter 10

Dyslipidemias in Chronic Kidney Disease

Joni J. Pagenkemper, MS, MA, RD

Cardiovascular disease (CVD) is the most frequent cause of death among patients with renal disease, regardless of treatment modality. Altogether, mortality from CVD in hemodialysis and peritoneal dialysis patients is approximately 9% per year, which is about 30 times the risk in the general population (1). This staggering data prompted the 1998 National Kidney Foundation (NKF) Task Force publication, *Controlling the Epidemic of Cardiovascular Disease in Chronic Renal Disease* (1). The Task Force concluded that patients with chronic kidney disease (CKD) should be considered in the highest risk category as a coronary heart disease (CHD) risk equivalent for risk factor management.

A number of other clinical recommendations followed in that report, which used as a foundation some of the strategies for prevention and treatment of CVD in the general population, namely, guidelines from the American Heart Association (2), the National Cholesterol Education Program (NCEP), and the Seventh Joint National Committee addressing high blood pressure (3). In 2001, the NCEP updated their Adult Treatment Panel (ATP III) guidelines (4).

All of these reports helped lay the foundation for the NKF Kidney Disease Outcomes Quality Initiative (K/DOQI) dyslipidemia guidelines (5), published in April 2003, which are intended to supplement the ATP III report and address specific recommendations for the evaluation and treatment of dyslipidemias in CKD. The guidelines apply to all stages of CKD (Stages 1 through 5) and kidney transplant recipients. For more information on the stage classifications of CKD (6), refer to Chapters 1 and 3 on pathophysiology and chronic kidney disease. Box 10.1 summarizes the K/DOQI clinical practice guidelines for managing dyslipidemias in CKD (5). Although adolescent guidelines are included in the report, the focus of this chapter is on adult assessment and treatment. Dietitians are encouraged to consult the full report in greater depth.

RISK FACTOR CLASSIFICATION OF DYSLIPIDEMIAS

The K/DOQI dyslipidemia guidelines recommend that the definitions of dyslipidemias for CKD should be consistent with those of the ATP III report (see Table 10.1) (4).

The updated guidelines of the ATP III apply to all CKD patients in Stages 1 through 4, with the following kidney-specific modifications (5):

- CKD is classified as a CHD risk equivalent, much like diabetes.
- Reduced kidney function may result in complications from lipid-lowering therapies.
- Treating proteinuria, if present in the kidney patient, may also be an effective treatment for dyslipidemias.

Box 10.1. Summary of K/DOQI Dyslipidemia Guidelines

Guideline 1:

- All adults and adolescents with CKD, and all kidney transplant recipients, should be evaluated for dyslipidemias.
- The assessment of dyslipidemias should include a complete lipid profile with total cholesterol, LDL, HDL, and TG.
- Evaluation should be done upon presentation (when patient is stable), at 2–3 months after a change in treatment or other conditions known to cause dyslipidemias, and at least annually thereafter.

Guideline 2:

- A complete lipid profile should be measured after an overnight fast whenever possible.
- Hemodialysis patients should have lipid profiles measured either before dialysis, or on days not receiving dialysis.

Guideline 3:

- CKD patients with dyslipidemias should be evaluated for remediable, secondary causes.

Guideline 4:

- For adults with fasting TG ≥ 500 mg/dL that cannot be corrected by removing an underlying cause, treatment with TLC and a TG-lowering agent should be considered.
- For adults with LDL ≥ 100 mg/dL, treatment should be considered to reduce LDL to < 100 mg/dL.
- For adults with LDL < 100 mg/dL, fasting TG ≥ 200 mg/dL, and non-HDL cholesterol (total cholesterol minus HDL) ≥ 130 mg/dL, treatment should be considered to reduce non-HDL cholesterol to < 130 mg/dL.

Guideline 5:

- For adolescents with fasting triglycerides ≥ 500 mg/dL that cannot be corrected by removing an underlying cause, treatment with TLC should be considered.
- For adolescents with LDL ≥ 130 mg/dL, treatment should be considered to reduce LDL to < 130 mg/dL.
- For adolescents with LDL < 130 mg/dL, fasting triglycerides ≥ 200 mg/dL, and non-HDL cholesterol (total cholesterol minus HDL) ≥ 160 mg/dL, treatment should be considered to reduce non-HDL cholesterol to < 160 mg/dL.

Abbreviations: CKD, chronic kidney disease; HDL, high-density lipoprotein; LDL, low-density lipoprotein; TG, triglycerides; TLC, therapeutic lifestyle changes.

Source: Adapted from National Kidney Foundation. K/DOQI clinical practice guidelines for managing dyslipidemias in chronic kidney disease patients. *Am J Kidney Dis.* 2003;41(Suppl 3):S22–S56, with permission from the National Kidney Foundation.

Other risk factors are important in the pathogenesis of atherosclerotic CVD (ACVD) and should be treated in CKD patients. Specifically, the aggressive treatment of hypertension early in the course of renal failure will delay the progression of renal disease and is considered the most potent intervention to decrease subsequent cardiovascular mortality in patients receiving dialysis (7). Therefore, modifiable conventional risk factors, including hypertension, cigarette smoking, glucose intolerance or diabetes control, and obesity should be assessed at initial presentation and at least yearly thereafter (5).

These modifiable risk factors should be managed according to existing guidelines, which are listed at the end of this chapter. Many of these guidelines promote diet and lifestyle changes as essential strategies for pre-

Table 10.1. Dyslipidemias as Defined in the Adult Treatment Panel III Guidelines

Dyslipidemia	*Level (mg/dL*)*
Total cholesterol	
Desirable	< 200
Borderline high	200–239
High	≥ 240
Low-density lipoprotein cholesterol	
Optimal	< 100
Near optimal	100–129
Borderline	130–159
High	160–189
Very high	≥ 190
Triglycerides	
Normal	< 150
Borderline high	150–199
High	200–499
Very high	≥ 500
High-density lipoprotein (HDL) cholesterol	
Low	< 40
Non-HDL cholesterol	
Normal	< 130

*To convert mg/dL to mmol/L, multiply triglycerides by 0.01129 and cholesterol by 0.02586.

Source: Adapted from Expert Panel on Detection, Evaluation, and Treatment of High Blood Cholesterol in Adults: executive summary of the Third Report of the National Cholesterol Education Program (NCEP) Expert Panel on Detection, Evaluation, and Treatment of High Blood Cholesterol in Adults (Adult Treatment Panel III). *JAMA*. 2001;285:2486–2497.

vention and treatment of these conditions, especially cardiovascular disease, high blood pressure, diabetes, and obesity.

ASSESSMENT OF DYSLIPIDEMIAS

Lipid abnormalities develop during the asymptomatic stages of CKD, become more pronounced with changes in proteinuria and declining glomerular filtration rate (GFR), and are not modified substantially by dialysis treatment or transplantation (8). Hemodialysis patients generally have a normal low-density lipoprotein (LDL) cholesterol, low high-density lipoprotein (HDL) cholesterol, and high triglyceride (TG) lipid profile. Data reported from the Dialysis Morbidity and Mortality Study indicate that only 20% of hemodialysis patients are meeting the normal lipid parameters outlined by the ATP III guidelines (5).

Peritoneal dialysis patients have higher total cholesterol and LDL levels than hemodialysis patients, and triglycerides are frequently elevated due to the continuous absorption of glucose from the dialysate. The propensity toward obesity and protein losses compounds the lipid abnormalities. Cross-sectional studies have found that only 15% of peritoneal dialysis patients have normal lipid levels according to the ATP III guidelines (4,5).

The prevalence of dyslipidemia in kidney transplant recipients is very high, with increases primarily in total and LDL-cholesterol. Triglycerides are often increased, but HDL is usually normal. Immunosuppressive medications, especially prednisone, cyclosporine, and sirolimus, are among some of the causes of dyslipidemias in kidney transplant recipients (5). (Refer to Chapter 7 for more detail on immunosuppressive medications.)

Acute medical conditions that may transiently lower lipid levels include severe infections, surgery, and an acute myocardial infarction after the first 24 hours (9,10). Acute pancreatitis may result in higher lipid levels. Illness, inflammation, and poor nutrition can frequently be confounding factors affecting the relationship of dyslipidemias and ACVD morbidity and mortality (11).

In the early 1990s, data from Lowrie and Lew showed a U-shaped curve for the association of cholesterol and mortality in more than 12,000 hemodialysis patients (12,13). However, adjusting for low serum albumin levels, the association between low cholesterol and increased mortality was reduced. In contrast, high serum cholesterol predicted mortality in those patients with normal serum albumin (14). Lower serum cholesterol levels have been associated with other markers of inflammation, primarily C-reactive protein (CRP), as well as interleukin-6 (IL-6), and tumor necrosis factor-alpha (TNFα) (15).

All major treatment decisions for dyslipidemias are based on levels of TG, LDL, and non-HDL cholesterol. The LDL in mg/dL is generally calculated using the Friedewald formula (16):

$$\text{LDL} = \text{Cholesterol} - \text{HDL} - (\text{TG} / 5)$$

This formula may not be accurate when TG are 400 mg/dL or more. In these situations, direct measurement of LDL is reasonably accurate when TG are in the range of 400 to 800 mg/dL.

The metabolic syndrome (characterized by central obesity, hypertension, insulin resistance, and hyperlipidemia) typically presents with a normal LDL, but it is characterized by increases in lipoprotein remnants that are more readily measured as non-HDL cholesterol (total cholesterol minus HDL) (4).

Regarding Guideline 2, nonfasting measurements may be the only practical alternative for some patients. It is better to obtain some lipid profile rather than no evaluation whatsoever. If the nonfasting lipid profile is normal, then no further assessment is needed at that time. However, if there is an abnormality, it is best to obtain a fasting lipid profile to guide treatment decisions. In peritoneal dialysis patients, it is probably most practical to draw blood in the morning, after an overnight fast (whenever possible), and with whatever peritoneal dialysis fluid is dwelling in the peritoneal cavity when the blood is drawn (5).

Patients with dyslipidemias should be evaluated for remediable, secondary causes, as summarized in Box 10.2 (5).

Box 10.2. Secondary Causes of Dyslipidemias

Medical Conditions

Nephrotic syndrome
Diabetes
Excessive alcohol consumption
Hypothyroidism
Liver disease

Medications

13–*cis*–retinoic acid
Anticonvulsants
Highly active anti-retroviral therapy
Diuretics
Beta-blockers
Androgens
Oral contraceptives
Corticosteroids
Cyclosporine
Sirolimus

Source: Reprinted from National Kidney Foundation. K/DOQI clinical practice guidelines for managing dyslipidemias in chronic kidney disease patients. *Am J Kidney Dis*. 2003;41(Suppl 3):S38, with permission from the National Kidney Foundation.

Appropriate corrective actions should be taken where possible. For example, CKD patients who still produce urine should have protein excretion measured, because levels more than 3 g in 24 hours can contribute to dyslipidemias (17). The physician may prescribe angiotensin II converting enzyme inhibitors (ACE inhibitors) or angiotensin II receptor blockers (ARBs) to help reduce protein excretion (6). In the case of diabetes, obtain a fasting blood glucose and glycated hemoglobin and then work on improving glycemic control (18).

TREATING DYSLIPIDEMIAS WITH THERAPEUTIC LIFESTYLE CHANGES

Box 10.3 includes the therapeutic lifestyle changes (TLC) for adults from the ATP III report with adaptations for chronic kidney disease as found in the K/DOQI dyslipidemia report (5).

Dietary Fats and Cholesterol

The ATP III promotes diet and lifestyle changes as essential strategies for reducing the risk of cardiovascular disease and as the cornerstone of treatment. Saturated fat and cholesterol remain the primary targets for the TLC diet (4). Medical nutrition therapy must be individualized based on the patient's metabolic profile and treatment goals. The patient is the one who decides what changes are reasonable and feasible to put into practice. Monitoring outcomes from the interventions will determine if improvements have been made and if further modifications are possible.

In any patient with CKD, it is important to assess for malnutrition and protein energy deficits. A low total cholesterol may signal malnutrition, in which case improving nutrition intake should be the primary goal. If the patient is well nourished, adding dietary modifications for dyslipidemia management can be safely undertaken.

A meta-analysis of 37 dietary intervention studies in free-living subjects (9,276 subjects in intervention groups and 2,310 subjects in control groups) published between 1981 and 1997 found that dietary interventions with 7% of energy from saturated fat and 200 mg/day of dietary cholesterol reduced total cholesterol from baseline by 13%, LDL by 16%, HDL by 7%, and TG by 8% ($P < .01$ for all) (19). Adding exercise resulted in greater decreases in total and LDL cholesterol and triglycerides and prevented the decrease in HDL

Box 10.3. Therapeutic Lifestyle Changes (TLC) for Adults With Chronic Kidney Disease

Diet*

Emphasize reduced saturated fat
- Saturated fat: < 7% of total calories
- Polyunsaturated fat: up to 10% of total calories
- Monounsaturated fat: up to 20% of total calories
- Total fat: 25%–35% of total calories
- Cholesterol: < 200 mg per day
- Carbohydrate: 50%-60% of total calories

Emphasize components that reduce dyslipidemia
- Fiber: 20–30 g per day; emphasize 5–10 g per day viscous (soluble) fiber
- Consider plant stanols/sterols 2 g per day
- Improve glycemic control

Emphasize total calories to attain/maintain standard NHANES body weight
- Match intake of overall energy (calories) to overall energy needs
- Body mass index 25–28 kg/m^2
- Waist circumference
  - Men < 40 inches (102 cm)
  - Women < 35 inches (88 cm)
  - Waist-Hip Ratio (Men < 1.0; women < 0.8)

*Consult a dietitian with expertise in chronic kidney disease.

Physical Activity

Moderate daily lifestyle activities
- Use pedometer to attain/maintain 10,000 steps per day
- Emphasize regular daily motion and distance (within ability)

Moderate planned physical activity
- 3–4 times per week 20–30 minute periods of activity
- Include 5–minute warm-up and cool-down
- Choose walking, swimming, supervised exercise (within ability)
- Include resistance exercise training
- Emphasize lean muscle mass and reducing excess body fat

Habits

Alcohol in moderation; limit one drink per day with approval of physician
Smoking cessation

Source: Reprinted from National Kidney Foundation. K/DOQI clinical practice guidelines for managing dyslipidemias in chronic kidney disease patients. *Am J Kidney Dis.* 2003;41(Suppl 3):S43, with permission from the National Kidney Foundation.

cholesterol. Exercise has also been shown to be essential for long-term maintenance of weight loss (20).

In patients with the metabolic syndrome, a higher intake of total dietary fat, mostly in the form of unsaturated fats, can help reduce triglycerides and increase HDL and improve postmeal glycemia. However, the high monounsaturated fat (MUFA) diets have not been shown to improve fasting glucose or hemoglobin A_{1C} levels (21).

Some studies seem to suggest that energy intake is the more critical factor in determining the effects of high-carbohydrate diets versus high-MUFA diets. If energy intake is reduced and a low-fat, high-carbohydrate diet is compared with a diet high in MUFA, there is no detrimental effect on triglycerides from the high-carbohydrate diet (22). Low-fat, high-carbohydrate diets consumed over long periods of time have been shown to not increase triglycerides and have led to modest weight loss and maintenance of weight loss better than other types of reduced-energy diets (23,24). In contrast, diets high in fat may lead to higher energy intakes and weight gain, which may be a concern. Therefore, the patient's metabolic profile and need to lose weight will determine the medical nutrition therapy recommendations.

In subjects with type 2 diabetes, the use of n-3 fatty acid supplements has beneficially reduced triglycerides with no detrimental effects on glycemic control (25,26). If supplements are used, the effects on LDL cholesterol should be monitored. Due to inconclusive results in the few studies that examined fish oil supplements in patients with CKD, the K/DOQI dyslipidemia guidelines made no recommendations regarding the use of n-3 supplements.

Dietary Fiber

Soluble fibers (especially beta-glucan and pectin) modestly reduce total cholesterol and LDL beyond what is observed from a diet low in saturated fat and cholesterol. Consuming 5 to 10 g of soluble fiber per day can reduce LDL an additional 3% to 5% (4,27,28). Foods high in fiber are often higher in potassium and phosphorus, so monitoring laboratory values is essential. Patients need to know how to read nutrition labels. Providing lists of acceptable high-fiber foods with tips on how to include their choices in a daily action plan will gradually help them meet their fiber goal (29). Adjustments in phosphate binders or potassium content of the dialysate may be needed to maintain normal serum potassium and phosphorus.

Functional fibers that are extracted from synthetic or natural sources can also be added when patients are unable to consume adequate fiber through their diet. Many of these come as tasteless powders that can be added to meals (in juices, water, applesauce, cooked cereals, etc). Soluble fiber examples are generic psyllium products and Metamucil (Proctor and Gamble, Cincinnati, OH 45202). Unifiber (Niche Pharmaceuticals, Inc, Roanoke, TX 76262) is a commonly used insoluble cellulose fiber. All provide 3 g of fiber per tablespoon or dose. Package inserts and labels should be reviewed before use to ensure the product contains low amounts of potassium, sodium, and magnesium.

High-fiber diets require additional fluid intake to avoid constipation and GI distress. This may be difficult for the anuric dialysis patient who is often limited to 1 L of fluid per day. Constipation is a chronic problem for dialysis patients who are restricted in the actual amount of fiber and fluid they may consume (5). Osmotic agents such as Miralax (Braintree Laboratories, Braintree, MA 02185), a polyethylene glycol powder taken orally in a 17–g dose mixed with 8 oz of water, may be needed on a short-term basis to relieve constipation. The laxative effect of Miralax works by the osmotic action of pulling water into the large bowel, which more than offsets the fluid intake required. This should be well tolerated even by dialysis patients with fluid restrictions. Miralax is a covered drug in some state kidney disease programs.

Plant Sterols and Stanols

Plant sterols are found in very small amounts in plant foods such as corn, soy, and other vegetable or plant oils. Plant stanols are created by the hydrogenation of plant sterols. Both function in a similar manner by competing with cholesterol for entry into the mixed micelles that must form during digestion for dietary fatty acids and cholesterol to be absorbed. By blocking the intestinal absorption of dietary and endogenous cholesterol, some cholesterol molecules become insoluble and are excreted in the stool (30). Intakes of 2 to 3 g of plant stanols/sterols per day are reported to decrease total and LDL cholesterol levels by 6% to 15%, with considerable variability in response among individuals (28,31).

There is no contraindication to the use of plant stanols/sterols in patients with CKD. Commercially, plant stanols/sterols are found in margarine spreads or salad dressings in either regular or light options under the trademark names of Benecol (McNeil Nutritionals, Fort Washington, PA 19034) or Take Control (Unilever Bestfoods, Engelwood Cliffs, NJ 07632). Benecol products have a 1.7–g stanol ester content per serving, and Take Control products have a 1,650–mg soybean extract content per serving. These products can be used in cooking, baking, or frying, with the exception of the light versions, which should only be used as spreads. Patients need to consider the expense of these commercial products on the market and the equivalent energy and fat content relative to traditional margarines used. Table 10.2 compares the commercial sterol/stanol products to margarine and light spreads based on a 1-tablespoon serving.

Soy Protein

Although the K/DOQI dyslipidemia guidelines make no recommendations regarding the use of soy protein, a high intake can cause small reductions in LDL cholesterol when it replaces animal protein within the context of low-saturated fat and low-cholesterol diet (28, 32). A hallmark meta-analysis study (33) concluded that a minimum of 25 g of soy protein daily reduces total serum cholesterol by 9.3%, LDL by 12.9%, and TG by 10.5%. This conclusion eventually let the US Food and Drug Administration (FDA) to release a health claim in the fall of 1999 about soy protein's ability to reduce the risk of heart disease (34).

Consuming 25 g of soy protein daily is difficult for most Americans. From a practitioner's point of view, the increasing number of soy products available in supermarkets does provide an alternative for vegetarian patients or those patients who have an altered

Table 10.2. Comparison of Commercial Plant Sterol/Stanol Esters With Margarine and Light Spread

Nutrient per 1-Tbsp Serving	*Margarine*	*Light spread*	*Benecol**	*Benecol Light**	*Take Control†*	*Take Control Light†*
Energy (kcal)	100	50	80	45	80	45
Total fat (g)	11	5–6	9	5	8	5
Saturated fat (g)	1–2	1	1	0.5	1	0.5
Polyunsaturated fat (g)	4–5	1–2.5	3	2	2	2
Monounsaturated fat (g)	2–3	0.5	4	2.5	4.5	2
Sodium (mg)	105	100–140	110	110	85	85

*Benecol and Benecol Light are registered trademarks of McNeil Nutritionals (Fort Washington, PA 19034; http://www.benecol.com).

†Take Control and Take Control Light are registered trademarks of Unilever Bestfoods (Engelwood Cliffs, NJ 07632; http://www.takecontrol.com).

Source: Data are from product literature.

taste or lack of desire for meat. Most soy foods are higher in sodium, potassium, and/or phosphorus, so other adjustments may be needed in the patient's meal plan and medical management to maintain acceptable laboratory values (35).

TREATMENT OF DYSLIPIDEMIAS INCLUDING LIPID-LOWERING AGENTS

Table 10.3 is a useful summary of the CKD adult dyslipidemia treatment recommendations from the K/DOQI report (5). For the rare adult patient with very high serum TG (> 500 mg/dL), triglyceride reduction is the principal focus of treatment to prevent pancreatitis. Once TG are less than 500 mg/dL attention should focus on LDL reduction. Initially, very high TG should be treated with TLC. However, the diet should have an even greater fat restriction, with total fat limited to 15% or less of total energy. If drug treatment becomes necessary, studies from the general population suggest that fibrates and nicotinic acid reduce TG by 20% to 50%. The risk of complications from these drugs, particularly myositis and rhabdomyolysis, is increased in CKD (4,5).

Some patients with LDL of 100 to 129 mg/dL may achieve the goal of LDL less than 100 mg/dL with TLC alone, and this should be attempted for 2 to 3 months before beginning drug treatment (4,5). However, because of the number of other nutritional concerns, it is important to consult a dietitian experienced in the care of patients with CKD.

Because TLC alone is usually insufficient to reduce LDL to the goal of less than 100 mg/dL, a statin (3-hydroxy-3-methylglutaryl coenzyme A reductase inhibitor) should be added, provided there is no evi-

Table 10.3. The Management of Dyslipidemias in Adults With Chronic Kidney Disease

Dyslipidemia	*Goal*	*Initiate*	*Increase*	*Alternative*
TG ≥ 500 mg/dL	TG < 500 mg/dL	TLC	TLC + fibrate or niacin	Fibrate or niacin
LDL 100–129 mg/dL	LDL < 100 mg/dL	TLC	TLC + low-dose statin	Bile acid sequestrant or niacin
LDL ≥ 130 mg/dL	LDL < 100 mg/dL	TLC + low-dose statin	TLC + maximum-dose statin	Bile acid sequestrant or niacin
TG ≥ 200 mg/dL and non-HDL ≥ 130 mg/dL	Non-HDL< 130 mg/dL	TLC + low-dose statin	TLC + maximum-dose statin	Fibrate or niacin

To convert mg/dL to mmol/L, multiply triglycerides by 0.01129 and cholesterol by 0.02586.

Abbreviations: HDL, high-density lipoprotein cholesterol; LDL, low-density lipoprotein cholesterol; TG, triglycerides; TLC, therapeutic lifestyle changes.

Source: Reprinted from National Kidney Foundation. K/DOQI clinical practice guidelines for managing dyslipidemias in chronic kidney disease patients. *Am J Kidney Dis*. 2003;41(Suppl 3):S40, with permission from the National Kidney Foundation.

dence of acute or chronic liver disease (4,5). Therapeutic lifestyle changes (TLC) should always be continued as an adjunct to statin therapy. The statins currently approved for use in the United States include atorvastatin, fluvastatin, lovastatin, pravastatin, and simvastatin. Starting at a low dose and titrating the dose upwards is the best strategy for finding the lowest dose that achieves the LDL goal of less than 100 mg/dL while minimizing adverse effects, as shown in Table 10.4 (5).

There is strong evidence from studies in the general population that statins reduce CHD events and all-cause mortality. The reduction in mortality and in CHD events is proportional to the reduction in LDL (3). There is also substantial evidence that statins are safe and effective in reducing LDL in kidney transplant recipients (36). Because statins are associated with hepatotoxicity, liver enzymes should be monitored. Patients should also be monitored for signs and symptoms of myopathies.

Table 10.4 shows lipid-lowering medication dose adjustments for reduced kidney function. Neither atorvastatin nor pravastatin require adjustments. Cyclosporine has been shown to increase the blood levels of virtually every statin that has been investigated. However, statins can be used safely with cyclosporine if the dose of the statin is reduced. Any medications known to increase the statin blood levels should be avoided or the statin should be reduced or stopped. Again, the K/DOQI dyslipidemia guidelines provide more detail about this and readers are encouraged to consult the report if further information is needed (5).

Table 10.4. Recommended Daily Statin Dose Ranges*

	Level of GFR (mL/min/1.73m²)		
Statin	*≥ 30*	*< 30 or dialysis*	*With Cyclosporine*
Atorvastatin	10–80 mg	10–80 mg	10–40 mg
Fluvastatin	20–80 mg	10–40 mg	10–40 mg
Lovastatin	20–80 mg	10–40 mg	10–40 mg
Pravastatin	20–40 mg	20–40 mg	20–40 mg
Simvastatin	20–80 mg	10–40 mg	10–40 mg

*Adult Treatment Panel III recommendations for GFR ≥ 30 mL/min/1.73m2. Most manufacturers recommend once-daily dosing, but give 50% of the maximum dose twice daily.

Source: Reprinted from National Kidney Foundation. K/DOQI clinical practice guidelines for managing dyslipidemias in chronic kidney disease patients. *Am J Kidney Dis.* 2003;41(Suppl 3):S48, with permission from the National Kidney Foundation.

Two new lipid-lowering agents have become available since the publication of the K/DOQI dyslipidemia guidelines. In August 2003, the FDA approved a new statin, rosuvastatin (Crestor, AstraZeneca Pharmaceuticals, Wilmington DE 19850) for use at doses ranging from 5 to 40 mg per day (37–40). Product information indicates dosing precautions should be used in patients with Japanese or Chinese ancestry (40). Rosuvastatin should be used with caution in patients at risk of renal impairment. In patients taking a 40–mg dose, increased proteinuria and microscopic hematuria have been observed, although the conditions are generally transient and not associated with worsening renal function. Co-administration of cyclosporine, warfarin, and gemfibrozil affect the bioavailability of rosuvastatin. Patients who take cyclosporine should limit their dose of rosuvastatin to 5 mg once daily. If used in combination with cholestyramine or gemfibrozil, the dose of rosuvastatin should be limited to 10 mg once daily. For patients with severe renal impairment (GFR < 30 mL/min/1.73 m^2) and not on hemodialysis, dosing of rosuvastatin should be started at 5 mg once daily and not exceed 10 mg once daily (41).

In October 2002, the FDA approved the drug ezetimibe (Zetia, Merck/ScheringPlough Pharmaceuticals, Wales, PA 19454) as a stand-alone lipid-lowering treatment and also for use with statin drugs for patients who require further reductions in LDL cholesterol (42). In contrast to statins, which inhibit cholesterol production in the liver, ezetimibe works locally by preventing the absorption of cholesterol in the intestines. Ezetimibe is not meant to replace statins but to complement them, adding one 10–mg ezetimibe tablet daily to a statin regimen (43). Product information indicates that co-administration of cholestyramine, gemfibrozil, and cyclosporine affect the bioavailability of ezetimibe. Patients who take cyclosporine with ezetimibe should be carefully monitored. Also, the safety and effectiveness of ezetimibe with fibrates has not been established, so combination therapy with fibrates is not recommended at this time (44). (Refer to Chapter 15 on medications for more detail about lipid-lowering agents.)

When adding a second lipid-lowering agent to a statin, it is best to avoid fibrates, but bile acid sequestrants (BAS) can safely be used. The BAS are contraindicated in patients with TG of 400 mg/dL or more. It is best to avoid taking the BAS at the same time as any other medications. This is particularly important for kidney transplant recipients on immunosuppressive medications. For patients with high TG, nicotinic acid can be considered as an alternative second agent with a statin. Contraindications to nicotinic acid include liver disease, severe gout, and peptic ulcer disease (5).

Non-HDL Cholesterol and High Triglycerides

Non-HDL cholesterol may be a target of treatment for patients who present with a lipid profile consistent with the metabolic syndrome of high TG and normal LDL (44). Increased TG has been identified as an independent risk factor for ACVD in the general population because TG frequently are the result of atherogenic remnant lipoproteins highly correlated with very-low-density lipoprotein (VLDL) cholesterol (45). Because a normal VLDL cholesterol is usually defined as less than 30 mg/dL, a reasonable goal for non-HDL cholesterol is 30 mg/dL more than the LDL goal of 100 mg/dL, namely 130 mg/dL. The ATP III recommends using non-HDL cholesterol as a target of therapy rather than TG because triglycerides have more day-to-day variability (4). Also, non-HDL cholesterol is a good surrogate marker for apolipoprotein B, the major atherogenic apolipoprotein, especially because standardized measures of apolipoprotein B are not readily available (4).

Potential causes of hypertriglyceridemia that may be targets of treatment include obesity, physical inactivity, excessive alcohol intake, a high-carbohydrate diet, type 2 diabetes, nephrotic syndrome, and some medications, including estrogens, beta blockers, corticosteroids, and the immunosuppressive agents cyclosporine and sirolimus (5). Appropriate TLC should first be implemented. Specifically, weight reduction and increased physical activity are the first-line therapies that will effectively reduce all of the risk factors associated with the metabolic syndrome (4).

Adding a statin will generally cause a 15% to 25% reduction in TG. If contraindicated, treating with a fibrate, specifically gemfibrozil as the fibrate of choice, should be considered for most CKD patients. Blood levels of gemfibrozil do not seem to be altered by decreased kidney function, in contrast to other fibrates (bezafibrate, clofibrate, and fenofibrate) (46). Data on ciprofibrate in CKD is unknown at this time. The K/DOQI dyslipidemia guidelines cite several of these studies in table format and in references (5). Nicotinic acid may be effective in reducing triglycerides, but adverse side effects such as flushing and hyperglycemia may make compliance more difficult. If insulin resistance and hyperglycemia are contributing to the elevated TG, then clinical judgment may contraindicate the use of nicotinic acid (47).

CKD METABOLIC ABNORMALITIES WITH CARDIAC IMPLICATIONS

Although not extensively addressed in the K/DOQI dyslipidemia report, other unique complications of CKD are anemia and calcium and phosphorus metabolic abnormalities that have cardiac implications and may contribute to the risk of ACVD in CKD.

Vascular calcification is now known to be a major risk factor for cardiovascular events and may be present in as many as 90% of ESRD patients with coronary artery disease (48). Nearly 60% of all dialysis patients demonstrate cardiac calcification on autopsy (49). Chronic dialysis patients have more frequent, more severe, and more rapidly progressive calcifications in their coronary arteries and valves than age-matched nondialysis patients with known or suspected cardiac disease (50). Even young CRF patients in their twenties are at risk for coronary and vascular calcifications (51). Calcification may lead to cardiac damage, resulting in conducting abnormalities and arrhythmia, left ventricular dysfunction, stenosis of the aortic and mitral valves, regurgitation, complete heart block, ischemia, congestive cardiac failure, and death (49–52). Electron beam computed tomography (EBCT), a new, noninvasive imaging technique, permits sensitive quantification of calcium deposits and can detect the early stages of calcification (53).

Consequently, prevention and treatment of hyperphosphatemia has taken on a new level of importance and priority because of its critical role in not only causing secondary hyperparathyroidism and metabolic bone disease, but in leading to vascular calcification and ultimately increased mortality (48,54). Use of the phosphate-binding agent sevelamer hydrochloride has significantly improved the lipid profile of hemodialysis patients, with a 30% mean decrease in LDL and an 18% mean increase in HDL (55).

Left ventricular hypertrophy (LVH) also has a high prevalence in patients with CKD. Treatment of both hypertension and anemia reduces the morbidity and mortality associated with LVH (1).

CONCLUSION

Dietitians play a critical role on the health care team to improve outcomes in all of these areas. They assist in protocols designed to meet K/DOQI anemia management guidelines, particularly in the area of iron therapy. They coordinate dietary and medical interventions to meet K/DOQI bone metabolism and disease management guidelines. Finally, they promote diet and lifestyle interventions effective in lowering blood pressure and reducing cardiovascular risk factors. The challenge of blending therapeutic lifestyle changes with the complexity of the renal diet, acknowledging the crucial role TLC plays in treatment, underscores the need for a dietitian with professional expertise in both cardiovascular and renal disease to effectively tailor the best dietary approach for each patient.

REFERENCES

1. Levey AS, Beto JA, Coronado BE, Eknoyan G, Foley RN, Kasiske BL, Klag MJ, Mailloux LU, Manske CL, Meyer KB, Parfrey PS, Pfeffer MA, Wenger NK, Wilson PWF, Wright JT. Controlling the epidemic of cardiovascular disease in chronic renal disease: what do we know? What do we need to learn? Where do we go from here? National Kidney Foundation Task Force on Cardiovascular Disease. *Am J Kidney Dis*. 1998;32:853–906.
2. Krauss RM, Eckel RH, Howard B, Appel LJ, Daniels SR, Deckelbaum RJ, Erdman JW, Kris-Etherton P, Goldberg IJ, Kotchen TA, Lichtenstein AH, Mitch WE, Mullis R, Robinson K, Wylie-Rosett J, St. Jeor S, Suttie J, Tribble DL, Bazzarre TL. AHA Dietary Guidelines: revision 2000: a statement for health-care professionals from the National Committee of the American Heart Association. *Circulation*. 2000;102:2284–2299.
3. US Department of Health and Human Services; National Institutes of Health; National Heart, Lung, and Blood Institute. *The Seventh Report of the Joint National Committee on Prevention, Detection, Evaluation, and Treatment of High Blood Pressure (JNC 7 Express)*. Bethesda, Md: National Heart, Lung, and Blood Institute; 2003. NIH Publication 03–5233.
4. Expert Panel on Detection, Evaluation, and Treatment of High Blood Cholesterol in Adults. Executive summary of the Third Report of the National Cholesterol Education Program (NCEP) Expert Panel on Detection, Evaluation, and Treatment of High Blood Cholesterol in Adults (Adult Treatment Panel III). *JAMA*. 2001;285:2486–2497.
5. National Kidney Foundation. K/DOQI clinical practice guidelines for managing dyslipidemias in chronic kidney disease patients. *Am J Kidney Dis*. 2003;41(Suppl 3):S1–S91.
6. National Kidney Foundation. K/DOQI clinical practice guidelines for chronic kidney disease: evaluation, classification, and stratification. *Am J Kidney Dis*. 2002;39(Suppl 1):S1–S266.
7. Morbidity and mortality of renal disease: an NIH Consensus Conference statement. *Ann Intern Med*. 1994;121:62–70.
8. Ma KW, Greene EL, Raij L. Cardiovascular risk factors in chronic renal failure and hemodialysis populations. *Am J Kidney Dis*. 1992;19:505–513.
9. Gore JM, Goldberg RJ, Matsumoto AS, Castelli WP, McNamara PM, Dalen JE. Validity of serum total cholesterol level obtained within 24 hours of acute myocardial infarction. *Am J Cardiol*. 1984; 54:722–725.
10. Ryder REJ, Hayes TM, Mulligan IP, Kingswood JC, Williams S, Owens DR. How soon after myocardial infarction should plasma lipid values be assessed? *BMJ*. 1984;289:1651–1653.
11. Sammalkorpi K, Valtonen V, Kerttula Y, Nikkila E, Taskinen MR. Changes in serum lipoprotein pattern induced by acute infections. *Metabolism*. 1988;37:859–865.
12. Lowrie EG, Lew NL. Death risk in hemodialysis patients: the predictive value of commonly measured variables and an evaluation of death rate differences between facilities. *Am J Kidney Dis*. 1990;15:458–482.
13. Lowrie EG, Lew NL. Commonly measured laboratory variables in hemodialysis patients: relationships among them and to death risk. *Semin Nephrol*. 1992;12:276–283.
14. Iseki K, Yamazato M, Tozawa M, Takishita S. Hypocholesterolemia is a significant predictor of death in a cohort of chronic hemodialysis patients. *Kidney Int*. 2002;61:1887–1893.
15. Bologa RM, Levine DM, Parker TS, Cheigh JS, Serur D, Stenzel KH, Rubin AL. Interleukin-6 predicts hypoalbuminemia, hypocholesterolemia, and mortality in hemodialysis patients. *Kidney Int*. 2002;61:1887–1893.
16. Friedewald WT, Levy RI, Fredrickson DS. Estimation of the concentration of low-density lipoprotein cholesterol in plasma, without use of the

preparative ultracentrifuge. *Clin Chem*. 1972;18: 499–502.

17. Kaysen GA, Don B, Schambelan M. Proteinuria, albumin synthesis and hyperlipidaemia in the nephrotic syndrome. *Nephrol Dial Transplant*. 1991;6:141–149.
18. American Diabetes Association. Clinical practice recommendations 2002. *Diabetes Care*. 2002; 25(Suppl 1):S1–S147.
19. Yu-Poth S, Zhao G, Ehterton T, Naglak M, Jonnalagadda S, Kris-Etherton PM. Effects of the National Cholesterol Education Program's Step I and II dietary intervention programs on cardiovascular disease risk factors: a meta-analysis. *Am J Clin Nutr*. 1999;69:632–646.
20. Maggio CA, Pi-Sunyer FX: The prevention and treatment of obesity: application to type 2 diabetes (technical review). *Diabetes Care*. 1997;20: 1744–1766.
21. Garg A. High-monounsaturated fat diets for patients with diabetes mellitus: a meta-analysis. *Am J Clin Nutr*. 1998;67(3 Suppl):577S-582S.
22. Heilbronn I, Noakes M, Clifton P. Effect of energy restriction, weight loss, and diet composition on plasma lipids and glucose in patients with type 2 diabetes. *Diabetes Care*. 1999;22:889–895.
23. Franz MJ. American Diabetes Association, National Cholesterol Education Program Adult Treatment Panel III, and American Heart Association nutrition guidelines: similar but not the same. *On the Cutting Edge: Diabetes Care and Education*. 2002;23:4–12.
24. Schaefer EJ, Lichtenstein AH, Lamon-Fava S, McNamara JR, Schaefer MM, Rasmussen H, Ordovas JM. Body weight and low-density lipoprotein cholesterol changes after consumption of a low-fat ad libitum diet. *JAMA*. 1995;274:1450–1455.
25. Friedberg CE, Janssen MJEM, Heine RJ, Grobbee DE. Fish oil and glycemic control in diabetes: a meta-analysis. *Diabetes Care*. 1998;21: 494–500.
26. Montori VM, Farmer A, Wollan PC, Dinneen SF. Fish oil supplementation in type 2 diabetes: a quantitative systematic review. *Diabetes Care*. 2000;23:1407–1415.
27. Brown L, Rosner B, Willett WW, Sacks F. Cholesterol-lowering effects of dietary fiber: a meta-analysis. *Am J Clin Nutr*. 1999;69:30–42.
28. Van Horn L, Ernst N. A summary of the science supporting the new National Cholesterol Education Program dietary recommendations: what dietitians should know. *J Am Diet Assoc*. 2001;101: 1148–1154.
29. Daigle NW. High-fiber foods. *J Ren Nutr*. 1996; 6:52–55.
30. Schryver T, Wrick KL. Plant sterol and stanol esters: phytochemical food ingredients for lowering serum cholesterol. *Dietitian's Edge*. 2000;1: 35–38.
31. Hallikainen MA, Uusitupa MIJ. Effects of 2 low-fat stanol ester-containing margarines on serum cholesterol concentrations as part of a low-fat diet in hypercholesterolemic subjects. *Am J Clin Nutr*. 1999;69:403–410.
32. Jenkins DJ, Kendall CW, Vidgen E, Mehling CC, Parker T, Seyler H, Faulkner D, Garsetti M, Griffin LC, Agarwal S, Rao AV, Cunnane SC, Ryan MA, Connelly PW, Leiter LA, Vuksan V, Josse R. The effect on serum lipids and oxidized low-density lipoprotein of supplementing self-selected low-fat diets with soluble-fiber, soy, and vegetable protein foods. *Metabolism*. 2000;49: 67–72.
33. Anderson JW, Johnston BM, Cook-Newell ME. Meta-analysis of the effects of soy protein intake on serum lipids. *N Engl J Med*. 1995;333:276–282.
34. Food and Drug Administration. Food labeling: health claims, soy protein and coronary heart disease. 64 *Federal Register* 206(1999) (codified at 21 CFR §101).
35. Pagenkemper JJ. Planning a vegetarian renal diet. *J Ren Nutr*. 1995;5:234–238.
36. Kasiske BL, Heim-Duthoy KL, Singer GG, Watschinger B, Bermain MJ, Bastani B. The effects of lipid-lowering agents on acute renal allograft rejection. *Transplantation*. 2001;72:223–227.
37. US Food and Drug Administration. FDA approves new drug for lowering cholesterol. August 12, 2003. Available at: http://www.fda.gov/bbs/topics. Accessed October 9, 2003.
38. Jones PH. Comparing HMG-CoA reductase inhibitors. *Clin Cardiol*. 2003;26(Suppl 1):I15–I20.
39. Davidson M, Ma P, Stein EA, Gotto AM Jr, Raza A, Chitra R, Hutchinson H. Comparison of effects on low-density lipoprotein cholesterol and high-density lipoprotein cholesterol with rosu-

vastatin versus atorvastatin in patients with type IIa or IIb hypercholesterolemia. *Am J Cardiol.* 2002;89:268–275.

40. Crestor (rosuvastatin calcium) tablets [prescribing information]. Revised ed. Wilmington, Del: AstraZeneca Pharmaceuticals; 2003.
41. Department of Health and Human Services, US Food and Drug Administration. FDA approval for Zetia (ezetimibe) tablets, 10 mg. October 2002. Available at: http://www.fda.gov. Accessed October 9, 2003.
42. Gagne C, Bays HE, Weiss SR, Mata P, Quinto K, Melino M, Cho M, Musliner TA, Gumbiner B. Efficacy and safety of ezetimibe added to ongoing statin therapy for treatment of patients with primary hypercholesterolemia. *Am J Cardiol.* 2002; 90:1084–1091.
43. Zetia (ezetimibe) tablets, 10 mg [prescribing information]. Revised ed. Wales, Pa: Merck/Schering Plough Pharmaceuticals; 2002.
44. Cui Y, Blumenthal RS, Flaws JA, Whiteman MK, Langenberg P, Bachorik PS, Bush TL. Non-high density lipoprotein cholesterol level as a predictor of cardiovascular disease mortality. *Arch Intern Med.* 2001;161:1413–1419.
45. Austin MA, Hokanson JE, Edwards KL. Hypertriglyceridemia as a cardiovascular risk factor. *Am J Cardiol.* 1998;81:7B–12B.
46. Lipscombe J, Lewis GF, Cattran D, Bargman JM. Deterioration in renal function associated with fibrate therapy. *Clin Nephrol.* 2001;55:39–44.
47. Gibbons LW, Gonzalez V, Gordon N, Grundy S. The prevalence of side effects with regular and sustained-release nicotinic acid. *Am J Med.* 1995; 99:378–385.
48. Block GA, Hulbert-Shearon TE, Levin NW, Port FK. Association of serum phosphorus and calcium x phosphate product with mortality risk in chronic hemodialysis patients: a national study. *Am J Kidney Dis.* 1998;31:607–617.
49. Llach F. Cardiac calcification: dealing with another risk factor in patients with kidney failure. *Semin Dial.* 1999;12:293–295.
50. Braun J, Oldendorf M, Moshage W, Heidler R, Zeitler E, Luft FC. Electron beam computed tomography in the evaluation of cardiac calcification in chronic dialysis patients. *Am J Kidney Dis.* 1996;27:394–401.
51. Goodman WG, Goldin J, Kuizon BD, Chun Y, Gales B, Sider D, Wang Y, Chung J, Emerick A, Greaser L, Elashoff RM, Salusky IB. Coronary-artery calcification in young adults with end-stage renal disease who are undergoing dialysis. *N Engl J Med.* 2000;341:1478–1483.
52. Guerin AP, London GM, Marchais SJ, Metivier F. Arterial stiffening and vascular calcifications in end-stage renal disease. *Nephrol Dial Transplant.* 2000;15:1014–1021.
53. Rumberger JA, Brundage BH, Rader DJ, Kondos G. Electron beam computed tomographic coronary calcium scanning: a review and guidelines for use in asymptomatic persons. *Mayo Clin Proc.* 1999;74:243–252.
54. Block GA, Port FK. Re-evaluation of risks associated with hyperphosphatemia and hyperparathyroidism in dialysis patients: recommendations for a change in management. *Am J Kidney Dis.* 2000;35:1226–1237.
55. Chertow GM, Burke SK, Dillon MA, Slatopolsky E. Long-term effects of sevalamer hydrochloride on the calcium x phosphate product and lipid profile of haemodialysis patients. *Nephrol Dial Transplant.* 1999;14:2907–2914.

ADDITIONAL RESOURCES

A clinical practice guideline for treating tobacco use and dependence: a US Public Health Service report. The Tobacco Use and Dependence Clinical Practice Guideline Panel, Staff, and Consortium Representatives. *JAMA.* 2000;283:3244–3254.

Goldstein LB, Adams R, Becker K, Furberg CD, Gorelick PB, Hademenos G, Hill M, Howard G, Howard VJ, Jacobs B, Levine SR, Mosca L, Sacco RL, Sherman DG, Wolf PA, del Zoppo GJ. Primary prevention of ischemic stroke: A statement for health-care professionals from the Stroke Council of the American Heart Association. *Circulation.* 2001;103:163–182.

Krauss RM, Eckel RH, Howard B, Appel LJ, Daniels SR, Deckelbaum RJ, Erdman JW, Kris-Etherton P, Goldberg IJ, Kotchen TA, Lichtenstein AH, Mitch WE, Mullis R, Robinson K, Wylie-Rosett J, St. Jeor S, Suttie J, Tribble DL, Bazzarre TL. AHA dietary guidelines: revision 2000: a statement for health-care professionals from the National Committee of the American Heart Association. *Circulation.* 2000;102:2284–2299.

Mosca L, Collins P, Herrington DM, Mendelsohn ME, Pasternak RC, Robertson R, Schenck-Gustafsson

K, Smith SC, Taubert KA, Wenger N. Hormone replacement therapy and cardiovascular disease: a statement for health-care professionals from the American Heart Association. *Circulation*. 2001; 104:499–503.

National Heart, Lung, and Blood Institute. *Clinical Guidelines on the Identification, Evaluation, and Treatment of Overweight and Obesity in Adults*. Bethesda, Md: National Heart, Lung, and Blood Institute; 1998.

The sixth report of the Joint National Committee on Prevention, Detection, Evaluation, and Treatment of High Blood Pressure. *Arch Intern Med*. 1997; 157:2413–2446.

Smith SC Jr, Blair SN, Bonow RO, Brass LM, Cerqueira MD, Dracup K, Fuster V, Gotto A, Grundy SM, Miller NH, Jacobs A, Jones D, Krauss RM, Mosca L, Ockene I, Pasternak RC, Pearson T, Pfeffer MA, Starke RD, Taubert KA. AHA/ACC scientific statement: AHA/ACC guidelines for preventing heart attack and death in patients with atherosclerotic cardiovascular disease: 2001 update: a statement for health-care professionals from the American Heart Association and American College of Cardiology. *Circulation*. 2001;104:1577–1579.

US Preventive Services Task Force: Aspirin for the primary prevention of cardiovascular events: recommendation and rationale. *Ann Intern Med*. 2002; 136:157–160.

Chapter 11

Pregnancy and Dialysis

Jean Stover, RD

Pregnancy in women with chronic kidney disease (CKD) is considered high risk whether it occurs in the early stages of the disease, while undergoing dialysis, or following kidney transplantation. Hypertension is the most prevalent life-threatening problem for women in all of these groups. There is also a higher risk for more rapid loss of kidney function among women who become pregnant when creatinine levels are 1.4 mg/dL or more. Women who become pregnant after a kidney transplant, however, do not have an increased risk as long as the function is well preserved (1).

Women with CKD generally do not become pregnant as frequently as those with normal kidney function. Women with CKD undergoing dialysis have a marked decrease in conception, with a pregnancy rate of 0.5% reported for this population in 1999. This compares with a rate of 9% for all women of child-bearing age in the United States in 1994 (1,2). Fertility usually returns for women with well-functioning kidney transplants, but immunosuppressive drug therapy, especially cyclosporine, has been known to result in the birth of babies who are small for gestational age. These drugs have not been associated with an increase in congenital anomalies, but all groups of women with CKD are at risk for premature births (1).

Given the circumstances outlined above, a woman with CKD who becomes pregnant presents many challenges to the health care team, as substantive research on the specialized medical and nutritional needs for this unique patient population is lacking. Thus, the health care team must work synergistically and monitor the patient's clinical indicators closely in order to increase the probability of successful maternal and fetal outcomes. Adequate nutrition, including vitamin and mineral therapy, is particularly important during pregnancy to promote a successful outcome. Also, the amount of dialysis treatment must be increased during pregnancy to more closely assimilate the function of normal kidneys during fetal development, and women undergoing dialysis must realize the time commitment involved. Although the survival rates of infants born to women undergoing dialysis are improving, the involvement of the multidisciplinary renal health care team and ongoing communication with the high-risk obstetrics team is of utmost importance.

NUTRITION MANAGEMENT GUIDELINES

Box 11.1 provides a summary of the nutrition management guidelines for pregnant dialysis patients (3–9). These guidelines apply to women who are pregnant while undergoing hemodialysis. They should be adapted for earlier stages of CKD and for pregnant women undergoing peritoneal dialysis. Nutrient recommendations for pregnant women with well-functioning kidney

Box 11.1. Suggested Management Guidelines for Pregnancy and Dialysis

Medical Nutrition Therapy

- Energy: 35 kcal/kg of ideal body weight (IBW) or standard body weight (SBW) + 300 kcal per day (2nd and 3rd trimesters).
- Protein: 1.2 g/kg IBW + 10 g per day (2nd and 3rd trimesters).
- Other nutrients: Possibly liberalize intake of potassium, phosphorus, sodium, and fluid with more dialysis time.

Medications

- Renal vitamin preparations and added minerals: Include at least 2 mg folic acid and 15 mg zinc per day.
- Vitamin D: Vitamin D analogs have been given intravenously to some pregnant dialysis patients; not clear if any harm to fetus.
- Calcium: Supplement as needed to keep serum calcium/phosphorus levels within normal limits for dialysis patients; 2 g per day has been suggested (when a 2.5 mEq/L dialysate is used). May need to give apart from meals if phosphorus decreases with more frequent dialysis.
- Iron: Intravenous iron may be given as iron sucrose without noted complications to maintain serum ferritin and transferrin saturation (TSAT) within goals for dialysis patients; some physicians prefer oral iron alone or included in vitamin preparations.
- Epoietin alpha may be given to maintain hemoglobin (Hgb) ≥ 10–11 mg/dL and hematocrit (Hct) 33%–36%; monitor Hgb and Hct weekly.
- Antihypertensives: Will be needed if patient is euvolemic but blood pressure is ≥ 140/90 mmHg. Avoid angiotensin converting enzyme inhibitors; methyldopa, labetelol and beta blockers are considered safe; calcium channel blockers, clonidine and alpha blockers are probably safe.

Dialysis Regimen

- A Kt/V of 1.5–1.7 per treatment has been recommended and ≥ 20 hours dialysis per week seems to provide the best outcomes. Frequent dialysis is also recommended to avoid hypertension or hypotension with less fluid weight gain and more gentle fluid removal.
- A 2.5 mEq/L calcium dialysate should be adequate, especially if providing frequent dialysis and oral calcium preparations; monitor calcium and phosphorus levels.
- May need a 3 mEq/L potassium dialysate, especially if dialysis is more frequent.

Source: Data are from references 3–9.

transplants are similar to the recommendations for pregnant women without CKD.

The following discussion includes the case study of a woman who became pregnant approximately 5 months after initiating regular hemodialysis treatments. The rationale for specific medical nutrition therapy and the use of specific medications and dialysis treatment alterations during pregnancy are presented.

CASE STUDY

TW is a woman with CKD due to glomerulonephritis, and a past medical history of hypertension. In June 2001, at age 30 years, she initiated hemodialysis for 3.5 hours, three times per week. She continued on hemodialysis, with hospitalizations for a catheter infection, clotted fistula, and symptoms of pancreatitis during the first few months of treatment. In October 2001, a 24–hour urine collection was done as an outpatient and calculated manually to extrapolate a total Kt/V of 1.57, with a KrU (urea clearance) of 3.79 mL/min. TW did not bring another 24–hour urine collection until January 2002, which showed similar results. Toward the end of that month, she reported that her last menses had been in mid-December 2001. A pregnancy test that measures serum levels of the beta subunit of human gonadotropin (hCG) was done and appeared to be positive. TW had already given birth to four children and felt that she had definite symptoms of pregnancy. However, because the small amounts of hCG produced by somatic cells are excreted by the kidney, in renal failure this test can appear positive by usual standards (3). Thus, a pelvic ultrasound was done on February 13, 2002, which confirmed a live intrauterine gestation corresponding to 9 weeks and 5 days, with a positive fetal heart rate of 166 beats per minute.

The renal health care team subsequently counseled TW about what her dialysis regimen would entail if she decided to proceed with the pregnancy. She decided to continue the pregnancy. Once this decision was made, TW was referred to the high-risk obstetrics clinic at the university hospital associated with the dialysis unit. The renal health care team reviewed the available literature on pregnancy for women with CKD undergoing dialysis and developed a plan. TW had brought another urine collection in February 2002, and her 24–urine volume had increased from approximately 900 mL to 1,900 mL, with a manually calculated KrU of 6 mL/min and an extrapolated total Kt/V of 1.97. Because this exceeded the recommended target Kt/V during pregnancy, which is in the range of 1.5 to 1.7 for each treatment, there was no immediate need to change TW's dialysis regimen (3). Also, TW's predialysis BUNs for the last 3 months were 22 mg/dL, 24 mg/dL, and 32 mg/dL, respectively, with reasonable intakes reported, and TW was reluctant to increase her dialysis to four times per week. She therefore continued to receive 3.5 hours of dialysis three times per week using a PSN 170 dialyzer (Baxter International, Inc, Deerfield, IL 60015) and dialysate containing 3 mEq/L potassium and 2.5 mEq/L calcium.

Medical Nutrition Therapy

TW was encouraged to consume adequate energy and protein, with special emphasis on protein. She is 71 inches tall with an ideal body weight (IBW) of 70 kg based on the Hamwi method. Her estimated dry weight (EDW) at the approximate time of conception in December 2001 was 98.5 kg, which was 140% of her IBW. Her body mass index (BMI) was calculated to be 30.3. Her energy needs were estimated to be 35 kcal/kg IBW (for dialysis) plus 300 kcal/day (for pregnancy in the second and third trimester) (4–6). Because TW was nearing her second trimester, her total daily energy needs were calculated to be approximately 2,800 kcal. Her daily protein needs were estimated to be 94 g: 1.2 g/kg IBW (for dialysis) plus 10 g/day (for pregnancy) (4–6). Frequent verbal recalls were done to estimate her intakes. She seemed to be eating well, maintaining a serum albumin of 3.8 g/dL for her first trimester of pregnancy. TW's EDW was increased from 98.5 kg (December 2001) to 101.5 kg (February 2002) to 103.5 kg (March 2002) to 104.5 kg (April 2002) to 106 kg (May 2002) when she had reached 24 weeks' gestation. Her serum albumin decreased to 3.6 g/dL (April 2002) and 3.4 g/dL (May 2002) just before she was transferred to the inpatient hospital dialysis unit. The plan was for her to remain at the hospital unit as an outpatient for the rest of her pregnancy to receive fetal monitoring on dialysis. At the time she was transferred, her predialysis BUN was only 15 mg/dL, but she had received back-to-back dialysis just before the monthly treatment laboratory values were drawn. It was suggested that she begin nutritional supplementation at this time because she had also easily gone below her EDW without becoming hypotensive and reported not always consistently eating well because of her busy schedule with dialysis treatments, obstetric appointments, and other tests and evaluations. Her decreasing serum albumin was a concern, but this is common during pregnancy. The expected decrease during the course of pregnancy is approximately 1 g/dL, even in women without CKD (7).

TW's diet was only mildly restricted in potassium even before she increased her dialysis time to 15 hours per week. In December 2001, her dialysis bath had been changed to a 3 mEq/L potassium concentration due to a serum potassium level of 3.6 mEq/L and reported decreased intakes. When the dialysis regimen was increased to 15 hours per week in April 2002, she was given permission to liberalize her diet even more in potassium, as well as in sodium, phosphorus, and fluid content. Fluid weight gains were minimal, and her serum potassium level in May 2002 just before transfer was 4.8 mEq/L with a calcium level of 9.0 mg/dL and a phosphorus level of 3.1 mg/dL. She was encouraged to continue her calcium carbonate tablets as prescribed (see Medications section), but to take them between meals because of the decreasing phosphorus level. Serum levels of sodium, potassium, carbon dioxide, and calcium/phosphorus were monitored weekly beginning at 20 weeks' gestation, now that dialysis was more frequent.

Medications

Changes in TW's medication regimen were made once the pregnancy was confirmed in February 2002, and she decided to proceed with it. Her renal multivitamin dose was doubled because of increased requirements for water-soluble vitamins during pregnancy, as well as increased losses anticipated with more intensive dialysis later in the pregnancy. Because folate deficiency has been linked to neural tube defects in infants born to women without CKD, assuring at least 2 mg of folic acid per day for pregnant women undergoing dialysis has been encouraged (3). Also, zinc supplementation was prescribed in an effort to prevent increased risks of fetal malformation, preterm delivery, low birth weight, and pregnancy-induced hypertension (7). The latter three factors are known to be risks for pregnant women with CKD. The recommended zinc supplementation for all women during pregnancy is at least 15 mg/day (7). TW was encouraged to buy zinc gluconate because anecdotal evidence suggests that it is well tolerated and inexpensive. She purchased a preparation with 50 mg zinc and was given permission to take this dose.

Because severe hypertension is the primary maternal risk during pregnancy for dialysis patients, the goal is to keep the blood pressure 140/90 mmHg or less. If the patient is euvolemic and the blood pressure is higher than this measurement, several antihypertensive drugs are considered acceptable. These include methyldopa, beta blockers, and labetelol. There is less experience with calcium channel blockers, clonidine, and alpha blockers, but these are considered safe. The class of antihypertensives contraindicated during pregnancy is the angiotensin-converting enzyme inhibitors. They have been associated with a fetal loss of 80% to 93% in animal studies, and in human studies these drugs have been linked to an ossification defect in the fetal skull, dysplastic kidneys, neonatal anuria, and death from hypoplastic lungs (3). TW's antihypertensive drugs were evaluated, and as a safety precaution, her amlodipine was changed to methyldopa.

Intravenous iron sucrose, which TW had been receiving before she became pregnant, was initially discontinued but then resumed within a week after her health care team reviewed current literature. Two European studies reported that intravenous iron sucrose was effective and safe when given to iron-deficient women without CKD during pregnancy (10,11). Other case studies and literature concerning pregnant women on dialysis reported giving this type of iron without mentioning any adverse effects (8).

Epoetin alpha has commonly been given to pregnant women on dialysis. In one literature review, no congenital anomalies in infants born to mothers who received this medication were reported (3). In animal studies, only very large doses of epoetin alpha (500 units/kg) seemed to produce such anomalies (3). Dialysis patients who become pregnant almost always exhibit a worsening of anemia and usually require larger doses of epoetin alpha to maintain a hemoglobin at 10 to 11 g/dL or more (3). TW's epoetin alpha dose was adjusted based on her biweekly hemoglobin levels, and was actually decreased in the first 6 weeks after confirmation of the pregnancy. Her hemoglobin was 12.1 mg/dL when her pregnancy was confirmed in February 2002, was 12.9 mg/dL in March 2002, and 11.7 g/dL in April 2002. At approximately 23 weeks' gestation, just before she was transferred to the hospital unit, TW's hemoglobin had decreased further to 10.6 g/dL. At that time, her epoetin alpha dose was increased and levels were then monitored weekly.

TW had been taking two calcium acetate tablets (667 mg each) three times daily with meals and one tablet with snacks, which was initially continued until March 2002. At that time, she asked to switch to another phosphate binder because she could not tolerate the calcium acetate. She was prescribed calcium carbonate (500 mg), at a dose of two tablets three times daily with meals. Calcium levels remained within acceptable limits, as mentioned previously. The calcium content of the dialysate remained at 2.5 mEq/L (as it had been prior to the pregnancy) until May 13, 2002. It was then changed to 3.5 mEq/L based on two out of three serum calcium levels of 8.4 and 8.5 mg/dL. Although the fetus requires 25 to 30 g of calcium for proper skeletal development, it is usually not necessary to increase the dialysate calcium content when calcium-containing medications are taken and more frequent dialysis is given. There is also some production of calcitriol by the placenta, which makes it important to frequently monitor serum calcium levels to avoid hypercalcemia (3). Because TW was only receiving 15 hours of dialysis, the higher dialysate calcium content was felt to be reasonable, and serum levels would continue to be monitored weekly.

Just before TW's pregnancy was confirmed, the paricalcitol injection she had been receiving was reduced for an intact parathyroid hormone (PTH) of 67 pg/mL. This medication was subsequently discontinued because it is not known whether this form of vitamin D crosses the placental barrier, and if so, whether it is harmful to the fetus. A review of the literature did not produce any convincing evidence that this therapy would be safe (despite the placenta calcitriol production). Also, because the PTH was less than the usual goal of 150 to 300 pg/mL, it was thought that even if PTH did increase significantly, there would only be a temporary period without treatment. TW's PTH was measured with the usual quarterly laboratory tests approximately 3 months after the paricalcitol injection was discontinued, and the level was found to be 544 pg/mL. Still, no treatment was given at that time.

Dialysis Regimen

In April 2002, TW had a calculated Kt/V of 1.29 and was persuaded to increase her dialysis time. She had initially been reluctant to do so, even though the renal health care team had explained to her that literature reports indicated that 20 hours per week during pregnancy produced the best fetal outcome. Because TW did have residual renal function, and her life was so hectic with four other children, it was agreed that at least 15 hours per week of dialysis would be a compromise. Accordingly, she increased her dialysis time to 3.75 hours, four times per week.

It is difficult to evaluate weight gain during pregnancy for a woman undergoing hemodialysis. The goals are to prevent maternal hypertension, as previously discussed, but also to abate severe hypotension, which could promote preterm labor and cause harm to the fetus. Therefore, gentle fluid removable is desirable, and this is more easily attained with more frequent dialysis sessions. TW's EDW had been approximately 98.5 kg in December 2001, the month in which she conceived. She seemed to gain weight rapidly at first, with her EDW increasing to 103.5 kg by early March 2002, 104.5 kg by April, and 106 kg in May. She did go below her EDW at times, but this target weight was not changed. As mentioned previously, she was transferred to the university hospital in-patient unit at 24 weeks' gestation for the remainder of her pregnancy. She was maintained on dialysis for 3.75 hours, four times per week.

TW telephoned periodically for the next few months to keep the renal health care team in the unit aware of her progress. In early July (at approximately 30 weeks' gestation), she went for a regular appointment in the high-risk obstetrics clinic and her cervix was found to be 5 cm dilated. She was subsequently admitted to the hospital for treatment to avoid preterm labor and delivery. At 34 weeks' gestation, she was discharged from the hospital because the fetus was felt to be more viable at that point if TW should go into labor. She did, in fact, go into labor, and deliver at just less than 35 weeks' gestation (with a normal vaginal delivery).

Interestingly, TW's EDW had decreased to approximately 101 kg at the time of delivery. The recommended weight gain for women in normal health with a BMI more than 30 is at least 6 kg for the entire pregnancy (6). TW had a net weight gain of only about 3 kg, but she did not complete a full-term pregnancy. Also, she may have lost weight during her month of hospitalization because she disliked the food and nutritional supplements offered. Her daughter, however, weighed 1,986 grams (4 lb, 6 oz) at birth, was 16 inches in length, and required no artificial ventilation. However, the infant was sent to the high-risk nursery after delivery because infants born to mothers with CKD have BUN and creatinine levels similar to maternal levels, which promote a solute diuresis requiring close monitoring of electrolyte and volume status (3).

Case Study Summary

TW returned to dialysis in the out-patient setting 3 days after delivery. Because of her busy lifestyle and dialysis schedule, she decided not to breastfeed. Her baby remained in the hospital approximately 10 days because of episodes of apnea. During this time, TW was hospitalized again for possible pulmonary embolism due to shortness of breath. Once ruled out, her dry weight was reduced to 91 kg, 7.5 kg less than she had weighed at the time of conception. The baby was discharged with an apnea monitor but was able to be removed from the monitor after several months and seems to be growing normally. She is underweight for her length, although TW thinks her daughter eats well. To help improve the baby's health, TW was referred for nutrition counseling arranged through her pediatrician.

It has been speculated that because TW had significant residual kidney function, it was possible for her to have a positive outcome with less dialysis than is usually recommended for women with CKD during pregnancy. Her dialysis time was never increased to more than 15 hours per week, even when hospitalized. Although Kt/V measurements may be difficult to interpret because of urea generation by the fetus, the goals are higher per treatment, as previously mentioned, and probably should be evaluated to ensure adequate dialysis. The literature does suggest, though, that an increase in dialysis time to 20 hours per week or more seems to improve pregnancy outcome (3).

CONCLUSION

There are some case reports of pregnancy in individuals with CKD undergoing peritoneal dialysis and continuing this mode of therapy until delivery. Conception seems to occur more frequently in hemodialysis patients than in patients undergoing continuous ambulatory peritoneal dialysis (3). It is quite difficult to manipulate peritoneal dialysis exchanges to achieve adequate dialysis and also prevent extreme abdominal discomfort as the pregnancy progresses. Chang and associates report that using tidal peritoneal dialysis with a cycling machine can improve both dialysis clearance and abdominal symptoms during pregnancy in CKD patients (12).

Although kidney transplantation seems to be the best treatment modality for women with CKD who want to have children, there are still increased risks of maternal and fetal morbidity during pregnancy (1,13). The collaboration between the kidney transplant and high-risk obstetrics health care teams in prenatal management continues to be very important to promote successful outcomes. Women with well-functioning kidney transplants should follow the same nutrition recommendations as for women without CKD.

REFERENCES

1. Hou S. Pregnancy in chronic renal insufficiency and end-stage renal disease. *Am J Kidney Dis.* 1999;33:235–252.
2. Darroch JE, Landry DJ, Oslak S. Pregnancy rates among U.S. women and their partners in 1994. *Fam Plann Persp*. 1999;31:122–126,136.
3. Grossman S, Hou S. Obstetrics and gynecology. In: Daugirdas JT, Blake PG, Ing TS, eds. *Handbook of Dialysis.* 3rd ed. Baltimore, Md: Lippincott Williams & Wilkins; 2000:624–636.
4. National Kidney Foundation. Kidney Disease Outcomes Quality Initiative (K/DOQI) clinical practice guidelines for nutrition in chronic renal failure. *Am J Kidney Dis.* 2000;35(suppl 2):S1–S140.
5. Monsen ER. The 10th edition of the Recommended Dietary Allowances: what's new in the 1989 RDAs? (abstract). *J Am Diet Assoc.* 1989; 89:1748–1752.
6. Wiggins KL. Nutrition care of adult pregnant ESRD patients. In: *Guidelines for Nutrition Care of Renal Patients.* 3rd ed. Chicago, Ill: American Dietetic Association; 2002:105–107.
7. Hyten FE. Nutrition and metabolism. In: Hyten F, ed. *Clinical Physiology in Obstetrics.* Oxford, England: Blackwell Scientific Publications; 1988:177.
8. Vidal LV, Ursu M, Martinez A, Sanchez Roland S, Wibmer E, Pereira D, Subiza K, Alonso W, Seijas L, Piazze S, Lisorio L, Falconi JP, Canessa R, Laborda L, Dibello N. Nutritional control of pregnant women on chronic hemodialysis. *J Ren Nutr.* 1998;8:150–156.
9. Molaison EF, Baker K, Bordelon MA, Brodie P, Powell K. Successful management of pregnancy in a patient receiving hemodialysis. *J Ren Nutr.* 2003:13:229–232.
10. Breymann C, Visca E, Huch R, Huch A. Efficacy and safety of intravenously administered iron sucrose with and without adjuvant recombinant human erythropoietin for the treatment of resistant iron-deficiency anemia during pregnancy. *Am J Obstet Gynecol.* 2001;184:662–667.
11. al-Momen AK, al-Meshari A, al-Nuaim L, Saddique A, Abotalib Z, Khashogji T, Abbas M. Intravenous iron sucrose complex in the treatment of iron deficiency anemia during pregnancy. *Eur J Obstet Gynecol Reprod Biol.* 1996;69:121–124.
12. Chang H, Miller MA, Bruns FJ. Tidal peritoneal dialysis during pregnancy improves clearance and abdominal symptoms. *Perit Dial Int.* 2002; 22:272–274.
13. Tan PK, Tan AS, Tan HK, Vathsala A, Tay SK. Pregnancy after renal transplantation: experience in Singapore General Hospital. *Ann Acad Med Singapore.* 2002;31:285–289.

Chapter 12

Nutrition Management of Chronic Kidney Disease in the Pediatric Patient

Julie Rock, MS, RD,
and Donna Secker, MSc, RD

Nutrient imbalances, particularly protein-energy malnutrition, are prevalent in children with chronic kidney disease (CKD). The leading causes of pediatric CKD, renal aplasia/hypoplasia/dysplasia and obstructive uropathy, are disorders that affect infants at birth (1,2). Infants and toddlers are at increased risk for malnutrition because they have low nutritional stores and high nutritional demands for rapid physical and brain growth. Adolescents are also at greater risk because of the high demands of growth during puberty. Growth delay and extremes in body mass index (BMI) are associated with an increased risk for morbidity and mortality in children with CKD (3,4). In addition, children who are chronically malnourished display behavioral changes such as irritability, apathy, and attention deficits, and children who are stunted often experience social disadvantages that adversely affect their development and quality of life (5). Although the causes of impaired growth and development in CKD are multifactorial, early and aggressive correction of nutritional imbalances leads to improvements (6,7).

The goal in nutrition management of the child with CKD is to promote optimal growth and development through maintenance of optimal nutritional status and prevention of malnutrition, uremic toxicity, and metabolic abnormalities. Optimizing nutritional status is an ongoing process that requires frequent monitoring and adjustments to the nutrition plan based on changes in age, development, anthropometrics, residual renal function (RRF), biochemistries, medications, renal replacement therapy (RRT), and psychosocial status. Input from the child and family/caretaker is important and is attained through frequent contact, friendly communication, and strong rapport. Consistent promotion of the benefits of dietary modification and provision of practical information and emotional support to children and their families can positively influence adherence and clinical outcomes and minimize stress around nutritional issues. Full compliance with all dietary restrictions is not always realistic. Priorities should be set on an individual basis, depending on the patient's goals, physical status, emotional needs, and social situation.

ASSESSMENT OF NUTRITIONAL STATUS

Compared with adults, children with kidney disease have very different requirements in terms of growth. Changes in their physical, social, emotional, and cognitive development require that children's nutritional needs be assessed on an ongoing basis (8,9). Although there are no widely accepted guidelines for nutrition assessment of children with CKD or posttransplant, guidelines do exist for children on dialysis (8). These guidelines can be adapted for nondialysis patients, with the intensity and frequency of assessment varying according to the child's age and stability of renal function. Recommended frequencies for assessing specific measures of nutritional status in children on dialysis are listed in Table 12.1 (8). These guidelines are minimum ones, and more frequent assessment is appropriate if the patient may benefit (8). In particular, infants and children with comorbid conditions may need closer follow-up (10,11). A thorough evaluation should also consider medical history, other biochemical parameters, hypertension, bowel habits, urine output, and fluid balance.

Dietary Evaluation

A thorough and accurate diet history will provide information for both quantitative and qualitative evaluation. A 3-day food record is preferred to the 24–hour dietary recall method and may be requested quarterly or as often as monthly, depending on age and the patient's nutritional status and goals. A variety of social and cultural factors influence food consumption and choices. A diet assessment should include food preparation and provision, location of meals, frequency of eating out, and consumption of nonfood items (pica).

Alterations in Normal Development

Healthy infants develop the physical and psychological readiness for solids by 4 to 6 months of age. Oral and gross motor skills steadily progress through infancy from the sucking reflex to improved ability to bite and chew. Skills for communicating a desire for food or the resulting satiety are quickly developed at this time and enhanced throughout childhood. The infant exhibits independent and exploratory behaviors, which are uncoordinated at first but lead to the ability to self-feed and hold a cup without help. Meals of various tastes and textures are then provided in a similar pattern to the rest of the family (12). Acute and chronic illnesses during infancy often disrupt normal infant development. Infants and toddlers with CKD often exhibit slow or no progression through the normal stages of acquired feeding skills. A lack of interest in solid foods is common, particularly when enteral feeds meet part or all of nutrient requirements. Unless there is severe developmental delay or medical contraindication, however, the goal should be to introduce solids and advance textures at the same age as for healthy children.

The overall physical presentation of the child should be observed. Macronutrient deficiencies manifest in loss of subcutaneous fat, muscle wasting, and/or growth failure. The appearance of children's hair, skin, teeth, and tongue, and the smell of their breath can aid in the detection of micronutrient deficiencies. Problems with wound healing may also suggest nutrient deficiencies. Serum zinc levels have been shown to be low in malnourished children, and a depressed dietary intake of zinc and copper has been observed in children receiving dialysis (8,13).

Table 12.1. Suggested Nutritional Parameters and Frequency of Measurement for Children on Dialysis

	Minimum Interval	
Nutritional Marker	*Age < 2 y*	*Age ≥ 2 y*
Dietary interview	Monthly	3–4 mo
Head circumference	Monthly	3–4 mo until age 36 mo
Recumbent length	Monthly	Not applicable
Standing height	Not applicable	3–4 mo
Standard deviation score (SDS) for length/height for chronological age	Monthly	3–4 mo
Estimated dry weight	Monthly	3–4 mo
Weight/height index	Monthly	3–4 mo
Serum albumin	Monthly	Monthly
Serum bicarbonate	Monthly	Monthly
Skinfold thickness	No agreement	3–4 mo
Midarm muscle circumference or area	3–4mo	3–4 mo

Source: Reprinted from National Kidney Foundation. Kidney Disease Outcomes Quality Initiative (K/DOQI) clinical practice guidelines for nutrition in chronic renal failure. *Am J Kidney Dis.* 2000;35(suppl 2):S111, with permission from the National Kidney Foundation.

Uremic consequences of renal disease may manifest in gastroesophageal reflux (GER) disorder, delayed gastric emptying, and frequent episodes of nausea and vomiting. Infants with CKD feed poorly, vomit easily, have taste alterations, and are at risk for chronic dehydration (14,15). Hormones involved in the modulation of hunger and satiety are significantly altered, further worsening anorexia (16). The resulting variations in spontaneous food intake from day to day make adequate oral consumption of nutrients unlikely (17).

Physical activity and clinical exercise evaluation are crucial components of the overall nutrition care plan. Many physiological and lifestyle factors contribute to sedentary behavior in children with CKD (18). In adults, anemia and cardiovascular abnormalities limit exercise capacity. Carnitine supplementation has been shown to improve exercise tolerance; however, the exact mechanism is not understood nor has supplementation been tested in children (18). Catabolism of lean body mass is an invariable consequence of CKD and uremia, especially when there is inadequate intake of energy and protein. Regular physical activity can counteract these adverse effects and increase protein utilization and muscle mass (19). Age-appropriate physical activity should be prescribed and encouraged often. Given that children with renal disease are often growth delayed and may have poor leg muscle mass, treadmill-based exercise and walking are the preferred methods of pediatric exercise testing (20).

Growth Measurement and Evaluation

Although growth failure has long been recognized in CKD, it is only now that these children are surviving to adulthood that severe short stature has emerged as a long-term sequelae of CKD in childhood (21). Various acute and chronic alterations of body composition place these children at a risk not seen in the general pediatric population (22). Growth deterioration has been observed during worsening kidney function (23), and these alterations are associated with an increased risk of mortality (4,24). A more complicated clinical course of dialysis has also been reported after growth failure during CKD (3).

The cause of growth retardation is multifactorial and includes the age of onset of disease, metabolic acidosis, electrolyte disturbances, renal osteodystrophy, repeated infections, abnormalities in the growth hormone/insulin-like growth factor axis, and insufficient caloric intake (3,25). Early and/or increased dialysis, correction of metabolic acidosis and renal bone disease, and early provision of estimated nutrient needs aid normal growth in children with CKD (9).

Measurement of growth parameters should be performed regularly by the same person, using standardized procedures and the same equipment (8). A recumbent length board and a wall-mounted stadiometer are essential for accurate results. Length or height, weight, and head circumference (for patients younger than 36 months of age) are the basic measurements. These are plotted by chronological age and sex on the childhood growth charts developed by the Centers for Disease Control and Prevention (CDC), which are available for downloading on the CDC Web site (26). Age corrected for prematurity (until 24 months) should be used for preterm infants.

With a skinfold caliper, additional assessment of fat stores and muscle mass can be obtained from measurements of triceps skinfold, mid-arm circumference, and mid-arm muscle circumference, and the measurements can then be compared with reference values of healthy children of the same age and sex (27). Reference values for these measurements can be found in references 8 and 27. Serial measurements allow the child to serve as his or her own standard of comparison (8). Evaluation of growth parameters can be accomplished using the child's chronological age or height age. Chronological age is the actual age of the child in months or years, and height age is the age at which the child would be at the 50th percentile for height on the growth chart. When values of chronological and height age are widely discrepant, comparison of growth parameters for height age may provide a more realistic assessment. Bone age is less frequently used and is based on epiphyseal maturation demonstrated by radiography of the hands and wrists.

Dry weight is difficult to determine because weight gain is expected in growing children. Rapid weight gain in the absence of significant energy intake must be thoroughly evaluated before it is assumed to be dry weight gain (8). Assessment of edema, blood pressure, and laboratory values used as markers of hydration, such as serum sodium and albumin, as well as a dietary interview, is useful in the estimation process. For children on maintenance dialysis (MD), tolerance of ultrafiltration should also be considered. For children on hemodialysis (HD), dry weight should be measured postdialysis; for children on peritoneal dialysis (PD), dry weight should be calculated as weight minus the weight of indwelling dialysate.

Additional tools allow close and precise monitoring of growth and body composition in this population. Height velocity is calculated over a period of 1 year (cm/year) and charted on growth velocity charts on which accelerations and decelerations in growth rate are revealed more accurately than on standard growth charts (28). These are available for downloading at the Serono Inc Web site (http://www.seronousa.com). On initial assessment, calculation of midparental height attempts to account for the inherited effect of genetics and predict a final adult height. Its long-term value shows growth potential and is used to estimate the severity of growth impairment and changes in growth potential imposed by treatment (25).

The following equations can be used to calculate midparental height:

For a boy:

$$\text{Midparental Height (cm)} = \frac{\text{Paternal Height (cm)} + \text{Maternal Height (cm)} + 12\text{ cm}}{2}$$

For a girl:

$$\text{Midparental Height (cm)} = \frac{\text{Paternal Height (cm)} - 12\text{ cm} + \text{Maternal Height (cm)}}{2}$$

BMI-for-age values are included on the growth charts developed by the CDC. Intended primarily as an aid in the diagnosis of overweight and underweight children, percentiles are given for ages 2 to 20 years (29). Bioelectrical impedance is a quick, noninvasive way of measuring body fat and can be useful in estimating estimated dry weight in patients with large fluid gains. Measurements are mainly determined by hydration of the arm and leg, rather than tissue composition of the trunk, and thereby are almost completely unaffected by presence of dialysate in the abdomen for PD patients (22).

Supraphysiologic doses of recombinant human growth hormone (rhGH) successfully improve linear growth and replete body compartments, specifically fat-free mass and total bone mineral mass in children with CKD or on MD (8,13,30). In addition to height velocity, body composition changes are regularly observed during the treatment phase and beyond. An increase in the uptake of amino acids and protein synthesis influence the number and size of muscle cells along with internal organ size. Body fat stores are reduced through mobilization of lipids, as evidenced by decreased triceps skinfold measurements. Additional benefits include improved bone mineralization as compared with height-matched controls (31) and increased head circumference in infants with CKD (32). Specific recommendations for the use of the rhGH in children on dialysis are outlined in the K/DOQI guidelines (8) and can be extrapolated to all children with CKD. These guidelines suggest that treatment with growth hormone be considered in children with growth potential (documented by open epiphyses) when the child's height for chronological age is less than 2.0 standard deviation scores (SDS) or their height velocity for chronological age is less than 2.0 SDS, and there is no other contraindication for rhGH use (8). Inadequate responses are seen in children with suboptimal calorie and protein intakes, acidosis, hyperphosphatemia, and secondary hyperparathyroidism (3,8). To take advantage of the benefits that rhGH offers growth-deficient children, it is imperative that children treated with rhGH are closely monitored and counseled regarding adequate nutrition and appropriately managed in respect to biochemical parameters (25).

Medications should be reviewed concurrently with biochemistries because normal serum electrolytes or stable blood pressure may be the result of drug therapy and/or dietary restriction, and may mask an altered biochemical state. Medications should also be considered in terms of potential drug-nutrient interactions, which could adversely affect nutritional status or drug efficacy (33,34).

Various conditions dictate re-evaluation of the nutrition care plan. These include estimated dry weight loss, decrease in BMI, lack of expected growth velocity, ongoing decrease in appetite, worsening gastrointestinal function, excessive interdialytic weight gain, deviations in nutritionally relevant biochemical parameters, continued poor compliance with diet, fluids and/or medications, or change in psychosocial situation (8).

FORMULATION OF THE DIETARY PRESCRIPTION

Differences among specific dietary recommendations for each treatment modality may be due to unique features of the RRT and associated drug therapy. To be efficient and avoid repetition, the remainder of this chapter has been organized so that for each topic common elements are discussed first, followed by any differences that pertain to the various stages of kidney disease and treatment modality.

Every CKD patient and appropriate family member or caretaker should receive intensive nutrition counseling based on an individualized plan of care and targeted at the appropriate education level of the child and family/caretaker (8). The nutrition care plan requires ongoing modification based on changes in the child's nutritional status, age, development, food preferences, renal function, biochemistries, medication regimen, psychosocial situation, and treatment modality.

The dietitian must establish rapport with both the child and the primary caretakers to enhance commitment to the nutrition regimen. The patient's age determines who becomes the focus of the dietitian's attention. With an infant, the parents or primary caretaker are responsible for food intake and should be instructed accordingly. With a child in grade school, the parents, primary caretaker, and the child should be involved in dietary management. The adolescent usually eats independently and needs to receive information directly; however, in most cases the parents provide and prepare the food and should also be informed of changes to the dietary prescription. Parents' desire to maintain control of the medical and nutrition regimen may conflict with the adolescent's growing independence (35). Family members and primary caretakers must be involved to have appropriate foods available and to provide support for food and fluid limitations as well as encouragement for nutrient consumption. Caregivers outside of the immediate family (eg, grandparents, babysitters, teachers) should be asked to be consistent in care to help the child follow his or her diet.

Messages from the nephrology team about the importance of nutrition intensify attention to food intake and may add to parental stress or the risk for feeding problems (eg, food refusal, self-induced vomiting) (36). Infants are typically satisfied with small volumes of oral feeds and many exhibit posttraumatic feeding disorders, gastrointestinal motility disorders, and/or GER (15,16,37). Toddlers and young children often have poor, fussy appetites and a preference for commercial fast foods. Parents frequently express frustration in feeding their infant or child, and they may pressure children to eat or give inappropriate attention to undesired behaviors and reward desired behavior with minimal interaction. Families need guidance and constant support to establish and consistently enforce limits about food and unacceptable conduct at mealtimes (36). Adolescents typically have poor and irregular eating habits, miss meals, drink lots of high-phosphorus fluids (ie, milk, colas), and patronize fast-food restaurants with their friends. Dietary instruction focused on cafeteria foods, fast foods, snacks, and alternative drinks can help an adolescent make relatively safe selections when eating away from home.

Tables 12.2, 12.3, and 12.4 outline nutrient recommendations for children with CKD, on MD, and posttransplant (38–43). These guidelines are based on recommendations for healthy children and should be used as a starting point (8). Recommendations may need modification during periods of catabolic stress, for patients significantly above or below their ideal body weight, or when a child's response to these recommendations is suboptimal. Restrictions are imposed only when clearly needed and should be individualized according to age, development, and food preferences (8). The use of chronological age is recommended for determining requirements and providing age-appropriate dietary recommendations (8). Revisions can be made based on the child's response. When chronological and height age are vastly different and a child has failed to meet goals for weight gain despite achieving requirements based on chronological age, basing requirements for energy and protein on height age may provide the additional "boost" required (22).

To increase energy intake and gain compliance, dietary modifications for children are typically less restrictive than for adults. Pediatric dietary restrictions usually take the form of a "low-nutrient *X* diet" (eg, low-sodium diet) with education provided on which foods are high in that nutrient and guidance about how to substitute for, or limit intake of, those foods. Depending on the response in the parameter relevant to that nutrient (eg, blood pressure; biochemical value), the restriction can be liberalized or tightened. Prescriptions for specific amounts of a restricted nutrient (eg, 3 mEq of nutrient *X* per kg) are rarely used in pediatrics. The specified amounts provided in Tables 12.2 through 12.4 can be used as general references for assessing an individual child's daily intake obtained from food records. If there is a range of values for a restriction, the upper end of the range should be considered initially and decreased if necessary (8,38–40).

Chronic Kidney Disease

The etiology of CKD in children can be congenital, hereditary, acquired, or metabolic; all causes can eventually lead to the need for RRT. For all etiologies, early referral to a pediatric nephrology team and active care helps limit or prevent growth failure, minimize bio-

Table 12.2. Daily Nutrient Recommendations for Children with Chronic Kidney Disease

Note: Restrictions should be implemented only where warranted and kept as liberal as possible to optimize energy intake and prevent malnutrition.

Pediatric dietary restrictions usually take the form of a "low-nutrient *X* diet" with education about avoiding or limiting foods high in that nutrient. Depending on the response in the parameter relevant to that nutrient (eg, blood pressure; biochemical value) the restriction can be liberalized or tightened.

Prescriptions for specific amounts of a nutrient (eg, 3 mEq nutrient *X*/kg) are rarely used in pediatrics. Amounts provided in the table can be used as references for assessment of daily intake obtained from food records.

				Adolescent	
Nutrient	*Infant, birth to 1 y*	*Toddler, 1–2 y*	*Child, 3–8 y*	*9–13 y*	*14–18 y*
Energy (kcal/kg/d)*					
Boys	Birth to 6 mo: 95 7–12 mo: 82	87	87	63	52
Girls	Birth to 6 mo: 87 7–12 mo: 75	82	82	60	44
Protein (g/kg/d)	Birth to 6 mo: 1.52† 7–12 mo: 1.1–1.5‡	0.88–1.10‡	0.76–0.95‡	0.76–0.95‡	Boys: 0.73–0.85‡ Girls: 0.71–0.85‡
Sodium (Recommendations for patients with edema or hypertension)	• No salt shaker and avoid salty foods (≥ 200 mg sodium/serving). • Infants and toddlers: restrict to 1–3 mEq/kg/d.§ • Children and adolescents: restrict to 87–174 mEq/d§ (2–4 g/d).				
Potassium (Recommendations for patients with hyperkalemia)	• Avoid foods with high potassium levels, such as bananas, chocolate, and orange juice. • Infants and toddlers: restrict to 1–3 mEq/kg/d.§ • Children and adolescents: restrict to 51–103 mEq/d§ (2–4 g/d).				
Calcium	• 100% of the DRI. • Monitor total calcium load, including calcium from phosphate binders.				
Phosphorus (mg/d) (Recommendations for patients with hyperphosphatemia)	Restrict to low-phosphorus formula and foods.	≤ 400–600		≤ 600–800	
Vitamins	• If needed, supplement to 100% of the DRI. • Supplement with vitamin D metabolite to prevent hyperparathyroidism and renal osteodystrophy.				
Trace minerals	• If needed, supplement to 100% of the DRI. • Iron supplementation is usually needed with erythropoietin therapy.				
Fluids	• Unrestricted unless warranted for fluid management (indications would be decreased urine output, edema, or hypertension). • If restriction is needed: Total Fluid Intake (TFI) = Insensible losses + Urine output + Other losses.				

*Energy recommendations are the estimated energy requirements (EERs). They are based on active physical activity levels (PAL) as the level recommended to maintain health and decrease risk of chronic disease and disability. EERs are presented in kcal/kg as determined by dividing the active PAL EER (total kcal/day) by the reference weight for each respective age.

†Protein recommendations are the adequate intake (AI) for ages birth to 6 months.

‡Protein recommendations are the range of estimated average requirement (EAR) to recommended dietary allowance (RDA) for ages 7 months to 18 years.

§For sodium and potassium, mEq = mmol.

Source: Data are from selected *Dietary Reference Intakes* publications (38–42).

Table 12.3. Daily Nutrient Recommendations for Children on Dialysis

Note: Restrictions should be implemented only where warranted and kept as liberal as possible to optimize energy intake and prevent malnutrition.

Pediatric dietary restrictions usually take the form of a "low-nutrient *X* diet" with education about avoiding or limiting foods high in that nutrient. Depending on the response in the parameter relevant to that nutrient (eg, blood pressure; biochemical value) the restriction can be liberalized or tightened.

Prescriptions for specific amounts of a nutrient (eg, 3 mEq nutrient *X*/kg) are rarely used in pediatrics. Amounts provided in the table can be used as references for assessment of daily intake obtained from food records.

				Adolescent	
Nutrient	*Infant, birth to 1 y*	*Toddler, 1–3 y*	*Child, 4–10 y*	*11–14 y*	*15–18 y*
Energy (kcal/kg/d)*	Birth to 6 mo: 108 7–12 mo: 98	102	4–6 y: 90 7–10 y: 70	Boys: 55 Girls: 47	Boys: 45 Girls: 40
Protein (g/kg/d)*					
for HD patients	Birth to 6 mo: 2.6 7–12 mo: 2.0	1.6	4–6 y: 1.6 7–10 y: 1.4	Boys: 1.4 Girls: 1.4	Boys: 1.7–1.8[†] Girls: 1.7–1.8[†]
for PD patients	Birth to 6 mo: 2.9–3.0 7–12 mo: 2.3–2.4	1.9–2.0	4–6 y: 1.9–2.0 7–10 y: 1.7–1.8	Boys: 1.3 Girls: 1.2	Boys: 1.4–1.5[†] Girls: 1.4–1.5[†]
Sodium (Recommendations for patients who are oliguric/anuric, edematous, or hypertensive)	• No salt shaker and avoid salty foods (≥ 200 mg Na/serving). • Infants and toddlers: restrict to 1–3 mEq/kg/d.[‡] • Children and adolescents: restrict to 87–174 mEq/day[‡] (2–4 g/d).				
Potassium (Recommendations for patients with hyperkalemia)	• Avoid foods with high potassium levels, such as bananas, chocolate, and orange juice. • Infants and toddlers: restrict to 1–3 mEq/kg/d.[‡] • Children and adolescents: restrict to 51–103 mEq/d[‡] (2–4 g/d).				
Calcium (mg/d)	• 100% of the DRI. • Monitor total calcium load, including calcium from phosphate binders.				
Phosphorus (mg/d) (Recommendations for patients with hyperphosphatemia)	Restrict to low-phosphorus formula and foods.	≤ 400–600		≤ 600–800	
Vitamins*	• If needed, supplement to 100% of the DRI for thiamin, riboflavin, pyridoxine, folic acid, and vitamin B-12, and 100% of the RDA for vitamins A, C, E, and K. • Supplement with vitamin D metabolite to prevent hyperparathyroidism and renal osteodystrophy.				
Trace minerals*	• If needed, supplement to 100% of the RDA for copper and zinc. • Iron supplementation is usually needed with erythropoietin therapy.				
Fluids	• Total fluid intake (TFI) = Insensible losses + Urine output + Ultrafiltration capacity + Other losses – Amount to deficit.				

*Future modification of K/DOQI guidelines will need to consider new recommendations for macronutrients, vitamins, minerals, and trace elements.

[†]Based on growth potential.

[‡]For sodium and potassium: mEq = mmol.

Source: Data are from K/DOQI guidelines (8) and selected *Dietary Reference Intakes* publications (38,40,41,43).

Table 12.4. Daily Nutrient Recommendations for Children With Kidney Transplants

Note: Restrictions should be implemented only where warranted and kept as liberal as possible to optimize energy intake and prevent malnutrition.

Pediatric dietary restrictions usually take the form of a "low-nutrient X diet" with education about avoiding or limiting foods high in that nutrient. Depending on the response in the parameter relevant to that nutrient (eg, blood pressure; biochemical value) the restriction can be liberalized or tightened.

Prescriptions for specific amounts of a nutrient (eg, 3 mEq nutrient X/kg) are rarely used in pediatrics. Amounts provided in the table can be used as references for assessment of daily intake obtained from food records.

				Adolescent	
Nutrient	*Infant, birth to 1 y*	*Toddler, 1–2 y*	*Child, 3–8 y*	*9–13 y*	*14–18 y*
Energy (kcal/kg/d)*					
Boys:	Birth to 6 mo: 95 7–12 mo: 82	87	87	63	52
Girls:	Birth to 6 mo: 87 7–12 mo: 75	82	82	60	44
Protein (g/kg/d)	• First 3 mo after transplant: 1.2–1.5 times the DRI. • After 3 mo posttransplant: DRI.				
Sodium (Recommendations for patients with edema or hypertension)	• No salt shaker and avoid salty foods (≥ 200 mg/serving). • Infants and toddlers: Restrict to 1–3 mEq/kg/d.† • Children and adolescents: Restrict to 87–174 mEq/d† (2–4 g/d).				
Potassium (Recommendations for patients with hyperkalemia)	• Restriction generally unnecessary. • Temporarily avoid foods with high potassium levels, such as bananas, chocolate, and orange juice, until serum levels are within normal range.				
Calcium (mg/d)	• 100% of the DRI.				
Phosphorus (mg/d)	• 100% of the DRI. • Supplementation is usually indicated initially for hypophosphatemia.				
Vitamins	• 100% of the DRI. • Supplementation is generally unnecessary, with the possible exception of vitamin D.				
Trace minerals	• 100% of the DRI. • Magnesium supplementation is usually indicated initially for hypomagnesemia.				
Fluids	• High fluid intake is encouraged.				

*Energy recommendations are the estimated energy requirements (EERs). They are based on active physical activity levels (PAL) as the level recommended to maintain health and decrease risk of chronic disease and disability. EERs are presented in kcal/kg as determined by dividing the active PAL EER (total kcal/day) by the reference weight for each respective age.

†For sodium, mEq = mmol.

Source: Data are from selected *Dietary Reference Intake* publications (38–42).

chemical and physiological consequences of uremia, enhance quality of life, and improve survival. Dietary restrictions are imposed only when indicated by progression of renal insufficiency and abnormalities in blood pressure and biochemical parameters.

Nephrotic Syndrome

Acquired nephrotic syndrome is a cause of CKD in children and is characterized by the presence of heavy proteinuria, hypoproteinemia, hyperlipidemia, and edema. Nutrition management includes sodium and fluid restrictions during active periods of proteinuria. Protein supplementation to account for urinary losses is not recommended because it has been shown to increase protein losses. Of the primary nephrotic syndromes in children, focal segmental glomerulosclerosis (FSGS), is the most common acquired cause of Stage 5 kidney disease in children. It is characterized by sclerosis of the glomeruli and nonresponsiveness to prednisone therapy. Only 20% to 30% of children with FSGS respond to steroid therapy, and one of every three children with FSGS progress to dialysis and/or transplant (2). Please refer to Chapter 1 for a description of the stages of CKD.

Dialysis

In contrast to the adult population requiring dialysis, the majority (65%) of pediatric patients are treated with peritoneal dialysis rather than hemodialysis (1). Several forms of PD are available, including continuous ambulatory peritoneal dialysis (CAPD), nocturnal or continuous cyclic PD (CCPD), tidal PD, and intermittent PD (IPD). Information on these different methods of PD can be found in Chapter 6.

Hemodialysis on children and adolescents is typically performed 3 times per week for 3 to 4 hours. Infants are usually "brittle" or unstable on HD, so PD is preferred. Food intake during HD may contribute to hypotension, cramps, or other gastrointestinal symptoms during dialysis (44). Children who consistently experience these symptoms during dialysis may experience fewer complications if food and fluids are not consumed before or during dialysis. Experience in using home nocturnal HD in children is limited; however, preliminary data suggest that dietary and fluid restrictions are not required and high-protein and high-phosphorus diets may be needed. Children who switch dialysis modality, or who have dialysis temporarily withheld for access problems, need teaching for required changes to their diet prescription.

Transplant

Renal transplantation is the preferred treatment of Stage 5 CKD in children. A well-functioning graft eases dietary and fluid restrictions required during the dialysis period. Ideally, a preemptive transplant is the treatment of choice and benefits patients by maintaining their quality of life and improving growth potential. Compared with dialyzed patients at the time of transplant, preemptive transplant patients had significantly less growth retardation (45).

High doses of posttransplant immunosuppressive medications lead to hypercaloric intake as well as alterations in nutritionally related biochemical parameters. As doses are weaned, the effects decrease and dietary restrictions and mineral supplementations can be liberalized or discontinued. Immunosuppressive drugs may also cause nausea, vomiting, constipation, diarrhea, or anorexia and these should be treated symptomatically.

A strong emphasis on growth and development continues after transplant. Normal adult height is the goal and is dependent on age and degree of height deficit at the time of transplant, corticosteroid dosages, and graft function (46,47). Catch-up growth is seen primarily in the youngest ages. Growth hormone has successfully accelerated growth in the transplant population, but its use remains controversial because deterioration of graft function after transplant has been observed (46). Nutrition management of patients with suboptimally functioning grafts should be based on relevant biochemical parameters and treatment modality initiated.

DIETARY MANAGEMENT

One of the most challenging aspects of living with kidney disease is modification of food and fluid intake. Necessary changes to the macro- and micronutrient content of a child's diet intrude on food preferences and have the potential to severely limit food choices when multiple restrictions are required or appetite is poor. Specific nutrients may be limited or encouraged, with changes occurring throughout the course of the disease. Nutrition specialists can ease the burden of successfully adopting diet alterations by providing practical suggestions for modifying or replacing favorite foods or fluids. To address individual problems, specialists must be familiar with infant and toddler feeding skills; infant formulas, enteral supplements and tube-feeding products; eating habits of children and adolescents; behavior modification techniques; and the nutrient content of popular homemade and commercial foods, snacks, and drinks, including those of different cultures.

Energy

Adequate intake of energy is important not only for weight gain and growth but also to prevent protein from being used as an energy source through gluconeogenesis. Energy recommendations for children with CKD have traditionally been based on requirements for healthy children because there is a lack of evidence to suggest that the requirements of children with CKD are greater than those of healthy children or that the growth of children with CKD improves if their intake exceeds these amounts. Therefore, the initial prescribed energy intake for infants, children, and adolescents with CKD or posttransplant should be the Dietary Reference Intakes (DRI) (39) for chronological age. Modifications can be made based on the child's response. Energy-malnourished children may require additional energy to "catch up" in growth and/or weight gain. The K/DOQI nutrition guidelines for MD were published prior to the release of the DRI report on macronutrients, and therefore recommend the earlier Recommended Dietary Allowances (RDA) (8); further updates to the guidelines will need to consider the newer DRI.

Infants who are anorexic or have GER frequently require supplementation with oral or tube feedings of fortified expressed breast milk or high-calorie formula. Depending on volumes, high-calorie breastmilk or formulas up to 2 kcal/mL (60 kcal/oz) may be needed to meet requirements (10,48). Gradual, stepwise increases in energy density of 2 to 4 kcal/oz theoretically improve tolerance. As energy density increases, oral intake may decrease and supplemental tube feeding may be needed. Infant formulas such as Good Start (Nestle Nutrition, Deerfield, IL 60015) or Similac PM 60/40 (Ross Products, Abbott Laboratories, Columbus, OH, 43215) contain less phosphorus and potassium and may be required by some infants to maintain normal serum levels. See Table 12.5 for the nutrient content of various infant feedings.

Good Start costs less than PM 60/40, is readily available where infant formulas are sold, and is 100% whey based, which increases the rate of gastric emptying. Often, it is not possible to increase the energy density of formula by concentration because of the increase in sodium, potassium, and phosphorus. The choice to add carbohydrate modules (Caloreen, Nestle Nutrition, Deerfield, IL 60015; Moducal, Mead Johnson Nutritionals, Evansville, IN 47721; Polycose, Ross Products, Abbott Laboratories, Columbus, OH 43215; Scandical, Axcan Scandipharm Inc, Birmingham, AL 35242), fat, or a combination of both (individual modules; Duocal, SHS International, Rockville, MD 20850) should be based on serum glucose and lipid profiles, the presence or absence of malabsorption or respiratory distress (carbohydrate metabolism increases carbon dioxide production), as well as cost to the family or caretaker. In addition, when making a formula with more than two to three increases in energy density, an attempt should be made to preserve a simi-

Table 12.5. Nutrient Content of Infant Feedings*

Product (Manufacturer)	*Energy (kcal/L)*	*Protein (g/L)*	*Fat (g/L)*	*Carbohydrate (g/L)*	*Osmolality (mOsm/kg H_2O)*	*Sodium (mg/L)*	*Potassium (mg/L)*	*Phosphorus (mg/L)*
Human milk (mean ± standard deviation)	720 ± 5	10.5 ± 2	39 ± 4	72 ± 2.5	290 ± 5	179 ± 39	524 ± 35	140 ± 22
Good Start Essentials Soy† (Nestle Clinical Nutrition)	678	19	34	74	200	235	778	423
Enfamil‡ (Mead Johnson)	676	14.2	35.8	73.7	300	183	729	358
Good Start Supreme‡ (Nestle Clinical Nutrition)	676	16.2	34.5	74	280	162	663	243
Isomil† (Ross Products)	676	16.6	36.9	68.3	230	300	730	510
Prosobee† (Mead Johnson)	676	20	36	68	200	243	825	502
Similac PM 60/40‡ (Ross Products)	676	15.8	37.6	69	280	160	580	190
Similac‡ (Ross Products)	676	14.5	36.5	72.3	300	190	730	390

*For the most current nutrient content, see product labels.

†Soy-based formula

‡Cow's milk-based formula

Source: Data are from manufacturers: Mead Johnson (Evansville, IN 47721), Nestle Clinical Nutrition (Deerfield, IL 60015), Ross Products (Abbott Laboratories, Columbus, OH 43215).

lar distribution of energy from carbohydrate and fat as in the base formula. Unless malabsorption is present, a "heart-healthy" oil such as corn, canola or safflower oil may be used. To prevent the oil from separating out during continuous tube feedings, an oil containing emulsified fat (Microlipid, Mead Johnson Nutritionals, Evansville, IN 47721) may be useful. See Table 12.6 for the nutrient content of various modular products.

Minimizing the number of restrictions in the diet and identifying favorite foods are the first steps to achieving energy goals for older children. Foods commonly found in the home will most likely have better acceptance than caloric supplements. Individuals with poor appetites may respond to small, frequent meals and snacks. Energy can be added to foods using heart-healthy margarines or oils, cream and other fats, melted cheese, sugars, syrups, or carbohydrate modules. Milkshakes and desserts made from whole-fat milk, cream, or nondairy products (Coffee Rich, Rich Products, Buffalo, NY 14214; Coffee Mate, Nestle USA, Glendale, CA 91203; Rice Dream, Imagine Foods, Garden City, NY 11530; Cool Whip, Kraft Foods Inc, Northfield, IL 60093) can be used. Low-calorie or calorie-free drinks should be avoided.

Supplemental nutrition support should be considered when a patient is not growing normally or fails to meet requirements for protein or energy. If intake is adequate and there is no sign of malnutrition, supplementation may cause obesity without improving linear growth. Oral supplementation is preferred, followed by tube feeding (8). Commercial supplements (eg, fruit-flavored beverages, milkshake-type drinks, puddings, bars) may be used; however, their phosphorus and potassium content may be too high. Nonrenal pediatric feedings designed for children older than 1 year (Kindercal, Mead Johnson Nutritionals, Evansville, IN 47721; Pediasure, Ross Products, Abbott Laboratories, Columbus, OH 43215; Resource for Kids, Novartis Nutrition, Minneapolis, MN 55440; Nutren Junior, Nestle Nutrition, Deerfield, IL 60015) have fairly high calcium and phosphorus content, which may prove problematic. See Table 12.7 for the nutrient content of these nonrenal pediatric feedings. Adult renal products designed to be energy dense, high or low in protein, and

Table 12.6. Nutrient Content of Modular Products*

Modular Product (Manufacturer)	*Energy (kcal)*	*Protein (g)*	*Fat (g)*	*Carbohydrate (g)*	*Sodium (mg)*	*Potassium (mg)*	*Phosphorus (mg)*
Carbohydrate (per 100g)							
Caloreen (Nestle Nutrition)	390	0	0	96	< 41	< 11.7	trace
Moducal (Mead Johnson)	375	0	0	95	70	5	trace
Polycose (Ross Products)	380	0	0	95	110	10	12
Scandical (Axcan Scandipharm)	538	0	38	62	350	307	185
Fat (per 100 mL)							
Corn oil	813	0	92	0	0	0	0
Microlipid (Mead Johnson)	449	0	51	0	0	0	0
Carbohydrate and fat (per 100 g)							
Duocal (SHS International)	492	0	73	22	≤ 20	≤ 5	≤ 5
Protein (per 100 g)							
Casec (Mead Johnson)	380	90	2	0	100	10	800
Resource Instant Protein Powder (Novartis Nutrition)	357	86	0	0	214	500	286

*For the most current nutrient content, please see product labels.

Source: Data are from manufacturers: Axcan Scandipharm (Birmingham, AL 35242), Mead Johnson (Evansville, IN 47721), Nestle Clinical Nutrition (Deerfield, IL 60015), Novartis Nutrition (Minneapolis, MN 55440), Ross Products (Abbott Laboratories, Columbus, OH 43215), SHS International (Rockville, MD 20850).

Table 12.7. Nutrient Content of Pediatric Formulas*

Formula (Manufacturer)	*Energy (kcal/L)*	*Protein (g/L)*	*Fat (g/L)*	*Carbohydrate (g/L)*	*Osmolality (mOsm/kg H_2O)*	*Sodium (mg/L)*	*Potassium (mg/L)*	*Phosphorus (mg/L)*	*Volume to meet RDA (mL)*
Compleat Pediatric (Novartis Nutrition)	1000	38	39	130	380	680	1500	1000	900†
Kindercal (Mead Johnson)	1060	30	44	135	310	370	1310	850	950†
Kindercal With Fiber (6.3 g dietary fiber/L) (Mead Johnson)	1060	30	44	135	345	370	1310	850	950†
Nutren Junior (Nestle Clinical Nutrition)	1000	30	42	128	350	460	1320	800	1000†
Nutren Junior With Fiber (Nestle Clinical Nutrition)	1000	30	42	128	350	460	1320	800	1000†
Pediasure (Ross Products)	1000	30	50	110	345	380	1310	800	1000‡ 1300§
Pediasure With Fiber (Ross Products)	1000	30	50	114	345	380	1310	800	1000‡ 1300§
Peptamen Junior (Nestle Clinical Nutrition)	1000	30	39	138	260–360	460	1320	800	1000†
Resource Just for Kids (Novartis Nutrition)	1000	30	50	110	390	380	1300	800	1000†
Resource Just for Kids with Fiber (Novartis Nutrition)	1000	30	50	110	390	590	1140	800	1000†
Vivonex Pediatric (Novartis Nutrition)	800	24	24	130	360	400	1200	800	1000‡ 1170§

*For the most current nutrient content, please see product labels.

†For children ages 1–10 y

‡For children ages 1–6 y

§For children ages 7–10 y

Source: Data are from manufacturers: Axcan Scandipharm (Birmingham, AL 35242), Mead Johnson (Evansville, IN 47721), Nestle Clinical Nutrition (Deerfield, IL 60015), Novartis Nutrition (Minneapolis, MN 55440), Ross Products (Abbott Laboratories, Columbus, OH 43215), SHS International (Rockville, MD 20850).

low in electrolytes and phosphorus (Nepro and Suplena, Ross Products, Abbott Laboratories, Columbus, OH 43215; NovaSource Renal, Novartis Nutrition, Minneapolis, MN 55440; Magnacal Renal, Mead Johnson Nutritionals 47721; Renalcal, Nestle Nutrition, Deerfield, IL 60015) are recommended for children older than 4 years but have been used successfully at diluted strength in children as young as 1 year. (See Table 13.1 in Chapter 13 for the nutrient content of these adult renal products.) Serum magnesium levels should be monitored carefully in toddlers who use these products because the magnesium content is significantly higher than in breastmilk or infant formulas. If necessary, these products can be mixed to provide the appropriate protein content for an individual child. The cost of products and lack of third-party reimbursement may deter use of supplements; involvement of a social worker is invaluable.

Enteral tube feeding should be considered when a child is unable to meet nutritional goals orally (8). Nasogastric, gastrostomy (G), and gastrojejeunostomy (GJ) tubes have all been used successfully to provide additional nutrition by intermittent bolus or continuous infusion (49,50). Reported complications associated with nasogastric and gastrostomy feeding include emesis, exit-site infection, leakage, and, for patients on PD, peritonitis. Choice of formula and feeding route is guided by age, biochemical values, fluid allowance, and consideration of financial costs to the family or caretaker. In most cases, minimizing the volume of feeds is necessary to maintain fluid balance, optimize feeding tolerance, and keep the duration of feeding times manageable within the child's daily schedule. To encourage daytime oral intake, continuous overnight feeds are generally preferred. Infants and toddlers who have been tube fed experience a difficult transition to oral feeding (51). Careful attention to oral stimulation and involvement of a multidisciplinary feeding program (8,52) enable most tube-fed children to meet their nutritional requirements orally without tube feeding posttransplant (51,53).

Chronic Kidney Disease

Progressive decline in renal function often causes anorexia and failure to achieve prescribed energy goals. Timely initiation of RRT may prevent malnutrition. This has been observed in adults; the initiation of dialysis increased dietary protein intake (DPI), lean body mass, and subjective global assessment rating in patients started on PD, and increased DPI and serum albumin in HD patients (54). Given the significance of these positive outcomes, timely initiation of dialysis may also provide the same benefits to the pediatric population as observed in adults.

Energy

Dialysis

The initial energy prescription for children on MD should be the RDA (43) for chronological age (8).

Peritoneal Dialysis

Children undergoing PD may experience early satiety or anorexia due to feelings of fullness from the indwelling dialysate exerting pressure on the stomach, or the negative effect of absorption of the dialysate glucose on the brain's appetite control center. Supplemental tube feeding may be required for those who are unable to meet their nutritional requirements orally; wherever possible, placement of G- or GJ-tubes should occur before starting PD to decrease the risk of peritonitis. Intraperitoneal dialysate glucose absorption in children on CAPD increases energy obtained by approximately 7 to 10 kcal/kg (55). Energy absorbed from the dialysate glucose should be included in the total energy intake (8). Please see Chapter 6 for equations to assist in estimating dialysate glucose absorption. Obesity is occasionally seen in adolescents, especially those on PD needing dialysate with high glucose concentrations for ultrafiltration. The use of dialysate containing icodextrin, a glucose polymer, in place of dextrose may improve fluid removal and prevent weight gain in these patients (56,57).

Hemodialysis

Children on HD are usually more uremic than those on peritoneal dialysis. Their appetite may vary between dialysis and nondialysis days because they often feel tired postdialysis or are more anorexic before their next dialysis session. Intradialytic parenteral nutrition (IDPN) is a noninvasive method of providing carbohydrate, protein, and lipids to undernourished patients via venous access during HD. Preliminary evidence of its safety and effectiveness in improving oral intake and weight gain, but not serum albumin, has been seen in a small numbers of malnourished children (58,59). IDPN is costly and its use should be limited to patients with severe malnutrition who cannot receive adequate nutrition enterally. Unlike supplemental tube feeding, which can occur daily, the supplemental benefits of IDPN are limited by the patient's weekly frequency of HD sessions. (Specific information on the content and administration of IDPN can be found in Chapter 14.)

Transplant

The combination of successful renal transplant and high-dose corticosteroids increase appetite and make weight control a challenge. The goal is to achieve and maintain BMI-for-age within recommended ranges. Large corticosteroid doses in the first 6 months after transplant increase insulin secretion, causing glucose uptake by fat cells, impaired glucose tolerance, glycosuria, and a relative resistance to insulin. The immunosuppressive agent tacrolimus causes diabetes in 10% to 20% of patients. Therefore, simple carbohydrates are eliminated from the diet in the immediate posttransplant period, and afterward as needed. Controlling total energy intake, participating in regular physical activity, and using behavior modification techniques aid in weight management.

Protein

Protein intake often exceeds recommended levels; however, protein malnutrition may occur in spite of adequate protein intake when energy intake is low. Protein intake may be insufficient because of anorexia, low meat intake, chewing problems, or a low-phosphorus diet (which limits protein-rich dairy foods). Requirements are increased by proteinuria, catabolism, peritonitis, and glucocorticosteroids. Protein breakdown and amino acid oxidation are also increased to buffer excess hydrogen ions during metabolic acidosis. If clinical evaluation suggests protein malnutrition (eg, dietary evaluation, hypoalbuminemia, low serum urea), protein intake should be increased.

Protein recommendations may be exceeded as long as serum urea and phosphate are acceptable (8). Approximately 60% to 70% of protein should be of high biological value because it minimizes urea production by reusing circulating nonessential amino acids for protein maintenance. Minced or chopped meat, chicken, fish, egg, tofu, or fat-free milk powder can be added to soups, pasta, or casseroles. Milk, milk products, or eggs can be substituted if meat is disliked; however, phosphorus intake will increase. Powdered protein modules (Casec, Mead Johnson Nutritionals, Evansville, IN 47721; Promod, Ross Products, Abbott Laboratories, Columbus, OH 43215; Resource Instant Protein Powder, Novartis Nutrition, Minneapolis, MN 55440) can be added to formula, strained foods, cereals, beverages, and moist foods. Protein-containing liquid or pudding supplements are other alternatives. Vegetarians, especially vegans, typically need specific dietary counseling to meet higher protein needs (60). (See Appendix C for more information on vegetarian diets.)

Chronic Kidney Disease

Children with progressive renal disease should be prescribed protein intakes according to the DRI (39). Restrictions in dietary protein have been noted to postpone the development of uremic symptoms and the start of dialysis in animals with advanced renal failure. Based on the premise that a higher protein intake induces hyperfiltration and glomerular hypertrophy, prospective clinical studies in both adults (61–63) and children (64) were conducted to determine whether a low-protein diet delays the progression of chronic renal failure. These studies failed to show a statistically significant benefit of reduced DPI on the decrease in renal function within a period of 2 to 3 years. Low-protein diets may also interfere with achievement of nutrition goals for children (17). Although adverse effects on growth were not observed in children (64), a small but progressive loss of lean body mass was seen in adults (54,65). Goals in CKD should focus on avoiding excessive protein intake for the purposes of preventing exacerbation of uremia and limiting dietary intake of phosphorus, which is commonly found in protein-rich foods. Earlier initiation of RRT with less restrictive diets is a strategy to consider in enhancing the quality of life of pediatric patients with CKD (54,64).

Dialysis

In addition to traditional methods of dietary evaluation, dietary protein intake can also be indirectly estimated from urea kinetics, provided the child is in nitrogen balance (8). In stable patients, the protein nitrogen appearance equals the dietary protein intake. In undernourished children with poor appetite, urea kinetic modeling can suggest if inadequate dialysis may be a factor. Patients with a low urea may seem to be well-dialyzed but may actually have a low Kt/V, indicative of underdialysis, and a poor protein intake. Currently, there is insufficient evidence to recommend routine use of urea kinetics in the nutrition assessment and management of children treated with MD (8).

Peritoneal Dialysis

The initial dietary protein intake for children on PD should be based on the RDA (43) for their chronological age plus an additional increment based on anticipated peritoneal losses (8). Losses are similar for CAPD, CCPD, and tidal dialysis but vary widely among individuals (66). Requirements are higher on a g/kg basis for infants and toddlers because protein losses are inversely related to body weight and peritoneal surface area. The K/DOQI nutrition guidelines for MD were published prior to the release of the DRI report on macronutrients, and therefore base protein recommendations on the RDA (8); future revisions to the K/DOQI nutrition guidelines will need to consider the newer DRI (39).

Children on PD have low concentrations of plasma proteins and albumin. Whether these are an indicators of nutritional status must be evaluated individually because many factors can affect serum albumin levels (67). Children should be advised to stop any previous efforts to avoid excessive protein intake. Children unable to maintain adequate oral or enteral protein intake may benefit from the use of amino acids as the osmotic agent in the dialysate to compensate for protein and amino acid losses and improve nitrogen balance (68,69). In most cases, one exchange per day is replaced with the amino acid solution. To avoid using the amino acids for energy, the solution has usually been given during the day when meals or snacks provide a source of energy. Giving the amino acids overnight via a cycler, coupled with the usual glucose solutions as an energy source, has been tried with good effect (68). Potassium supplementation is often needed when intraperitoneal amino acid (IPAA) therapy is used. Routine use of IPAA is impractical due to high costs.

Hemodialysis

Children on HD should have their initial dietary protein intake based on the RDA (43) for chronological age and an additional increment of 0.4 g/kg/day for dialysis protein losses (8). Future revisions to the K/DOQI nutrition guidelines will need to consider the newer DRI (39). Predialysis urea levels more than 35 mmol/L (> 100 mg/dL) can occur for a variety of reasons, including excessive protein intake, adequate protein but insufficient energy intake, catabolism (eg, infection), inadequate dialysis, and recirculation of blood secondary to the condition of the vascular access. Persistently low urea levels (ie, < 18 mmol/L or < 50 mg/dL) may indicate overall inadequate protein and energy intake. Serum levels of proteins may not be decreased unless dietary intake has been inadequate for an extensive period.

Transplant

Large steroid doses along with stress of surgery markedly increase protein catabolism. Additional alterations of protein metabolism include decreased anabolism through diminished uptake of amino acids in muscle tissue and increased liver uptake of amino acids. To counteract these effects in the immediate posttransplantation period, protein is recommended at 1 to 1.5 times the DRI. Successful renal transplant promotes an increase in food intake, and achieving adequate protein intake is rarely a concern. After approximately 3 months, reducing protein intake to the DRI is appropriate.

Fat

Fats are a crucial source of energy for growing children; however, high-calorie diets or tube feedings may influence lipid profiles. Hypercholesterolemia and hypertriglyceridemia are present in most children on dialysis or posttransplant (70,71). The main abnormality of lipoprotein metabolism is thought to be decreased lipoprotein catabolism (70). Tube feeding can provide an appropriate energy intake with a balanced fat and carbohydrate profile did not adversely affect serum lipids (72).

Dialysis

In children on MD, glucose uptake from dialysis or increased protein losses through dialysate may affect lipid profiles. Dietary manipulation to adhere to lipid-lowering recommendations has proven difficult in adults and resulted in decreased energy intakes with minimal change in lipid profiles (73). For children, diet therapy has been directed at modifying the diet to include healthful foods without limiting energy intake below requirements, increasing intake of complex carbohydrates vs simple sugars, using unsaturated fats, and avoiding saturated fats and *trans* fatty acids (70). Lipid-lowering drugs have been reserved for children with atherogenic lipoprotein profiles (70); however, given the more recent concerns about future cardiovascular disease, more aggressive treatment may be warranted, especially for children on long-term MD (21).

Carnitine deficiency may contribute to hypertriglyceridemia because carnitine is produced by the kidney and is essential for transporting long-chain fatty acids across the mitochondria to be oxidized to provide energy for muscle and other cells. Supplementation in children with normal serum carnitine levels significantly increased carnitine levels but did not affect levels of triglycerides (74,75).

Transplant

Disorders of lipid metabolism have also been described after transplantation, usually as an adverse effect of immunosuppressant medications (76). Dietary modification remains the first line of therapy for hyperlipidemia in transplant patients, although some patients may need pharmacotherapy to reach target levels (76). Lowering total caloric intake and the percentage of calories from fat also benefit weight management.

Vitamins and Minerals

CKD alters the status of many vitamins and minerals (34). When the volume or variety of dietary intake is limited by anorexia or dietary restrictions, the risk for deficiencies is increased. Vitamin D supplementation should be provided for exclusively breastfed infants, especially those at highest risk for development of vitamin D-deficiency rickets (ie, infants who are born to vitamin D-deficient mothers, have limited exposure to sunlight, or are dark skinned). Vitamin D metabolites are initiated based on serum parathyroid hormone (PTH) and calcium and phosphorus levels. (See Chapter 16 for additional information.) Fluoride supplementation should be considered for children living in regions with low fluoride levels in the water source when fluoride intake from other sources is also low. Children on recombinant erythropoietin (rHuEPO) therapy to treat renal anemia usually require large amounts of supplemental iron. Iron supplements are prescribed based on levels of serum ferritin and transferrin saturation. (See Chapter 17 for guidelines on rHuEPO and supplemental iron therapy.)

Chronic Kidney Disease

When estimated intake is considerably less than the DRI (38,40–42), vitamin and iron supplementation may be indicated, taking care to avoid excess amounts of vitamins A and C.

Dialysis

Children on dialysis have additional risk of vitamin and mineral deficiencies associated with increased losses through dialysis and increased needs (34). The K/DOQI guidelines (8) recommend that dietary intake should achieve 100% of the DRI for thiamin, riboflavin, pyridoxine, vitamin B-12, and folic acid (41), and 100% of the RDA for vitamins A, C, E, and K, copper, and zinc (43). Future revisions to the K/DOQI nutrition guidelines will need to consider the newer DRIs (38,40). Supplementation of water-soluble vitamins, zinc, and copper should be considered when intake alone is less than recommended levels or when monitoring reveals laboratory or clinical evidence of deficiency (8). Blood levels of fat-soluble vitamins A and E are usually normal or elevated even without supplementation; therefore, supplementation is generally avoided (34). In the absence of a pediatric supplement, a renal B and C vitamin preparation specifically formulated for adult dialysis patients is used. (See Chapter 15 for a comparison of renal multivitamin products.) These preparations are designed to contain 100 mg or less of vitamin C to avoid complications of retention of oxalate, a vitamin C metabolite for which the kidney is the only route of excretion. A crushed tablet can be used for infants and children who have difficulty swallowing intact tablets or are tube fed; alternatively, a regular liquid vitamin B and C product can be used, where available. A vitamin D metabolite or analog is required to promote calcium homeostasis and treat or prevent renal osteodystrophy (77,78). The type of vitamin D selected and the dosage used depends on the individual's needs; adjustments are made based on serum calcium, phosphorus, and PTH levels. Vitamin K deficiency is possible, especially for those who have poor dietary intakes and receive frequent antibiotics. Vitamin K status plays a role in bone health and therefore is of interest. Children of all ages usually require large amounts of supplemental oral or intravenous iron if they are receiving rHuEPO therapy.

Hyperhomocsyteinemia, a risk factor for vascular disease, is a feature of CKD and is associated with low folate status compared with normal children (79,80). Vascular disease associated with CKD is aggressive and starts early; therefore, efforts to prevent it are important. Supplementation with folic acid increases serum folate and red cell folate levels and reduces homocysteine levels. Long-term study is needed to determine whether this reduces risk of cardiovascular disease (81,82).

Transplant

Multivitamin supplementation is generally not necessary after a successful renal transplant because dietary restrictions are lifted and appetite significantly improves. Vitamin D supplementation may be needed until levels of serum calcium, phosphorus, and PTH normalize. Hypomagnesemia occurs early in patients treated with cyclosporine or tacrolimus and supplements are usually required initially. The prevalence of hypomagnesemia decreases with time, with only approximately 25% of long-term cyclosporine-treated recipients remaining on magnesium supplements (83). Low magnesium levels have been linked to hyperlipidemia in adult transplant recipients and in a small, uncontrolled trial, magnesium replacement reduced elevated total and low-density lipoprotein cholesterol levels (83). This has not been studied in children.

Calcium and Phosphorus

Normal levels of serum calcium and inorganic phosphate must be maintained to prevent hyperparathyroidism, renal osteodystrophy, and poor growth (77,78). Treatment of secondary hyperparathyroidism and hyperphosphatemia is initiated early in CKD, based on serum calcium, phosphorus, and PTH levels. Normal values for serum phosphorus are higher for infants and young children, reflecting needs for bone mineralization. Therapy includes active forms of vitamin D, a low-phosphorus diet, and phosphate binders (typically calcium-containing) taken with feeds or meals. Nonbreastfed infants who are hyperphosphatemic require a low-phosphorus formula (Similac PM 60/40; Good Start), which may be continued after 1 year of age to delay introducing phosphorus-rich cow's milk. Milk and milk products are limited to 240 mL/day, in combination with daily limits of eggs, cheese, and peanut butter and avoidance of other high-phosphorus foods. Nondairy, edible oil creamers and frozen nondairy desserts can be used in place of milk and ice cream. Labels rarely state phosphorus content.

Dietary phosphorus control complicates efforts to achieve adequate protein intake because protein and phosphorus are often found in the same foods. The lowest quantity of phosphorus intake in proportion to the quantity and quality of protein comes from animal-flesh proteins (average: 11 mg phosphorus/g protein). Eggs, dairy products, legumes, and lentils have higher phosphorus to protein ratios (average: 20 mg phosphorus/g protein). As a result, phosphorus control is more difficult in vegetarians. Vegetarians may need higher dosages of phosphorus binders to control serum phosphorus levels and meet dietary protein recommendations. (See Appendix C for more information on vegetarian diets.)

Intestinal phosphorus absorption can be minimized with phosphate binders (calcium carbonate or calcium acetate, but not calcium citrate because it increases aluminum absorption from the gut) given with meals or snacks. Phosphate binder dosages should be matched to the phosphate content of each feeding and taken with the formula, meal, or snack to maximize binding. Children and caregivers can be taught to adjust the timing of binders to coincide with meals or snacks containing the most phosphorus. Recent awareness of the harmful consequences of hypercalcemia and a high serum calcium × phosphorus product have led clinicians to carefully evaluate calcium supplementation and calcium loads. To avoid soft tissue calcification in hypercalcemic children, a nonabsorbable, calcium- and aluminum-free phosphorus binder, such as sevalamar hydrochloride (Renagel; Genzyme Corp, Cambridge, MA 02142), can be used.

Because calcium and phosphorus commonly occur together in foods, the calcium content of the diet may be low. To supplement calcium, a calcium product is prescribed between meals to maximize calcium absorption. Iron supplements should not be taken at the same time as calcium-containing products because they compete with calcium for absorption and limit the binding of phosphorus.

Dialysis

All forms of dialysis are poor in clearing phosphate, so hyperphosphatemia continues to be treated with a low-phosphorus diet and phosphate binders taken with meals.

Transplant

Calcium requirements are increased posttransplant in association with corticosteroid therapy, which reduces intestinal calcium absorption and increases calcium resorption. Calcium is prescribed to meet 100% or more of the DRI, and serum levels are routinely monitored. Supplementation may be necessary for those unable to meet their needs through diet. Hypophosphatemia is common in the early transplantation period because of impaired renal phosphate reabsorption; its prevalence decreases after several months, but mild hypophosphatemia may persist indefinitely for more than 50% of recipients (83). Liberal dietary intake of dairy products is encouraged and early supplementation is often needed.

Sodium

Sodium is directly linked to fluid balance. The need for sodium restriction varies with the primary kidney disease and residual renal function. Infants and children with salt-wasting syndromes such as obstructive uropathy, renal dysplasia, tubular disease, or polycystic kidney disease may need sodium supplements to avoid sodium depletion, decrease in extracellular volume, and impaired growth (84). Children with glomerular disease or those who have oliguria or anuria typically need sodium and fluid restrictions to control fluid balance and hypertension. Serum sodium reflects water balance and not total body sodium; hence, it is not an indicator of the need to limit sodium intake. Salty snacks, processed luncheon meats and cheeses, packaged entrees, and foods from fast-food restaurants are typically hardest for children to avoid. Medications such as sodium polystyrene sulfonate (Kayexalate, Sanofi-Synthelabo Inc, New York, NY 10016), NaCl, and Na_2HCO_3 add to sodium intake. Children and their caregivers should be taught to read ingredient lists and nutrient content charts on food labels to identify salty foods (85). Foods containing 200 mg of sodium or more per serving are considered salty. Salt substitutes contain potassium in place of sodium and should be avoided if a potassium restriction is needed.

Chronic Kidney Disease

Dietary sodium is restricted only for children who have a history of hypertension or edema.

Dialysis

Sodium and fluid allowances are more liberal in PD compared with HD (or IPD) because dialysis is continuous and the dialysate dextrose concentration can be varied to regulate fluid removal.

Transplant

Corticosteroids, cyclosporine, and tacrolimus enhance sodium retention and cause hypertension. The reported prevalence of hypertension in children is 79% 1–month posttransplant and decreases by 25% at 2 years (83). Sodium restriction is prescribed for hypertensive children and is liberalized as hypertension subsides with decreases in immunosuppressant doses. Nonpharmacological antihypertensive therapies include weight control and exercise, which complement dietary measures.

Potassium

Potassium metabolism is directly linked to muscle function and elevated serum levels can produce cardiac arrhythmias or arrest. Potassium is less frequently listed on food labels and cannot be tasted. Foods containing 200 mg potassium or more per serving are considered excessive. High-potassium foods favored by children, such as french fries, potato chips, chocolate, tomato products, bananas, and orange juice should be avoided. In cases when children are not hyperkalemic, they may be encouraged to try some of these foods, on a limited and well-controlled basis, in order to boost calories or dietary intake. Potassium exchange resins (eg, kayexalate) may be necessary. When a dietary source of hyperkalemia cannot be identified, nondietary causes should also be investigated, including: constipation; hemolyzed blood sample; metabolic acidosis; inadequate dialysis; medications such as potassium-sparing diuretics, cyclosporine or tacrolimus, or angiotensin converting enzyme inhibitors; and tissue destruction due to infection, chemotherapy, surgery, or catabolism (86). Serum bicarbonate should be monitored and corrected when levels are less than 22 mEq/L (8).

Chronic Kidney Disease

A potassium-restricted diet is usually not necessary in early stages of CKD. As chronic kidney disease advances, the potassium excretion capacity of each nephron increases as does the potassium secretion in the bowel. Restrictions are typically not necessary until the GFR falls to less than 10% of normal or dialysis is initiated.

Dialysis

Because PD occurs daily and, in most types of PD, continually, children on PD seldom need dietary potassium restriction once they reach full maintenance dialysate exchange volumes (ie, ≥ 1.1 L). Occasionally, children on PD may require potassium supplementation to maintain normal serum levels. In contrast, the majority of children on HD need to carefully follow a low-potassium diet.

Transplant

In transplant recipients, hyperkalemia may result from cyclosporine or tacrolimus therapy, especially when cyclosporine or tacrolimus blood levels are outside the target range. Dietary potassium restriction is initiated only as serum levels dictate.

Fluids

Polyuric infants and children require high fluid intakes to prevent chronic dehydration and poor growth. Children with a history of edema or hypertension may need fluid restriction; the prescribed total fluid intake (TFI) is based on insensible fluid losses (400 mL), measured 24–hour urine output, and other losses (eg, vomiting, diarrhea, drainage). Liquids and foods that are liquid at room temperature (eg, gelatin, ice, Popsicles, ice cream) are considered in the TFI.

Chronic Kidney Disease

Fluid restriction is rarely needed during CKD. Additional fluids are needed if the infant or child is polyuric.

Dialysis

For children on MD, fluid restrictions should also consider ultrafiltration capacity. Nutrition should never be compromised by fluid restrictions. More frequent dialysis is warranted if more volume for enteral feeds is needed to meet nutritional goals. Children on PD rarely need fluid restrictions because dialysate with a higher glucose concentration may be used to increase ultrafiltration. On HD, goals for intradialytic (fluid) weight gain are individualized based on body size and tolerance of fluid removal, and, except for the smallest patients, are typically approximately 1 to 1.5 kg for 2–day between-dialysis intervals and 1.5 to 2 kg for longer, 3–day intervals.

Transplant

High fluid intakes are encouraged posttransplant to maintain good perfusion of the transplanted kidney and avoid cyclosporine or tacrolimus toxicity, which can occur if patients become underhydrated (83). Patients are given an individualized minimum daily total fluid intake based on such factors as estimated needs, laboratory hydration indicators, and usual physical activity. This is gradually lowered over time. Individuals are encouraged to drink water rather than calorie-containing beverages.

SUMMARY

Nutritional management of infants and children with CKD is a challenging process that requires frequent alterations in the nutrition care plan in response to changes in the child's age and stage of development, as well as changes in medical status and therapy. Continued promotion of the benefits of diet and fluid modification, and provision of practical information relevant to the individual child, go a long way toward successful adaptation to these changes by the child and family/caretaker and optimization of the child's nutritional status, growth, development, and health.

REFERENCES

1. Neu AM, Ho PL, McDonald RA, Warady BA. Chronic dialysis in children and adolescents. The 2001 NAPRTCS annual report. *Pediatr Nephrol.* 2002;17:656–663.
2. Chan JCM, Williams DM, Roth KS. Kidney failure in infants and children. *Pediatr Rev*. 2002;23: 47–60.
3. Furth SL, Stablein D, Fine RN, Powe NR, Fivush BA. Adverse clinical outcomes associated with short stature at dialysis initiation: a report of the North American Pediatric Renal Transplant Cooperative Study. *Pediatrics*. 2002;109:909–913.
4. Wong CS, Gipson DS, Gillen DL, Emerson S, Koepsell T, Sherrard DJ, Watkins SL, Stehman-Breen C. Anthropometric measures and risk of death in children with end-stage renal disease. *Am J Kidney Dis*. 2000;36:811–819.

5. Morel P, Almond PS, Matas AJ, Gillingham KJ, Chau C, Brown A. Long-term quality of life after kidney transplantation in childhood. *Transplantation.* 1991;52:47–53.
6. Ledermann SE, Shaw V, Trompeter RS. Long-term enteral nutrition in infants and young children with chronic renal failure. *Pediatr Nephrol.* 1999;13:870–875.
7. Warady BA, Belden B, Kohaut E. Neurodevelopmental outcome of children initiating peritoneal dialysis in early infancy. *Pediatr Nephrol.* 1999; 13:759–765.
8. National Kidney Foundation Kidney Disease Outcomes Quality Initiative. Clinical practice guidelines for nutrition in chronic renal failure. *Am J Kidney Dis.* 2000;35(6 Suppl 2):S1–140.
9. Tom A, McCauley L, Bell L, Rodd C, Espinosa P, Yu G, Yu J, Girardin C, Sharma A. Growth during maintenance hemodialysis: impact of enhanced nutrition and clearance. *J Pediatr.* 1999;134:464–471.
10. Spinozzi NS, Nelson PA. Nutrition support in the newborn intensive care unit. *J Ren Nutr.* 1996; 6:188–197.
11. Coleman JE, Norman LJ, Watson AR. Provision of dietetic care in children on chronic peritoneal dialysis. *J Ren Nutr.* 1999;9:145–148.
12. Groh-Wargo SL, Antonelli K. Normal nutrition during infancy. In: Queen PM, Lang CE, eds. *Handbook of Pediatric Nutrition.* Gaithersburg, Md: Aspen Publishers; 1993:107–144.
13. Sedman A, Friedman A, Boineau F, Strife C, F., Fine R. Nutritional management of the child with mild to moderate chronic renal failure: final report of the growth failure in children with renal disease study. *J Pediatr.* 1996;129(suppl):S13–S18.
14. Van Dyck M, Sidler S, Proesmans W. Chronic renal failure in infants: effect of strict conservative treatment on growth. *Eur J Pediatr.* 1998; 157:759–762.
15. Ruley EJ, Bock GH, Kerzner B, Abbott AW, Majd M, Chatoor I. Feeding disorders and gastroesophageal reflux in infants with chronic renal failure. *Pediatr Nephrol.* 1989;3:424–429.
16. Ravelli AM. Gastrointestinal function in chronic renal failure. *Pediatr Nephrol.* 1995;9:756–762.
17. Wingen AM, Mehls O. Nutrition in children with preterminal chronic renal failure. Myth or important therapeutic aid? *Pediatr Nephrol.* 2002;17: 111–120.
18. Fitts SF. Physical benefits and challenges of exercise for people with chronic renal disease. *J Ren Nutr.* 1997;7:123–128.
19. Castaneda C, Gordon PL, Uhlin KL, Levey AS, Keyayias JJ, Dwyer JT, Fielding RA, Roubenoff R, Singh MF. Resistance training to counteract the catabolism of a low-protein diet in patients with chronic renal insufficiency. *Ann Intern Med.* 2001;135:965–976.
20. Sabath RJ. Exercise evaluation of children with end-stage renal disease. *Adv Ren Replace Ther.* 1999;6:189–194.
21. Warady BA, Alexander SR, Watkins S, Kohaut E, Harmon WE. Optimal care of the pediatric end-stage renal disease patient on dialysis. *Am J Kidney Dis.* 1999;33:567–583.
22. Schaefer F, Wuhl E, Feneberg R, Mehls O, Scharer K. Assessment of body composition in children with chronic renal failure. *Pediatr Nephrol.* 2000;14:673–678.
23. Norman LJ, Coleman JE, Macdonald IA, Tomsett AM, Watson AR. Nutrition and growth in relation to severity of renal disease in children. *Pediatr Nephrol.* 2000;15:259–265.
24. Furth SL, Hwang W, Yang C, Neu AM, Fivush BA, Powe NR. Growth failure, risk of hospitalization and death for children with end-stage renal disease. *Pediatr Nephrol.* 2002;17:450–455.
25. Abitbol C, Chan JC, Trachtman H, Strauss J, Greifer I. Growth in children with moderate renal insufficiency: measurement, evaluation and treatment. Final report of the Growth Failure in Children with Renal Diseases Study. *J Pediatr.* 1996; 129(suppl):S3–S8.
26. Centers for Disease Control and Prevention. 2000 CDC Growth Charts: United States. Available at: http:///www.cdc.gov/growthcharts. Accessed May 6, 2003.
27. Frisancho AR. New norms of upper limb fat and muscle areas for assessment of nutritional status. *Am J Clin Nutr.* 1981;34:2540–2545.
28. Tanner JM, Davies PW. Clinical longitudinal standards for height and height velocity for North American children. *J Pediatr.* 1985;107:317–329.
29. Roberts SB, Dallal GE. The new childhood growth charts. *Nutr Rev.* 2001;59:31–36.
30. Johnson VL, Wang J, Kaskel FJ, Pierson RN. Changes in body composition of children with

chronic renal failure on growth hormone. *Pediatr Nephrol.* 2000;14:695–700.
31. Van Dyck M, Gysells A, Proesmans W, Nijs J, Eeckels R. Growth hormone treatment enhances bone mineralisation in children with chronic renal failure. *Eur J Pediatr.* 2001;160:359–363.
32. Van Dyck M, Proesmans W. Growth hormone therapy in chronic renal failure induces catch-up of head circumference. *Pediatr Nephrol.* 2001;16: 631–636.
33. Mason NA, Boyd SM. Drug nutrient interactions in renal failure. *J Ren Nutr.* 1995;5:214–222.
34. Chazot C, Kopple JD. Vitamin metabolism and requirements in renal disease and renal failure. In: Kopple J, Massry S, eds. *Nutritional Management of Renal Disease.* Baltimore, Md: Williams & Wilkins; 1997:415–477.
35. Davis MC, Tucker CM, Fennell RS. Family behavior, adaptation, and treatment adherence of pediatric nephrology patients. *Pediatr Nephrol.* 1996;10:160–166.
36. Arts-Rodas D, Benoit D. Feeding problems in infancy and early childhood: identification and management. *Paediatr Child Health.* 1998;3: 21–27.
37. Benoit D, Coolbear J. Post-traumatic feeding disorders in infancy: behaviors predicting treatment outcome. *Infant Mental Health J.* 1998;19:409–421.
38. Institute of Medicine. *Dietary Reference Intakes for Vitamin C, Vitamin E, Selenium, and Carotenoids.* Washington, DC: National Academy of Sciences; 2000.
39. Institute of Medicine. *Dietary Reference Intakes for Energy, Carbohydrates, Fiber, Fat, Protein and Amino Acids (Macronutrients).* Washington, DC: National Academy of Sciences; 2002.
40. Institute of Medicine. *Dietary Reference Intakes for Vitamin A, Vitamin K, Arsenic, Boron, Chromium, Copper, Iodine, Iron, Manganese, Molybdenum, Nickel, Silicon, Vanadium, and Zinc.* Washington, DC: National Academy of Sciences; 2002.
41. Institute of Medicine. *Dietary Reference Intakes for Thiamin, Riboflavin, Niacin, Vitamin B-6, Folate, Vitamins B-12, Pantothenic Acid, Biotin, and Choline.* Washington, DC: National Academy of Sciences; 1998.
42. Institute of Medicine. *Dietary Reference Intakes for Calcium, Phosphorous, Magnesium, Vitamin D, and Fluoride.* Washington, DC: National Academy of Sciences; 1997.
43. Food and Nutrition Board. *Recommended Dietary Allowances.* Washington, DC: National Research Council; 1989.
44. Strong J, Burgett M, Buss ML, Carver M, Kwankin S, Walker D. Effects of calorie and fluid intake on adverse events during hemodialysis. *J Ren Nutr.* 2001;11:97–100.
45. Harada H, Seki T, Nonomura K, Chikaraishi T, Takeuchi I, Morita K, Usuki T, Watarai Y, Togashi M, Hirano T, Koyanagi T. Pre-emptive renal transplantation in children. *Int J Urology.* 2001;8: 205–211.
46. Qvist E, Marttinen E, Ronnholm K, Antikainen M, Jalanko H, Sipila I, Holmberg C. Growth after renal transplantation in infancy or early childhood. *Pediatr Nephrol.* 2002;17:438–443.
47. El Haggan W, Vendrely B, Chauveau P, Barthe N, Castaing F, Berger F, de Precigout V, Potaux L, Aparicio M. Early evaluation of nutritional status and body composition after kidney transplantation. *Am J Kidney Dis.* 2002;40:629–637.
48. Yiu VW, Harmon WE, Spinozzi N, Jonas M, MS. K. High-calorie nutrition for infants with chronic renal disease. *J Ren Nutr.* 1996;6:203–206.
49. Watson AR, Coleman JE, Warady BA. When and how to use nasogastric and gastrostomy feeding for nutritional support in infants and children on CAPD/CCPD. In: Fine RN, Alexander SR, Warady BA, eds. *CAPD/CCPD in Children.* Boston, Mass: Kluwer Academic Publishers; 1998:281–300.
50. Coleman JE. Supplemental tube feeding. In: Warady BA, Alexander SR, Fine RN, Schaefer F, eds. *Pediatric Dialysis.* Boston, Mass: Kluwer Academic Publishers; 2004.
51. Dello Strologo L, Principato F, Sinibaldi D, Appiani AC, Terzi F, Dartois AM, Rizzoni G. Feeding dysfunction in infants with severe chronic renal failure after long-term nasogastric tube feeding. *Pediatr Nephrol.* 1997;11: 84–86.
52. Schauster H, Dwyer J. Transition from tube feedings to feedings by mouth in children: Preventing eating dysfunction. *J Am Diet Assoc.* 1996;96: 277–281.
53. Ledermann SE, Spitz L, Moloney J. Gastrostomy feeding in infants and children on peritoneal dialysis. *Pediatr Nephrol.* 2002;17:246–250.

54. Mehrotra R, Nolph KD. Treatment of advanced renal failure: low-protein diets or timely initiation of dialysis? *Kidney Int.* 2000;58:1381–1388.
55. Salusky IB, Fine RN, Nelson P, Blumenkrantz MJ, Kopple JD. Nutritional status of children undergoing continuous ambulatory peritoneal dialysis. *Am J Clin Nutr.* 1983;58:599–611.
56. de Boer AW, Schroder CH, van Vliet R, Willems JL, Monnens LAH. Clinical experience with icodextrin in children: ultrafiltration profiles and metabolism. *Pediatr Nephrol.* 2000;15:21–24.
57. Wolfson M, Piraino B, Hamburger RJ, Morton AR, for the Icodextrin Study Group. A randomized controlled trial to evaluate the efficacy and safety of icodextrin in peritoneal dialysis. *Am J Kidney Dis.* 2002;40:1055–1065.
58. Goldstein SL, Baronette S, Vital Gambrell T, Currier H, Brewer ED. nPCR assessment and IDPN treatment of malnutrition in pediatric hemodialysis patients. *Pediatr Nephrol.* 2002;17:531–534.
59. Krause I, Shamir R, Davidovits M, Frishman S, Cleper R, Gamzo Z, Poraz I, Eisenstein B. Intradialytic parenteral nutrition in malnourished children treated with hemodialysis. *J Ren Nutr.* 2002; 12:55–59.
60. Pagenkemper J. Planning a vegetarian renal diet. *J Ren Nutr.* 1995;5:234–238.
61. Klahr S, Levey AS, Beck GJ, Caggiula AW, Hunsicker L, Kusek JW, Stricker G, for the Modification of Diet in Renal Disease Study Group. The effects of dietary protein restriction and blood pressure control on the progression of chronic renal disease. *N Engl J Med.* 1994;330:877–884.
62. Kasiske BL, Lakatua JDA, Ma JZ, Louis TA. A meta-analysis of the effects of dietary protein restriction on the rate of decline in renal function. *Am J Kidney Dis.* 1998;31:954–961.
63. Levey AS, Green T, Beck GJ, Caggiula AW, Kusek JW, Hunsicker LG, Klahr S, for the Modification of Diet in Renal Disease Study Group. Dietary protein restriction and the progression of chronic renal disease: what have all of the results of the MDRD study shown? *J Am Soc Nephrol.* 1999;10:2426–2439.
64. Wingen AM, Fabian-Bach C, Schaefer F, Mehls O, for the European Study Group for Nutritional Treatment of Chronic Renal Failure in Childhood. Randomised multicentre study of a low-protein diet on the progression of chronic renal failure in children. *Lancet.* 1997;349:1117–1123.
65. Kopple JD, Levey AS, Greene T, Chumlea WC, Gassman JJ, Hollinger DL, Maroni BJ, Merrill D, Scherch LK, Schulman G, Wang SR, Zimmer GS. Effect of dietary protein restriction on nutritional status in the Modification of Diet in Renal Disease Study. *Kidney Int.* 1997;52:778–791.
66. Quan A, Baum M. Protein losses in children on continuous cycler peritoneal dialysis. *Pediatr Nephrol.* 1996;10:728–731.
67. Secker D, Pencharz PB. Nutritional therapy for children on CAPD/CCPD: theory and practice. In: Fine RN, Alexander SR, Warady BA, eds. *CAPD/CCPD in Children.* Boston, Mass: Kluwer Academic; 1998:567–603.
68. Canepa A, Verrina E, Perfumo F, Carrea A, Menoni S, Delucchi P, Gusmano R. Value of intraperitoneal amino acids in children treated with chronic peritoneal dialysis. *Perit Dial Int.* 1999; 18(Suppl 2):S435–S440.
69. Qamar IU, Secker D, Levin L, Balfe JA, Zlotkin S, Balfe JW. Effects of amino acid dialysis compared to dextrose dialysis in children on continuous cycling peritoneal dialysis. *Perit Dial Int.* 1999;19:237–247.
70. Querfeld U. Disturbance of lipid metabolism in children with chronic renal failure. *Pediatr Nephrol.* 1993;7:749–757.
71. Murakami R, Momota T, Yoshiya K, Yoshikawa N, Nakamura H, Honda M, Ito H. Serum carnitine and nutritional status in children treated with continuous ambulatory peritoneal dialysis. *J Pediatr Gastroenterol Nutr.* 1990;11:371–374.
72. Kari JA, Shaw V, Vallance DT, Rees L. Effect of enteral feeding on lipid subfractions in children with chronic renal failure. *Pediatr Nephrol.* 1998; 12:401–404.
73. Saltissi D, Morgan C, Knight B, Chang W, Rigby R, Westhuyzen J. Effect of lipid-lowering dietary recommendations on the nutritional intake and lipid profiles of chronic peritoneal dialysis and hemodialysis patients. *Am J Kidney Dis.* 2001;37: 1209–1215.
74. Zachwieja J, Duran M, Joles JA, Allers PJ, van de Hurk D, Frankhuisen JJ. Amino acid and carnitine supplementation in haemodialysed children. *Pediatr Nephrol.* 1994;8:739–743.
75. Warady BA, Borum P, Stall C, Millspaugh J, Taggart E, Lum G. Carnitine status of pediatric patients on continuous ambulatory peritoneal dialysis. *Am J Nephrol.* 1990;10:109–114.

76. Hines L. Can low-fat/cholesterol nutrition counseling improve food intake habits and hyperlipidemia of renal transplant patients? *J Ren Nutr.* 2000;10:30–35.
77. Kuizon BD, Salusky IB. Diagnosis and treatment of renal bone diseases in children undergoing CAPD/CCPD. In: Fine RN, Alexander SR, Warady BA, eds. *CAPD/CCPD in Children.* 2nd ed. Boston, Mass: Kluwer Academic Publishers; 1998:199–217.
78. Salusky IB. Management of renal bone disease. In: Warady BA, Alexander SR, Fine RN, Schaefer F, eds. *Pediatric Dialysis.* Boston, Mass: Kluwer Academic Publishers; 2004.
79. Merouani A, Lambert M, Delvin EE, Genest J Jr, Robitaille P, Rozen R. Plasma homocysteine concentration in children with chronic renal failure. *Pediatr Nephrol.* 2001;16:805–811.
80. Litwin M, Abuauba M, Wawer ZT, Grenda R, Kuryt T, Pietraszek E. Folate, vitamin B12, and sulfur amino acid levels in patients with renal failure. *Pediatr Nephrol.* 2001;16:127–132.
81. Bennett-Richards K, Kattenhorn M, Donald A, Oakley G, Varghese Z, Rees L, Deanfield JE. Does oral folic acid lower total homocysteine levels and improve endothelial function in children with chronic renal failure? *Circulation.* 2002;105:1810–1815.
82. Schroder CH, de Boer AW, Giesen AM, Monnens LA, Blom H. Treatment of hyperhomocysteinemia in children on dialysis by folic acid. *Pediatr Nephrol.* 1999;13:583–585.
83. Kasiske BL, Vazquez MA, Harmon WE, Brown RS, Danovitch GM, Gaston RS, Roth D, Scandling JD, Singer GG. Recommendations for the outpatient surveillance of renal transplant recipients. *J Am Soc Nephrol.* 2000;11:1–86.
84. Rodriguez-Soriano J, Arant BS. Fluid and electrolyte imbalances in children with chronic renal failure. *Am J Kidney Dis.* 1986;7:268–274.
85. Secker D. Achieving nutritional goals for children on dialysis. In: Warady BA, Alexander SR, Fine RN, Schaefer F, eds. *Pediatric Dialysis.* Boston, Mass: Kluwer Academic Publishers; 2004.
86. Beto J, Bansal VK. Hyperkalemia: evaluating dietary and nondietary etiology. *J Ren Nutr.* 1992;2: 28–29.

Chapter 13

Enteral Nutrition in Kidney Disease

Pamela Charney, MS, RD, CNSD

Most would agree that a significant number of individuals with chronic kidney disease (CKD) have some degree of nutritional deficiency. Malnutrition may be related to adverse outcomes in this population (1). Various treatments for malnutrition are available, ranging from diet supplementation to total parenteral nutrition. Oral and enteral nutrition are effective treatments in this population. When enteral nutrition is used in individuals with CKD, feedings must be carefully monitored to prevent complications.

ORAL NUTRITIONAL SUPPLEMENTATION

Dietary management of the individual with CKD may be complicated by factors associated with both the disease and its treatment. Renal failure leads to alterations in metabolism and nutrient handling. Uremia can cause anorexia and altered taste acuity. Other factors associated with poor oral intake in these individuals include psychosocial factors, fatigue, and unduly restricted diets (2,3). Therefore, skillful management should optimize food choices and taste. Nutrition therapy should be individualized, avoiding unnecessary restrictions (4). In the past, severely restricted diets were ordered in hopes of preventing a buildup of toxins, a practice that may have contributed to the development of malnutrition in some cases. Because repleting lost nutrient stores in patients with CKD can be difficult, it is important to monitor dry weight, oral intake, and other indicators of nutritional status and intervene as early as possible. When warranted, diet restrictions should be minimized. Many high-calorie foods also contain substantial amounts of phosphorus and potassium; however, rather than restrict these foods, it is important to monitor overall intake and lab results (5). In the case of phosphorus, binder prescriptions may need to be adjusted, and dialysis prescriptions can be altered to allow for a higher dietary phosphorus intake.

In some cases, it may be necessary to use modules containing concentrated sources of one or more nutrients to increase the energy or protein density of foods. Modules can be purchased as powders or liquids that can be added to foods. The patient should be encouraged to sample different modules to determine the best acceptability. When a patient is not meeting nutritional requirements with protein- and calorie-enhanced foods, then oral nutritional supplements may be used. Commercial formulas are convenient and easy for patients who may often be fatigued. It is important to note the nutrient content of these formulas because formulas differ in their levels of nutrients. (See Tables 13.1 and 13.2 for specific formula information.)

Consumption of liquid supplements may not lead to a significant increase in energy and protein intake because the supplements may merely replace foods in the diet (6). However, in a study by Caglar et al, substantial

Table 13.1. Renal and Calorie-Dense Formulas

Formula (Manufacturer)	*Energy (kcal/mL)*	*Protein (g/L)*	*Fat (g/L)*	*Carbohydrate (g/L)*	*Osmolality (MOsm/kg)*	*Sodium (mg/L)*	*Potassium (mg/L)*	*Phosphorus (mg/L)*	*Volume to Meet Dietary Reference Intake (mL):*
Suplena (Ross Laboratories)	2.0	30	96	255	600	790	1120	730	950
Renalcal (Nestle Clinical Nutrition)	2.0	34	82	290	600	—	—	—	1000 to meet DRI for vitamins
Magnacal Renal (Novartis)	2.0	75	101	200	570	800	1270	800	1000
Nepro (Ross Laboratories)	2.0	70	96	222	665	830	1056	660	960
Nutra-Renal (Nestle Clinical Nutrition)	2.0	70	104	205	650	740	1256	700	750
Two-Cal HN (Ross Laboratories)	2.0	83	90	219	730	1460	2450	1055	950
Deliver 2.0 (Novartis)	2.0	75	101	200	640	800	1690	1010	1000
Ensure Plus (Ross Laboratories)	1.5	55	53	200	600	1141	2325	800	1600
Boost Plus (Novartis)	1.5	59	58	200	720	720	1610	1310	945
Nutren 1.0 (Nestle)	1.0	40	38	127	370 (vanilla)	876	1248	668	1500

— indicates amount is negligible.

Source: Data are from manufacturer Web sites: http://www.nestleclinicalnutrition.com; http://www.ross.com; http://www.novartis.com. All sites were accessed June 11, 2004.

improvement in Subjective Global Assessment scores was achieved after consumption of a supplement providing 350 to 475 kcal during hemodialysis treatments (7). There was no change in body weight during 6 months of follow-up in this study. Subjects in this study were provided with the supplement during dialysis treatment to improve compliance (7). It is important to monitor intake of supplements as well as other foods to ensure that oral supplements do not replace foods (8). Whenever possible, patients should be encouraged to meet nutrient requirements through food intake.

ENTERAL NUTRITION

Individuals who are unable to meet estimated nutrient requirements via voluntary oral intake but who have a functional gastrointestinal (GI) tract may be fed via enteral feeding tube. Current guidelines recommend initiating some form of nutrition support after a period of inadequate intake from a few days to 2 weeks, depending on the patient's overall condition and premorbid nutritional status (9). Compared with parenteral nutrition, enteral nutrition (EN) is more physiologic, easier

Table 13.2. Characteristics of Oral Supplements/Enteral Formulas

Type	*Examples*	*Characteristics*	*Indications*
Oral liquid supplements	Milkshakes, Instant Breakfast,* Ensure,† Nutren,* Boost‡	Flavored for oral consumption. May contain milk. Most contain 1 kcal/mL and moderate protein levels.	Inability to meet requirements via diet alone.
Standard enteral formulas	Nutren 1.0,* Osmolite,† Isocal,‡ Boost‡	1 kcal/mL, moderate protein content. Most meet DRI for nutrients in < 1500 mL.	Most patients requiring enteral feeding.
Fluid-restricted formulas	Nutren 2.0,* Magnacal,‡ TwoCal HN,† Boost Plus‡	1.5–2.0 kcal/mL, moderate protein content.	Used in patients with fluid restriction.
Fiber-containing	Jevity,† Ultracal,‡ Nutren with fiber*	1.0 kcal/mL, moderate protein. Type and amount of fiber may vary.	May help normalize bowel function in some patients.
Elemental and peptide-based	Vivonex,‡ Peptamen,* Vital HN,† Criticare HN‡	1.0 kcal/ml, moderate protein content. Protein source and type may vary.	Used for patients with malabsorption and extreme GI dysfunction. Very unpalatable, but may be used orally in some patients.
Glucose intolerance	Glucerna,† Diabetisource,‡ Choice DM‡	Usually 1 kcal/mL but can vary, moderate protein. Lower carbohydrate content than standard formulas.	Controversial, no well-controlled clinical trials support use, but may be effective in some enterally fed patients with difficult to control blood sugar.
Specialized for chronic kidney disease (CKD)	CKD (predialysis): Suplena,† Renalcal* On dialysis: Nepro,† Magnacal,‡ NutriRenal*	Protein and electrolytes modified. 2 kcal/mL.	Useful in patients with difficult-to-control serum electrolyte levels.

*Manufactured by Nestlé Nutrition. http://www.nestleclinicalnutrition.com. Accessed March 11, 2004.
†Manufactured by Ross Products. http://www.ross.com. Accessed March 11, 2004.
‡Manufactured by Novartis. http://www.novartis.com. Accessed June 11, 2004.

to maintain, and less expensive, and it presents less risk to the patient (10). A variety of newer techniques make it possible to provide enteral nutrition to all but the most challenging patients.

Tube Selection

The type of feeding tube and site of feeding will be determined by the patient's clinical status. Practitioner experience and comfort level with the tubes used will guide choice of tube. Nasogastric or nasoenteral feeding tubes are commonly used when less than 4 to 6 weeks of enteral feedings are anticipated. Various tubes are available that can be placed at the bedside with appropriate training. The most common nasoenteric tubes are 8 to 10 French, which refers to the inner diameter of the tube. Tubes larger than 10 French tend to be uncomfortable and not well tolerated, whereas those less than 8 French may be prone to clogging. Smaller bore feeding tubes (8 French and smaller) can be used with appropriate attention to flushing schedules, avoidance of medication administration via tube, and use of nonviscous formulas administered with a pump. Concentrated formulas with more than 1.0 kcal/mL may be too viscous to flow easily through smaller bore tubes and may require a feeding pump. Tubes are available with or without weights and stylets. It is important to remember that once removed, stylets should never be reinserted because this might cause perforation of the tube by the stylet. Radiologic confirmation of tube placement is recommended prior to beginning feedings.

Long-term feedings can be accomplished via either surgical or nonsurgical enterostomy tube placement. Gastrostomy feedings are commonly used in long-term care for those patients with adequate gastric emptying capacity. There are also double-lumen tubes available that can be used to simultaneously decompress gastric contents and feed into the small intestine. Surgical gastrostomies are commonly placed during another operative procedure. Nonsurgical long-term tube placement can be accomplished via percutaneous endoscopic gastrostomy (PEG). PEG feedings are used less frequently in peritoneal dialysis (PD) patients than in hemodialysis (HD) patients because the initial placement of PEG tubes in PD patients has been reported to be associated with an increase in infectious complications (11). However, a pre-existing PEG tube placed before initiation of PD can be used. There are many different tubes available depending on patient needs and therapy chosen. Surgically placed button gastrostomies are often used in children or active patients who require skin-level access.

Gastric feedings may be contraindicated in patients with disorders of gastric emptying or who may be at increased risk for aspiration. In these cases, jejunostomy tubes are often successfully used. Like gastrostomy tubes, jejunostomies can be placed either surgically or endoscopically. Standard polymeric formulas can be used when feeding into a jejunostomy tube; there is no need for hydrolyzed protein when using these tubes.

ENTERAL FORMULA CHOICE

There are hundreds of commercially prepared enteral formulas available for patients with CKD. Several formulas have been developed specifically for use when CKD dictates fluid and electrolyte restriction. Retail cost per 240 mL of formula can vary from less than $1 for standard, intact protein formulas to more than $5 for specialized "immune enhancing" formulas. Health care facilities often enter into buying contracts that can offer significantly reduced prices at the cost of a more limited formulary. Because cost containment is becoming an important component of health care, it is important to choose the most cost-effective formula that will meet the patient's needs. Tables 13.1 and 13.2 present some commonly used formulas and indications for their use.

Delivery Systems

Until 20 to 30 years ago, enteral formulas were homemade in facility kitchens with little control for bacterial contamination or consistency of nutrient content. The development of canned, sterile, nutritionally complete enteral formulas lessened the dependence on homemade feedings and allowed for more consistency in nutrient content as well as improved food safety. When proper handling techniques and hang times are observed, bacterial contamination of feedings can be kept to a minimum.

The advent of closed-system feedings, in which formulas are purchased in ready-to-hang containers, minimizes contamination. Closed system formulas have the advantage of a longer hang time than traditional open systems. Although closed systems offer the benefit of longer hang time (often more than 24 to 36 hours) and require less nursing time for tube feeding management, there is no option for formula additives or changing formulas if needed. This can lead to formula waste. Hang time for formulas used in open systems should be no longer than 4 to 6 hours, with shorter hang times allowed for formulas that have been manipulated by addition of modular components or medications. Manufacturers should be contacted for advice about appropriate hang times for various feedings.

Nutrient Considerations

Individuals with CKD receiving dialysis often must limit fluid intake. While most standard enteral formulas contain 1 kcal/mL and approximately 875 mL free water per liter of formula, there are calorie-dense formulas available that contain from 1.5 to 2.0 kcal/mL and thus less free water. By using a 2.0 kcal/mL formula 2,000 kcal can be provided in 1,000 mL volume (approximately 780 mL free water), which is adequate to meet the needs of the typical CKD patient.

In the past, it was common practice to use formulas containing only the essential amino acids plus histidine in individuals with CKD requiring enteral feedings. These formulas also contained minimal electrolytes. Amino acid requirements may be altered during acute illness so that formulas containing only the essential amino acids plus histidine may be deficient in one or more amino acids required for recovery. There is no evidence that enteral formulas containing only essential amino acids improve renal function or reduce the need for dialysis in the ill patient with CKD; therefore, such formulas are not routinely used. Further controversy surrounds the use of intact protein, hydrolyzed protein, or free amino acid formulas. The normal GI tract has a large functional reserve, such that intact protein formulas are well tolerated even in face of significant GI impairment. When GI disease precludes the use of intact protein formulas, those containing hydrolyzed proteins are generally well tolerated. The need for a formula containing a high percentage of free amino acids is debatable because dipeptides and tripeptides seem to be better absorbed and used.

Current recommendations for protein intake for the patient with CKD depend on the dialytic modality. Although the National Kidney Foundation Kidney Disease Outcomes Quality Initiatives (K/DOQI) guidelines (9) provide recommended levels of protein intake, some controversy remains regarding the most appropriate recommendations for protein intake for patients with CKD. Low-protein diets may be used in an attempt to preserve residual renal function prior to initiation of dialysis. Both HD and PD lead to the loss of amino acids and protein, with a larger amount lost in patients receiving PD. To account for these losses, patients on dialysis should be provided more than the dietary reference intake (DRI) for protein for healthy adults. There is little information about changes in protein requirements during acute illness in the patient with ESRD. A higher protein intake, with adjustments made based on the need for and type of dialytic therapy, may be beneficial in some critically ill patients (12). Patients receiving continuous renal replacement therapy (CRRT) in an ICU setting may require higher protein diets. Many formulas available offer a higher protein content. (See Chapter 4 for a discussion of acute renal failure.)

Electrolyte and Mineral Considerations

Other important considerations in choosing enteral formulas for patients with CKD include the electrolyte and mineral content of the formula. Changes in patient condition and effectiveness of dialytic therapy may require adjusting electrolyte intake during illness. Electrolyte content of formulas varies widely. Most standard formulas are designed to provide adequate but not excessive amounts of potassium, sodium, and phosphorus. These formulas may be well tolerated by the patient with CKD who is stable and adequately dialyzed. Special renal formulas are also available that contain lower amounts of these electrolytes. All sources of electrolytes, including diet, enteral formulas, medications, and intravenous fluids, should be assessed. Often, particularly in home care or in stable patients, dietary intake can vary.

The onset of feeding after a period of minimal or no nutritional intake can trigger a shift in potassium and phosphorus from the extracellular to intracellular space. This shift can lead to a precipitous and potentially fatal drop in serum levels of these electrolytes, a condition known as refeeding syndrome. Zealous restriction of electrolytes in patients with risk factors for refeeding (elderly, alcoholism, chronic starvation) may have disastrous results, including extreme hypophosphatemia, hypokalemia, and hypomagnesemia, potentially leading to cardiac and respiratory arrest (13,14).

ADMINISTRATION OF ENTERAL FEEDINGS

The choice of feeding administration method will vary from patient to patient and may be guided by patient condition, need for time away from feeding pumps and apparatus, and feeding tolerance. Continuous feedings are most frequently used as an initial regimen in the acute care setting. Feedings are often initially given over 24 hours until patient tolerance has been established. Once feedings are well tolerated, feeding time can be decreased with an increase in rate. There is no need to dilute enteral formulas because formula osmolality is not high enough to lead to osmotic diarrhea. In most patients, it is possible to initiate full-strength feedings at 30 to 50 mL/hour, depending on patient condition and requirements.

Feeding Schedules

Cyclic feedings are often used during attempts to transition from enteral to oral diet. Feedings are administered nocturnally and are stopped 1 to 2 hours prior to the first meal of the day. This allows for a longer period free from feedings and is thought by some to promote development of sensations of hunger, which may stimulate increased voluntary oral intake.

Intermittent feedings are often used in long-term care, rehabilitation settings, and home care because the feeding schedule leaves time off of feedings for therapies, work, or other activities. Intermittent feeding schedules can more closely mimic regular meal times and are more physiologic. Intermittent feeding schedules vary widely and can include from four to six or more feedings spaced throughout the day. The transition from continuous to intermittent feedings can be achieved in several ways. One method is to simply start with many small intermittent feedings throughout the day with a short interval between feedings. Over the course of several days, the interval between feedings is increased and the volume of each feed is increased so that a constant volume of feeding is provided. As tolerance to intermittent feedings is established, the total volume of the formula for a 24-hour period can be divided into the number of feedings desired and infused over 20 to 60 minutes (15,16). Rapid infusion of feedings using syringes or bolus feedings are not usually recommended, although may be tolerated in some stable patients.

Creative feeding schedules are often used for patients receiving hemodialysis. Total volume of formula required to meet needs and a feeding schedule that accommodates dialysis should be determined to ensure that calorie goals are met. To optimize GI tolerance and prevent aspiration, the head of the bed should be elevated to 30 to 45 degrees during enteral feedings. Hypotensive complications during dialysis may require that the head be lowered. Therefore, enteral feeding may not be possible during dialysis. Additionally, patients with diabetes mellitus may need altered medication schedules on dialysis days.

Monitoring Enteral Feedings

Complications of enteral feeding can be classified as mechanical, biochemical, or gastrointestinal. Feeding tubes should be monitored carefully for evidence of dislodgement. Elevating the head of bed to 30 to 45 degrees can help prevent reflux and aspiration pneumonia. Aspiration pneumonia is a potentially deadly condition caused by aspiration of gastric contents into the bronchial tree. Enteral formulas are not the only cause of aspiration, and normal adults "silently" aspirate during sleep with no adverse consequences. Several methods have been used to detect aspiration of gastric contents, including addition of blue dye to formula, auscultation over the epigastric area, and glucose reagent testing of aspirates. None of these methods has proven to be uniformly effective; thus, monitoring and prevention remain the most effective treatment (17). Addition of blue dye to feedings is no longer recommended due to possible lethal complications in critically ill patients (18).

Administration of medications via feeding tube must be carefully monitored to avoid tube clogging. Frequent and thorough flushing of tubes with warm water is the best method to ensure tube patency. There is no evidence that the use of cola drinks, cranberry juice, or other liquids prevents tube clogging. Whenever possible, liquid forms of medications should be given because crushed medications given via feeding tube are a frequent cause of tube occlusion. Consult a pharmacist to assess the most appropriate dose, form, and route of delivery of medications for patients receiving enteral feedings. Additionally, any acidic medication given via tube must be diluted because the acidity of the medication may curdle the enteral formula and potentially lead to tube clogging. Warm water flushes should be used before and after giving medications via feeding tubes. Because water used to flush tubes can contribute significantly to the fluid intake of the CKD patient who may require a fluid restriction, it is important to communicate with other health care providers to ensure the most efficient medication schedule. In patients requiring fluid restriction, the volume of water used for tube flushing should be monitored and kept to the minimum required for tube patency.

Complications

Hyperglycemia is probably the most common biochemical complication of enteral feeding. Approximately two thirds of all dialysis patients also have either type 1 or type 2 diabetes (19,20), so the clinician caring for the enterally fed CKD patient will most likely encounter abnormalities in blood glucose control. Both renal failure and acute illness are associated with abnormalities in glucose control, including peripheral insulin resistance, decreased insulin clearance, and uptake of glucose from dialysate solutions that may lead to hyperglycemia. Critical illness is also associated with multiple metabolic abnormalities, including increased gluconeogenesis, which can make glucose control even more problematic. Hyperglycemia has been implicated in poor wound healing as well as increased infectious complications after surgery, making it imperative that hyperglycemia be identified and aggressively treated (21).

When initiating enteral feedings in patients with preexisting type 1 diabetes or type 2 diabetes requiring insulin, a proportion of previous insulin requirements can be given as subcutaneous regular insulin to maintain blood glucose as close to normal as possible. Sliding scale insulin may be needed by acutely ill patients who did not require insulin before starting enteral feedings, but a continuous insulin infusion allows for more proactive control of blood glucose levels. Oral hypoglycemic agents may be used for managing blood glucose in stable type 2 diabetic patients or those in home or extended care settings.

Other metabolic abnormalities seen in patients with CKD include alterations in phosphorus, potassium, magnesium, and sodium. As mentioned previously, it is important to become familiar with the electrolyte contents of commonly used formulas. Patients with CKD who are receiving electrolyte-restricted formulas should be closely monitored for both increased and decreased levels of these electrolytes. Phosphate binder prescriptions can be altered to address hyperphosphatemia. Dialysis prescriptions can be altered to account for some changes in electrolyte levels that cannot be addressed by changing feedings. If oral electrolyte supplementation must be given in addition to feedings, they should be well diluted before adding because these solutions are hyperosmolar and may lead to an osmotic diarrhea.

Diarrhea is the most common GI complication of enteral feedings and has been reported to occur in a large percentage of patients receiving enteral nutrition support (22). Various causes for diarrhea have been cited, including rapid administration of formula, hypoalbuminemia, cold formulas, medications such as antibiotics and those with extremely high osmolarities, and hypertonic formulas. Of these, the most likely cause is medication, with hypertonic elixirs causing osmotic diarrhea and antibiotics causing changes in gut flora (23). Various treatments have been used, including the addition of soluble fiber to formulas, with varying results (24).

CONCLUSION

Malnutrition is a common complication of CKD and can lead to increased risk for morbidity and mortality in this population. Enteral nutrition is a safe and effective therapy for patients with CKD. Indications for enteral nutrition in patients with CKD are no different from those in any other patient population. Enteral feedings in patients with CKD does provide some unique challenges in terms of alterations in nutrient needs as well as the metabolic and nutritional implications of renal replacement therapy. Although special attention must be paid to the nutrient composition of feedings, standard enteral formulas are appropriate for most patients with CKD unless there are difficult to control serum electrolyte levels.

REFERENCES

1. Benabe JE, Martinez-Maldonado M. The impact of malnutrition on kidney function. *Miner Electrolyte Metab.* 1998;24:20–26.
2. Mehrotra R, Kopple JD. Nutritional management of maintenance dialysis patients: why aren't we doing better? *Ann Rev Nutr.* 2001;21:343–379.
3. Zimmerer JL, Leon JB, Covinsky KE, Desai U, Sehgal AR. Diet monotony as a correlate of poor nutritional intake among hemodialysis patients. *J Ren Nutr.* 2003;13:72–77.
4. Chertow GM. Modality specific nutrition support in ESRD: weighing the evidence. *Am J Kidney Dis.* 1999;33:193–197.
5. Madigan SM, O'Neill S, Clarke J, L'Estrange F, MacAuley DC. Assessing the dietetic needs of different patient groups receiving enteral tube feeding in primary care. *J Hum Nutr Diet.* 2002; 15:179–184.
6. Wilson MMG, Purushothaman R, Morley JE. Effect of liquid dietary supplements on energy intake in the elderly. *Am J Clin Nutr.* 2002;75:944–947.
7. Caglar K, Fedje L, Dimmitt R, Hakim RM, Shyr Y, Ikizler TA. Therapeutic effects of oral nutritional supplementation during hemodialysis. *Kidney Int.* 2002;62:1054–1059.
8. Cuppari L, Medeiros FAM, Papini HF, Neto MC, Canziani MEF, Martini L, Ajzen H, Draibe SA. Effectiveness of oral energy-protein supplementation in severely malnourished hemodialysis patients. *J Ren Nutr.* 1994;4:127–135.
9. National Kidney Foundation. K/DOQI clinical practice guidelines for nutrition in chronic renal failure. *Am J Kidney Dis.* 2000;35(suppl):S48–S50.
10. Kopple JD. Therapeutic approaches to malnutrition in chronic dialysis patients: the different modalities of nutritional support. *Am J Kidney Dis.* 1999;33:180–185.
11. Fein PA, Madane SJ, Jorden A, Babu K, Mushnick R, Avram MM, Grosman I. Outcome of percutaneous endoscopic gastrostomy feeding in pa-

tients on peritoneal dialysis. *Adv Perit Dial.* 2001;17:148–152.
12. Kopple JD. Dietary protein and energy requirements in ESRD patients. *Am J Kidney Dis.* 1998;32(suppl):S97–S104.
13. Solomon SM, Kirby DF. The refeeding syndrome: a review. *JPEN J Parenter Enteral Nutr.* 1990;14:90–97.
14. Brooks MJ, Melnik G. The refeeding syndrome: an approach to understanding its complications and preventing its occurrence. *Pharmacotherapy.* 1995;15:713–726.
15. Charney PJ. Enteral nutrition: indications, options, and formulations. In: *The Science and Practice of Nutrition Support: A Case-Based Core Curriculum.* Dubuque, Iowa: Kendall Hunt Publishing; 2001:141–166.
16. Minard G, Lysen L K. Enteral access devices. In: *The Science and Practice of Nutrition Support: A Case-Based Core Curriculum.* Dubuque, Iowa: Kendall Hunt Publishing; 2001:167–188.
17. Metheny NA, Dahms TE, Stewart BJ, Stone KS, Edwards SJ, Defer JE, Clouse RE. Efficacy of dye-stained enteral formula in detecting pulmonary aspiration. *Chest.* 2002;122:276–281.
18. Maloney JP, Ryan TA, Brasel KJ, Binion DG, Johnson DR, Halbower AC, Frankel EH, Nyffeler M, Moss M. . Food dye use in enteral feedings: a review and a call for a moratorium. *Nutr Clin Pract.* 2002;17:169–181.
19. Locatelli F, Canaud B, Eckardt KU, Stenvinkel P, Wanner C, Zoccai C. The importance of diabetic nephropathy in current nephrological practice. *Nephrol Dial Transplant.* 2003;18:1716–1725.
20. Excerpts from the United States Renal Data Systems 2002 Annual Report: atlas of end stage renal disease in the US. *Am J Kidney Dis.* 2003;41(4 Suppl 2):S7–S254.
21. van den Berghe G, Wouters P, Weekers F, Verwaest C, Bruyninckx F, Schetz M, Vlasselaers D, Ferdinande P, Lauwers P, Bouillon R. Intensive insulin therapy in critically ill patients. *New Eng J Med.* 2001;345:1359–1367.
22. Lebak KJ, Zimmaro DB, Savik K, Patten-Marsh KM. What's new on defining diarrhea in tube-feeding studies? *Clin Nurs Res.* 2003;12:174–204.
23. Eisenberg P. An overview of diarrhea in the patient receiving enteral nutrition. *Gastroenterol Nurs.* 2002;25:95–104.
24. Schultz AA, Ashby-Hughes B, Taylor R, Gillis DE, Wilkins M. Effects of pectin on diarrhea in critically ill tube-fed patient receiving antibiotics. *Am J Crit Care.* 2000;9:403–411.

Chapter 14

Parenteral Nutrition in Kidney Disease

M. Patricia Fuhrman, MS, RD, CNSD, FADA

Parenteral nutrition (PN) is an alternative feeding modality when the gastrointestinal (GI) tract is inaccessible or enteral nutrition is insufficient to meet the patient's nutrient requirements. The following discussion is divided into six sections: general guidelines for PN in kidney disease, acute renal failure (ARF), chronic kidney disease (CKD), peripheral parenteral nutrition, intradialytic parenteral nutrition, and intraperitoneal parenteral nutrition.

PARENTERAL NUTRITION AND KIDNEY DISEASE

Fluid and electrolyte management in conjunction with adequate energy and protein are the mainstay of providing PN to patients with ARF or CKD. The nutrition assessment of patients for PN should include determining indications and contraindications for PN, identifying the route of infusion (central or peripheral), calculating macronutrient and micronutrient requirements, identifying metabolic derangements, and setting nutritional goals and measurable desired outcomes. Indications for PN are a nonfunctioning or nonaccessible GI tract. PN may also be indicated when a patient's nutrient needs cannot be met with either oral diet or tube feeding (1). Contraindications for PN include lack of intravenous (IV) access and poor prognosis (1).

Nutritional requirements depend on comorbidities, activity level, and dialysis modality. Table 14.1 provides general PN recommendations for patients with kidney disease (1–8). These guidelines should be individualized according to the needs and tolerance of each patient. Calculations for energy requirements should be based on the patient's edema-free weight or dry weight. Protein requirements are often based on the patient's ideal body weight. Total calories from all energy sources, amino acids, dextrose, and lipids, should be included in calculating PN energy requirements (2,9,10).

COMPONENTS OF PARENTERAL NUTRITION

Macronutrient components of PN solutions are amino acids, dextrose, and lipids. The most concentrated form of each should be used in PN so that the total volume can be minimized when necessary. The calorie contribution of each PN component is shown in Table 14.2 (2). Keep in mind that 70% dextrose (D_{70}) provides 2.38 kcal/mL and the most commonly used 20% lipid solution provides 2 kcal/mL, making dextrose the most concentrated source of PN calories. A 30% lipid solution can further increase PN calorie concentration by providing 3 kcal/mL. However, this lipid solution is not available at all facilities. The most concentrated source of amino acids is a 20% solution, which provides 0.8 kcal/mL.

Table 14.1. Suggested Composition of PN Solution for Adults with Acute Renal Failure or Chronic Kidney Disease

Component	*Recommendations*
Macronutrients	
Energy	• 25–35 kcal/kg/d based on estimated dry body weight
Amino acids	• Mixture of essential and nonessential amino acids. • Predialysis: 0.6–1.0 g/kg/d. • Chronic dialysis: 1.2–1.3 g/kg/d. • CRRT: at least 1 g/kg/d. • Acute renal failure on CRRT: 1.5–2.0 g/kg/d.
Dextrose	• Consider all sources of dextrose (IVF, dialytic therapy). • Provide maximum of 4–6 mg/kg/min in critically ill.
Lipids	• Include propofol infusion in lipid sources. • < 1g/kg or 20%–30% of total kcal. • PPN lipid content should not exceed 60% total kcal.
Fluid	• Volume depends on patient tolerance/requirements.
Electrolytes	• Amounts vary per patient tolerance. • Higher requirements may occur with CRRT.
Minerals	
Sodium	40–60 mEq/L
Potassium	10–40 mEq/L
Phosphorus	5–10 mmol/L
Calcium	5–10 mEq/L (Calcium acetate contains less aluminum.)
Magnesium	5–10 mEq/L
Chloride & acetate	Proportions vary depending on acid/base status.
Vitamins	
A	3300 IU/d
D	200 IU/d
E	10 IU/d
K	150 µg/d
C	200 mg/d
Thiamin (B-1)	6 mg/d
Riboflavin (B-2)	3.6 mg/d
Niacin (B-3)	40 mg/d
Pyridoxine (B-6)	6 mg/d
Cyanocobalamin (B-12)	5 µg/d
Folacin	600 µg/d
Pantothenic acid	15 mg/d
Biotin	60 µg/d
Trace Elements	
Zinc	2.5–4 mg/d
Copper	0.5–1.5 mg/d
Chromium	10–15 mg/d
Manganese	0.15–0.8 mg/d
Selenium	40–120 µg/d

Abbreviations: CRRT, continuous renal replacement therapy; IVF, intravenous fluids; PN, parenteral nutrition; PPN, peripheral parenteral nutrition.

Source: Data are from references 1–8.

Table 14.2. Calorie Contribution of Parenteral Nutrition Components

Parenteral Nutrition Component	*kcal/g*	*kcal/mL*
Dextrose	3.4	
70% dextrose		2.38
50% dextrose		1.85
Amino acids	4	
10% amino acids		0.4
15% amino acids		0.6
20% amino acids		0.8
Lipids	10	
10% lipids		1.1
20% lipids		2.0
30% lipids		3.0

Source: Data are from reference 2.

Amino Acids

There is no scientific evidence to support the practice of providing only essential amino acids to patients with kidney disease. Amino acid solutions should contain a mixture of essential and nonessential amino acids (11,12). An imbalance of amino acids can contribute to poor appetite and decreased protein synthesis (13). Prerenal azotemia can occur when a patient is given a high nitrogen load with insufficient energy and fluid (2). The amount of amino acids in PN is determined by the dialysis modality and the patient's comorbidities.

Carnitine is an amino acid involved in fatty acid transport and metabolism. Carnitine status in dialysis patients is negatively impacted by dietary restriction of meat and dairy products, reduced endogenous synthesis by the kidney, and increased loss via dialysis (14,15). Carnitine is not a standard component of PN solutions, and plasma levels have been found to be decreased in surgical patients within 4 weeks of receiving carnitine-free PN (16). Several studies in long-term hemodialysis patients have demonstrated increased serum carnitine levels with supplementation of 1 to 20 mg L-carnitine per kg/day (17–19). Interestingly, in a multicenter trial, carnitine was shown to reduce intradialytic hypotension and muscle cramps, improve exercise capacity and sense of well-being, and possibly improve lean body mass (18,19). The beneficial effects of carnitine seem to extend beyond its role in lipid metabolism.

Dextrose

Dextrose is the primary energy source in PN. Delivery of adequate dextrose to meet energy requirements without precipitating or worsening hyperglycemia can be challenging. Adverse effects of hyperglycemia can include hypercapnia, hepatic steatosis, cholestasis, hypermetabolism, lipogenesis, and immune dysfunction (20,21). Maintaining serum glucose levels within normal limits has been associated with a reduction of mortality, morbidity, polyneuropathy, bacteremia, inflammation, and anemia (22,23). Total glucose provision should not exceed 3 to 5 mg/kg per minute (20,24). To control hyperglycemia, patients with diabetes may need 0.1 units of insulin or more per gram of dextrose in the PN solution. Insulin can be provided as needed either as an insulin drip, subcutaneous injection, or an additive to PN to maintain glycemic control between 100 to 150 mg/dL (25).

Lipids

Lipids are a source of energy and essential fatty acids. Two percent to four percent of total energy as lipid is sufficient to prevent essential fatty acid deficiency (EFAD). Additional lipids can be added to offset the adverse effects of providing a high proportion of total energy as glucose. Thirty percent or less of the total energy as lipid is generally provided in PN. However, lipids are also associated with adverse effects of immunosuppression and hyperlipidemia (26). Serum triglyceride levels should be monitored in patients receiving lipid-containing solutions whether as propofol or as lipid-containing PN. Lipids in PN should be discontinued if serum triglycerides exceed 400 mg/dL during lipid infusion (1). If hypertriglyceridemia persists despite omission of lipids for more than 2 weeks, the patient should receive a minimum of 500 mL of 10% lipid twice per week to prevent EFAD (2).

Lipids also contain vitamin K, phosphorous, and egg phospholipid. The vitamin K content is variable from 0 to 290 μg/L depending on the oils used in the emulsion (27). The international normalized ratio (INR) should be monitored in PN patients receiving anticoagulation therapy. Lipids contain 7.5 mmol phosphate per 500 mL. If a patient develops refractory hyperphosphatemia despite elimination of phosphate as an additive in PN, it may be necessary to discontinue lipids for a day or two. Patients with an egg allergy should not receive lipids.

Although there is a slight risk of a patient experiencing an anaphylactic reaction to lipids, there is no evidence supporting giving the first dose of PN without lipids. If there is a risk of lipid intolerance, a test dose of 1 mL lipid per minute can be given for 15 to 30 minutes. An allergic reaction to lipids may include nausea, vomiting, headache, fever, flushes, sleepiness, pain in the chest and back, slight pressure over the eye, dizziness, and irritation at the infusion site (3).

Potential non-PN Sources of Energy

It is important to consider all potential sources of energy when determining the PN prescription. Carbohydrate sources of calories include intravenous fluids (IVF), medications, and renal replacement therapy (RRT) modalities, particularly hemodiafiltration and peritoneal dialysis. Propofol, a sedative used in the intensive care unit (ICU), is mixed in a 10% lipid solution that provides 1.1 kcal lipid/mL. Blood products and albumin infusions are additional sources of nitrogen and protein. However, the consistency of the provision of additional calories and protein must be considered before adjusting the PN. Often, medications, IVF, and blood product infusions are a temporary source of nutrients and do not have a significant impact on overall delivery of nutrition.

Fluid, Electrolytes, and Minerals

The volume of PN provided will be determined by the fluid allowance, urine and stool output, and total fluid volume required for medication and electrolyte management. Serum sodium levels often reflect hydration status rather than sodium status. The patient's clinical status and potential sources and losses of fluid and sodium must be determined before adjusting the PN solution.

Electrolyte and mineral metabolism is altered with renal failure. Serum phosphorus, potassium, and magnesium serum levels can increase as renal function declines. Phosphorus is not well dialyzed and often requires restriction in the PN solution to control serum phosphorus levels. Table 14.1 lists the amounts of electrolytes commonly added to PN for patients with renal failure. The amounts of electrolytes added to PN should be individualized to meet the patient's needs.

Acid-Base Balance

Acid-base balance can be managed to some extent with PN. Bicarbonate cannot be added to the PN because it can form insoluble calcium and magnesium salts within the solution (28). Acetate is added to PN solutions and is quickly metabolized to bicarbonate by the liver. Patients with metabolic acidosis may require an increased proportion of acetate to chloride. However, the absolute amount of acetate and chloride that can be added to PN solutions depends on the amount of sodium and potassium added because chloride and acetate are given as sodium and potassium salts.

Vitamins and Trace Elements

Micronutrient losses occur with acute and chronic dialysis (29). Water-soluble vitamins lost during dialysis are generally replaced with an oral vitamin B complex plus vitamin C supplement in the chronic dialysis patient. Vitamins A, D, and B-12 are protein-bound with lesser amounts lost during dialysis (29). As with any patient population, suspected and documented vitamin deficiencies and excesses should be treated accordingly. Standard dosages of multivitamins for PN as established by the American Medical Association Nutrition Advisory Committee and amended in 2000 are recommended for patients with CKD and for patients with ARF (Table 14.1) (4,5). The current injectable adult multivitamin preparation contains 150 μg vitamin K. The combined vitamin K content of the injectable multivitamin and the lipid solution is within the recommendation of 2 to 4 mg vitamin K per week (30). It is important to monitor patients for potential coagulopathy during PN infusion containing vitamin K.

Injectable multivitamins contain vitamin A. Vitamin A is not a component of oral vitamin supplements for patients with CKD and is indirectly restricted in the renal diet through the limitation of fruit and vegetable intake. In the short term, there is minimal risk of vitamin A toxicity with a daily injectable multivitamin because, in all likelihood, the patient on PN is not consuming an oral diet. Therefore, the injectable multivitamin is the only exogenous source of vitamin A. However, patients on long-term PN should be monitored for potential vitamin A toxicity (6).

Trace elements are protein bound, which reduces loss with dialytic therapy. Chromium, molybdenum, and selenium are primarily excreted in the urine (31);

therefore, losses are less in patients who are oliguric and anuric. CKD patients on PN should receive a daily trace element preparation (7). Iron is not a component of standard trace element preparations. The compatibility of iron dextran with lipid-containing PN is controversial. The addition of iron dextran once weekly to lipid-free PN may help prevent iron-deficiency anemia (2). Patients should receive a test dose of iron dextran before it is added to PN. There is concern that iron supplementation could stimulate microorganism proliferation, especially in patients with infections (32). The incorporation of less antigenic iron products such as iron sucrose and iron gluconate in PN has not been studied.

Administration of Parenteral Nutrition

PN should be initiated with a modest amount of calories and the full amount of protein to meet the patient's estimated protein needs. Infusion of 1,000 to 1,200 kcal containing 200 to 250 g of dextrose for the first 24 hours allows the clinician to identify tolerance to the PN components and manage potential shifts in fluid and electrolytes with introduction of PN (2). Another option is to limit the initial PN infusion to 1 L of solution with a proportional distribution of total calories as dextrose (50%), lipid (30%), and amino acids (20%). Laboratory abnormalities should be corrected before increasing to the caloric goal.

PN can be discontinued when the patient is able to meet 60% of estimated energy requirements from tube feeding or oral diet (33). Discontinue PN by reducing the rate by half for 1 hour before stopping the infusion. Although there have been reports of patient tolerance of abrupt discontinuation of PN, there is always the risk of rebound hypoglycemia in susceptible patients. Tapering the PN infusion can be beneficial in preventing rebound hypoglycemia (33–37). If PN infusion is stopped abruptly, consider providing 10% dextrose at half the previous PN infusion rate to prevent potential rebound hypoglycemia until PN can be resumed.

Monitoring Patients on Parenteral Nutrition

Table 14.3 provides guidelines for monitoring patients while they receive PN therapy (2,6,38). Parameters should be monitored more often in patients who are sicker and more unstable. Depending on the patient's comorbidities and other metabolic and physical problems and therapies, other parameters may need to be followed in addition to those listed. Long-term complications of PN include biliary disease, catheter-related infections, hyperoxaluria, hepatic disease, intestinal hypoplasia, and metabolic bone disease. Long-term PN therapy complications are addressed elsewhere (2,39).

Because aluminum is excreted by the kidneys, patients with renal failure should be monitored for potential aluminum toxicity (31). Sources of aluminum include medications, such as antacids, phosphate binders, and sucralfate, IVF, and PN components (40,41). Calcium and phosphate salts are major sources of aluminum in PN. It is important to be aware of all potential sources of aluminum and to minimize the total amount given to the patient. Effective July 26, 2004, all small and large volume parenteral nutrition products must provide the aluminum content on the label (42–44). The amount of aluminum listed on the label will be the maximum amount in the parenteral product at expiration.

ACUTE RENAL FAILURE

Nutrition management of the patient with ARF focuses on the underlying disease or injury with consideration given to the impact of the reduction or loss of renal function. Patients who develop ARF often present with a multitude of comorbidities, such as trauma, sepsis, cardiovascular disease, liver disease, and multisystem organ failure. Malnutrition negatively impacts renal function (45) and has been reported to increase mortality, morbidity and health care costs (46). Hemodynamic instability, impaired GI motility, volume overload, and oliguria contribute to difficulties providing consistent and adequate nutrition support.

Despite improvements in intensive care medical management, the mortality rate for patients requiring dialysis for ARF has been reported to range from 10% to 50% (47) and as high as 40% to 80% (48,49). Mortality is higher for patients with ARF in an ICU (72%) than those on a standard hospital floor (32%) (50).

Malnutrition in Acute Renal Failure

As stated previously, severe malnutrition has been linked to increased mortality in patients who develop ARF (46). The extent of preexisting malnutrition and risk of iatrogenic malnutrition are dependent on the duration and severity of the underlying disease and adequacy of nutrition. During times of severe metabolic

Table 14.3. Guidelines for Monitoring Patients on Parenteral Nutrition

Parameter	*Acute PN*	*Chronic PN*	*IDPN*	*IPN*
Weight	Daily	Every dialysis	Every dialysis	Daily
Intake and output	Daily	Daily	Daily	Daily
Appetite changes	Daily if consuming oral diet	Weekly if consuming oral diet	Weekly	Weekly
Diet records	Not applicable	Every 3–6 mo, if consuming oral diet	Every 3–6 mo	Every 3–6 mo
Subjective Global Assessment	Daily	Every 6 mo	Every 6 mo	Every 6 mo
Anthropometrics	Not applicable	Monthly	Monthly	Monthly
BUN/electrolytes	Daily until stable, then 2–3 times per week	Monthly	Every dialysis until stable, then monthly	Monthly
Calcium, phosphorus, magnesium	Daily until stable, then 2–3 times per week	Long-term—monthly	Every dialysis until stable, then monthly	Monthly
Glucose	Initially 4–6 times per day and then as needed according to glycemic control	Weekly (more often with insulin therapy and hyperglycemia). Long-term—monthly	Prior to, during, and following treatment	Daily
Triglycerides	Initially and then weekly	Monthly	6 hours after first treatment then monthly	Monthly
Liver enzymes and bilirubin	Initially and then weekly	Monthly	Monthly	Monthly
CBC*	Daily until stable, then 2–3 times per week.	Monthly	Monthly	Monthly
Vitamin D, calcium, phosphorus, aluminum, and PTH†	Not applicable	Monthly	Monthly	Monthly
Hepatic proteins	Weekly	Monthly	Monthly	Monthly

Abbreviations: BUN, blood urea nitrogen; CBC, complete blood count; IDPN, intradialytic parenteral nutrition; IPN, intraperitoneal parenteral nutrition; PN, parenteral nutrition; PTH, parathyroid hormone.

*Monitor for catheter-related infections and anemia.

†Monitor for metabolic bone disease.

Source: Data are from references 2,6,38.

stress, nutrient provision is often nil or sorely inadequate. Inadequate and inconsistent provision of nutrients contributes to poor wound healing, decreased immunocompetence, and catabolism of lean body mass.

Nutrition support can help sustain the patient during dialytic, medical, and surgical treatment in order to support recovery. The route of nutrition support is selected based on the GI function of the patient. A study by Fiaccadori et al found that enteral nutrition, although often problematic, provided adequate nutrients to acutely ill renal failure patients (51). The indications for PN for patients with ARF are the same as for other critically ill patients (1).

Nutrient Requirements and Components of PN in ARF

Nutrient requirements are primarily determined by the type and severity of the underlying disease, preexisting nutritional status, and type of dialytic therapy (52–54). Tables 14.1 and 14.3 provide general guidelines for providing PN and monitoring PN patients with ARF. The most concentrated source of dextrose, amino acids, and lipids should be used to maximize calories in a limited total volume. Estimated energy and protein requirements in critically ill patients with ARF on continuous renal replacement therapy (CRRT) range from

25 to 35 kcal/kg per day and from 1.5 to 2.0 g protein/kg per day, respectively (8). Requirements should be estimated using edema-free weight. Recent research indicates that this protein recommendation may be controversial and the clinician must carefully evaluate and monitor the patient. (See Chapter 4 for further information and discussion on CRRT.)

Amino Acids

The additional requirement for conditionally essential amino acids along with aberrations of amino acid metabolism during critical illness necessitates the infusion of essential and nonessential amino acids in patients with ARF (55). ARF and critical illness contribute to accelerated muscle catabolism and ineffective use of amino acids for protein synthesis, resulting in negative nitrogen balance. Protein requirements can range from 1.0 to 2.0 g/kg depending on the extent of injury and illness and provision of and type of dialytic therapy. Protein losses vary with the type of renal replacement therapy: 4 to 13 g/treatment (HD) (56); 5 to 10 g/day (PD) (57); 9 to 14 g/day (CRRT) (58). In the absence of RRT, noncatabolic patients should receive approximately 1 g protein per kg dry body weight (57). Despite aggressive provision of nutrition support, negative nitrogen balance and protein catabolism often persist in patients with ARF. Excessive protein provision may increase urea and nitrogenous waste production, resulting in worsening uremia and increasing dialysis requirements (59).

The synthesis, retention, and availability of carnitine may be impaired in the patient with ARF on dialysis receiving PN for longer than 1 month. However, studies are lacking about the short-term effect of ARF on carnitine status, and there are currently no established recommendations for supplementation of carnitine in PN for ARF patients.

Carbohydrate

Nutrient requirement is not synonymous with nutrient tolerance. Hyperglycemia, a problem in critically ill patients, can be aggravated by concomitant ARF. Increased gluconeogenesis, insulin resistance, and glucose uptake from dialysate along with decreased insulin clearance, decreased responsiveness to insulin, and decreased glycogen synthesis impact glycemic control (20,53,60). Serum glucose levels should be less than 200mg/dL during initiation of PN and less than 150 mg/dL after a stable PN solution and infusion rate has been established (25).

The use of dianeal as the osmotic gradient in CRRT results in uptake of glucose (288 to 316 g/24 hours) and increased serum glucose levels (135 to 278 mg/dL) (20,61). Figure 14.1 provides calculations that can be used to estimate glucose uptake during CRRT when dianeal is used (62,63). Lactate can also provide a metabolic fuel (25 mL/minute provides 500 kcal/day) (64). These additional sources of energy can complicate glycemic control in critically ill patients with ARF. PN solutions may need to be adjusted to compensate for the increased energy load.

Lipid

Lipid metabolism is adversely affected by critical illness and ARF (65). ARF impairs lipolysis with a resulting increase in serum triglycerides and a reduction in serum cholesterol, particularly high-density lipoprotein (HDL) cholesterol. Trauma patients given hypocaloric PN without lipids (27 kcal/kg) had fewer nosocomial infections and a shorter ICU stay than those given PN with lipids (34 kcal/kg) (66). It remains unclear if the absence of lipids, the avoidance of overfeeding, or the combination of the two resulted in better outcomes. Lipid infusion in the critically ill ARF patient should be less than 1 g/kg per day (every 500 mL lipid contains 100 g fat) (2).

Fluid

Fluid management often becomes the focus of patient management in ARF. This can result in the need to restrict PN solutions to 1,000 to 1,500 mL per day (6). The need for this severe of a volume restriction is often short term until ARF resolves or dialysis is initiated. CRRT permits adequate provision of nutrients without fluid volume limitations. Urine output as well as the patient's overall intake and output should be closely monitored.

Electrolytes and Minerals

Electrolyte and major mineral requirements will be impacted by the underlying disease, urine output, and type of dialytic therapy. Adjustments in PN should be based on the etiology of the derangement and not simply on serum levels. Provision of potassium, magnesium, and phosphorus in PN is often limited with

Formula 1:

Dialysate Flow Rate (mL/hr) × 24 h
× Dialysate Glucose (g/mL) × 3.4 kcal/g Dextrose
× % Uptake

Example 1 43% uptake with 1.5% dialysate at 999 mL/h

999 mL/h × 24 h × 0.015 g/mL × 3.4 kcal/g dextrose
× 0.43 = 526 kcal/24 h

Example 2 45% uptake with 2.5% dialysate at 999 mL/h

999 mL/h × 24 h × 0.025 g/mL × 3.4 kcal/g dextrose
× 0.45 = 917 kcal/24 h

Formula 2:

$Glucose_{added} = (Glucose_{in} - Glucose_{out}) \times BFR \times k$

Where: $Glucose_{added}$ is quantity (g/d) of glucose absorbed across dialysis membrane; $Glucose_{in}$ is serum glucose level (mg/dL) in blood returning to patient; $Glucose_{out}$ is serum glucose level (mg/dL) of blood coming from patient to dialyzer; BFR is blood flow rate (200 mL/min) through the dialysis cartridge; k is conversion factor (0.0144).

Example $Glucose_{in}$, 369 mg/dL; $Glucose_{out}$, 317 mg/dL; BFR, 200 mL/min

$Glucose_{added} = (369 - 317) \times 200 \times 0.0144 = 150$ g/day

---

Figure 14.1. Two formulas for determining energy (kcal) provision from dianeal. Formula 2 adapted from reference 62; reprinted with permission from the American Society for Parenteral and Enteral Nutrition (ASPEN) from the following: *Nutrition in Clinical Practice* (NCP); V. 14; No. 3; p.121; Adjustment of nutrition support with continuous hemodiafiltration in a critically ill patient. ASPEN does not endorse the use of this material in any form other than its entirety.

ARF, but with CRRT patients may require supplementation to maintain electrolyte and mineral balance.

Hypocalcemia with decreased serum ionized calcium occurs with elevated calcitonin levels during ARF and sepsis. Provision of supplemental calcium in a patient with hyperphosphatemia increases the risk of precipitation of calcium phosphate in the blood with subsequent deposition of calcium phosphate crystals in soft tissue. The risk of precipitating calcium phosphate within the PN solution places limits on the amounts of calcium and phosphate that can be safely added to PN. Patients with ARF on CRRT may require supplementation of magnesium and calcium beyond that which can be safely added to PN (67). In this case, supplemental electrolytes and minerals should be provided orally or IV as needed.

Metabolic acidosis causes impaired protein metabolism and contributes to muscle wasting and catabolism in ARF (68,69). Patients often require a higher proportion of acetate salts compared to chloride salts in the PN. Treatment of metabolic acidosis may require the provision of sodium bicarbonate as a separate IV infusion. Hyperkalemia associated with metabolic acidosis will correct with treatment with acetate and bicarbonate. If the patient is hypokalemic with metabolic acidosis, correction of acidosis should include potassium supplementation.

Vitamins and Trace Elements

Vitamin and mineral issues can become complex in the patient with ARF. Metabolic derangements that occur with ARF may compromise nutrient adequacy, availability, and use (70). The inflammatory process and certain medications can contribute to increased requirements for vitamins A, C, E, and folate (70). Patients with ARF are at risk for deficiencies of fat-soluble vitamins, with the notable exception of vitamin K (71). Critically ill patients with and without CRRT were found to have reduced serum levels of vitamins C and E, selenium, and zinc (72). Critically ill patients seem to have increased selenium requirements, but recommendations for supplementation are inconclusive (72,73). The amount of zinc in standard PN trace element preparations seems adequate to compensate for zinc losses with CRRT (67). The standard PN preparations of vitamins and trace elements are currently recommended for patients with ARF (Table 14.2) (4,5,7).

As mentioned previously, iron can be added to non-lipid-containing PN. However, it is important to note that critically ill patients sequester free iron in ferritin and reduce its availability for microorganism proliferation. Supplementation of iron could increase the risk of infection in susceptible patients (32,73). Critically ill patients with ARF are at risk for hemosiderosis because of multiple blood product transfusions and decreased erythropoiesis (32). Therefore iron supplementation should be reserved for critically ill patients with a suspected or documented iron-deficiency anemia.

CHRONIC KIDNEY DISEASE

As with ARF, patients with CKD may require PN if they are unable to tolerate adequate amounts of nutrients enterally. Micronutrient composition of the PN solution should be individualized based on the patient's requirements and tolerances. In most cases, patients receive the standard multivitamin and trace element preparations (4,5,7). Table 14.1 provides general guidelines for PN composition for patients with CKD.

Table 14.3 provides guidelines for monitoring patients on PN. Monitoring should be done routinely and serially so that changes in the various parameters can be noted and adjustments made in the PN solution. Parameters must be checked more often for the critically ill patient than for the stable patient.

PERIPHERAL PARENTERAL NUTRITION

Peripheral parenteral nutrition (PPN) is infused via a peripheral vein and is generally recommended for no longer than 14 days. Peripheral vein infusions are limited to 700 to 900 mOsm/L (74). This limits the amount of hypertonic solutions, such as dextrose and amino acids, that can be given peripherally. Lipids are fairly isotonic and provide approximately 50% to 60% of total calories in PPN. The American Society for Parenteral and Enteral Nutrition recommends that lipids provide no more than 60% of total calories (1). Lipids should be restricted to less than 30% of total calories in patients with an inflammatory process (1). Chronic dialysis is associated with an inflammatory process and may indicate the need to reduce total fat provided in PN (75,76). Sterile water is used as a component of PPN to dilute the osmolality of the dextrose and amino acids. This can result in a final volume of 2 to 3 L per day. The large volume, high fat content, and inadequate energy and protein content limit the usefulness of PPN for patients with either ARF or CKD.

INTRADIALYTIC PARENTERAL NUTRITION

Intradialytic parenteral nutrition (IDPN) is the provision of nutrients through the venous drip chamber of the hemodialysis machine. Components of IDPN formulations are shown in Table 14.4 (77). Vitamins and trace elements are not usually added to IDPN because the additives could be lost in the dialysate. However, vitamins can be added during the last 30 minutes of IDPN if the patient does not tolerate oral multivitamin supplementation. IDPN alone is insufficient to meet the estimated energy and protein requirements of the patient, but it does enable the clinician to provide a consistent amount of energy and protein with each dialysis session as a supplement to the patient's enteral intake. Criteria used to justify the use of IDPN in hemodialysis patients include chronic GI problems such as nausea, vomiting, diarrhea, and anorexia; weight loss of 10% to 15% over 6 months; a weight of less than 90% of ideal body weight; triceps skinfold values less than 6 mm (males), less than 12 mm (females); serum albumin of 3.4 g/L or less; and a protein catabolic rate less than 0.8 g/kg/day (3,78). According to the 2000 National Kidney Foundation Kidney Disease Outcomes Quality Initiative (K/DOQI), IDPN may be beneficial in patients who are malnourished or unable to consume adequate energy and protein to meet nutrient requirements, who are unable to tolerate oral feedings or tube feedings, and who are able to meet their needs with the combination of oral or tube feeding intake plus IDPN (38).

Administration and Management of IDPN

Amino Acids

As with all PN formulations given to patients with CKD, IDPN should contain an amino acid formulation that contains essential and nonessential amino acids. The amount of amino acids that can be given will depend on the total volume to be infused. However, a 15% amino acid solution enables the clinician to provide 75 g of protein in 500 mL.

Dextrose

Glycemic control is a major concern with infusion of IDPN. Patients often require insulin in the PN bag as well as subcutaneously. Peripheral glucose should be checked prior to starting IDPN and hourly during infusion, with insulin given as needed to main-

Table 14.4. Types of Intradialytic Parenteral Nutrition Solution

Characteristics	*Prescription*	*Total Volume*	*Formula Composition*	*kcal*
Lipid-free	250 mL D_{50} 250 mL 10% AA	500 mL	125 g dextrose 25 g protein	525
Increased kcal, higher protein, with lipids	250 mL D_{50} 550 mL 10% AA 250 mL 20% lipid	1050 mL	125 g dextrose 55 g protein 50 g fat	1145
High protein, lipid free	500 mL D_{50} 550 mL 10% AA	1050 mL	250 g dextrose 55 g protein	1070
High protein, lipid free, limited volume	250 mL D_{50} 550 mL 10% AA	800 mL	125 g dextrose 55 g protein	815
High protein, high kcal (use D_{70} to limit volume)	250 mL D_{70} 500 mL 15% AA 250 mL 20% lipid	1000 mL	175 g dextrose 75 g protein 50 g fat	1395

Abbreviations: AA, amino acids; D_{50}, 50% dextrose; D_{70}, 70% dextrose.

Source: Reprinted from Malnutrition in chronic kidney disease. In: McCann L, ed. *Pocket Guide to Nutrition Assessment of the Patient With Chronic Kidney Disease.* 3rd ed. New York, NY: National Kidney Foundation; 2002:9–17; with permission from the National Kidney Foundation.

tain serum glucose levels less than 200 mg/dL (25). The amount of glucose infused over 24 hours should be 3 to 5 mg/kg per minute or less to maintain glycemic control and avoid exceeding the oxidative capacity of the liver to metabolize glucose (24). Insulin therapy with 5 units of regular insulin per 1,000 mL of IDPN has been recommended when serum glucose levels exceed 300 mg/dL (3). Insulin can be increased by 2 units for each treatment until satisfactory glycemic control is achieved (3).

The recent evidence of reduced mortality and morbidity with serum glucose levels less than 110 mg/dL during PN suggests the importance of maintaining tight glycemic control (22,23). It is currently unknown what the adverse effects are of maintaining hyperglycemia for 3 to 4 hours during dialysis three times per week in a patient with CKD and its associated comorbidities. However, the impact of tight glycemic control in IDPN has not been studied, and there is concern that tight glycemic control in CKD patients could increase the risk of lethal hypoglycemia (79).

Infusion of glucose can promote an intracellular shift of electrolytes. Serum levels of potassium, magnesium, and phosphorus should be monitored. One hour after stopping IDPN infusion, the patient's peripheral glucose level should be rechecked to monitor for potential rebound hypoglycemia. If the patient can consume oral nutrients, a snack should be provided.

Lipid

Hyperlipidemia during IDPN infusion can also be problematic in the hemodialysis patient. Lipid provision is often maximized, but lipid infusion should not exceed 2.5 g/kg per day or provide more than 60% of total calories (3). Serum triglycerides should be monitored prior to the first infusion and again 6 to 24 hours after the first infusion to determine adequacy of lipid clearance. A serum triglyceride level more than 250 mg/dL 6 hours after the infusion is completed indicates poor lipid clearance. Some clinicians defer the addition of lipids in IDPN for the first week of therapy to determine overall tolerance to PN without the confounding factor of lipid intolerance or an anaphylactic lipid reaction. Allergic reactions to lipids include nausea, vomiting, headache, fever, flushing, sleeplessness, back and chest pain, slight pressure over the eye, dizziness, and irritation at the site of infusion.

Infusion and Monitoring of IDPN

There are no definitive guidelines about how to initiate IDPN. It is generally safe to start with about half the goal volume and 25 to 55 g protein, and progress to goal depending on glycemic control and patient tolerance of the infusion. Predialysis electrolytes, magnesium, and phosphorus as well as peripheral glucose levels and serum triglyceride levels should be monitored while the patient is being treated with IDPN. Table 14.3 provides guidelines for monitoring patients while providing IDPN. The frequency of monitoring and the parameters to follow will depend on each patient's metabolic condition and comorbidities. The company providing the IDPN may also provide monitoring and administration guidelines.

Therapeutic Benefit and Cost-Effectiveness of IDPN

IDPN has been reported to improve weight, appetite, and survival in malnourished hemodialysis patients (13,80–82). However, studies have not examined if similar results could be achieved with intensive dietary counseling in conjunction with oral diet or tube feeding. There is also debate about the parameters used to determine the presence of malnutrition and the impact of nutrition intervention in the dialysis population. Serum hepatic proteins and body weight are affected by factors other than nutrition that could skew interpretation of the patient's nutritional status and the effect of IDPN (53,83).

An evidence-based analysis of the effectiveness of IDPN demonstrated that all but one of the studies supporting the efficacy of IDPN are level "C" data, meaning the research studies were not well designed, randomized, or controlled (84). This means that support for IDPN is primarily based on expert opinion and editorial consensus rather than strong scientific evidence. The cost of IDPN has been estimated at $30,000 per year per patient (84). Coupling this with the 3 to 9 months it may take to see any benefit of treatment as well as the number of patients that would be needed to demonstrate a measurable benefit of IDPN, the cost of producing the evidence becomes staggering.

Current reimbursement criteria for IDPN under the Centers for Medicare and Medicaid Services is identical to coverage for PN (85). Few dialysis patients meet the criteria required; therefore, third-party reimbursement for the costs of IDPN is limited. Overall, there is insufficient evidence to promote widespread use of IDPN in patients with CKD (84). According to the ASPEN 2002 Clinical Guidelines, IDPN should only be given when the patient experiences GI failure or another unusual circumstance in which PN and enteral nutrition are not feasible (1).

INTRAPERITONEAL PARENTERAL NUTRITION

Nutrient losses via the peritoneal membrane during peritoneal dialysis are greater than losses that occur during hemodialysis. In 1980, the peritoneal cavity was successfully used as an "artificial gut" for absorption of glucose, amino acids, and lipids (86). Glucose and amino acids were better absorbed via the peritoneal membrane than lipids. Most of the current research on intraperitoneal parenteral nutrition (IPN) focuses on the use of amino acids in place of glucose as the osmotic gradient during peritoneal dialysis. The amino acids serve not only as a dialysate to cleanse the blood of toxins, but also as a way to counter the loss of 5 to 15 g of amino acids per day through the peritoneal membrane. The substitution of a 1.1% weight/volume concentration of amino acids for one to two glucose exchanges per day can also reduce the absorption of excess calories from the glucose dialysate. This could potentially reduce adverse effects caused by hyperglycemia in patients with diabetes mellitus and hypertriglyceridemia (87). Commercially available amino acid solutions have also been developed that contain primarily essential amino acids with specific nonessential amino acids known to be conditionally essential in peritoneal dialysis patients (88). According to the K/DOQI guidelines, IPN is indicated for patients who are malnourished and consume inadequate energy and protein, who cannot tolerate adequate oral diet or tube feeding to meet estimated needs, who can meet their needs with the combination of IPN plus oral diet or tube feeding, and who have difficulty with glycemic and lipid control related to carbohydrate content of the dialysate (38).

Formulas and Administration of IPN

Amino acid solutions of 1.1% and 2% weight/volume have been used for IPN. Two liters of an amino acid solution are used in place of one or two glucose exchanges per day. It is important for the patient and caregiver to be trained in aseptic technique when handling the amino acid solutions. Ideally, the IPN should be supplied by a company with personnel familiar with the composition and administration of IPN. Table 14.3 provides guidelines for monitoring patients while receiving IPN. The clinical status and comorbidities of each patient will dictate if any additional parameters should be routinely followed.

Effectiveness of IPN

Studies have shown improvement in nitrogen balance (89,90), weight (90), anthropometrics (91), hepatic protein levels (86–90), lipid levels (90,92), and amino acid profile (89–91,93) with IPN. The ultrafiltration effect of a 1% weight/volume amino acid solution has been reported to be equivalent to 1.5% to 2.5% dextrose solution (3). A reduction in serum phosphorus and potassium levels have also been reported with IPN (91). Jones et al compared the amino acids provided in the dialysate with the amino acids and protein lost in the peritoneal dialysate effluent in 20 hospitalized peritoneal dialysis patients (94). Replacement of one glucose exchange with an amino acid solution resulted in a net gain of amino acids (absorption > losses) over 24 hours (94). However, using an amino acid solution for peritoneal dialysis is also associated with an increased risk of metabolic acidosis that could increase protein catabolism in patients with renal failure (89–93). A study by Young et al demonstrated only modest nutritional benefit when eight patients had one glucose exchange per day substituted with amino acids for 12 weeks (92). As with IDPN, insurance reimbursement is problematic and evidence-based recommendations are currently not available.

CONCLUSION

The burdens of PN must be weighed against potential benefits. ARF patients and CKD patients must be closely monitored to reduce the risk of complications associated with PN infusion. It is important to analyze the desired outcomes vs those achievable by PN support modalities. PN should be reserved for the renal failure patient unable to receive sufficient nutrients enterally, either orally or by feeding tube, to maintain weight and functional status.

REFERENCES

1. ASPEN Board of Directors and The Clinical Guidelines Task Force. Guidelines for the use of parenteral and enteral nutrition in adult and pediatric patients. *JPEN J Parenter Enteral Nutr.* 2002;26(suppl):1SA–138SA.
2. Fuhrman MP. Complication management in parenteral nutrition. In: Matarese LE, Gottschlich MM, eds. *Contemporary Nutrition Support Practice: A Clinical Guide.* 2nd ed. Philadelphia, Pa: WB Saunders Co; 2003;242–262.
3. American Dietetic Association. *A Clinical Guide to Nutrition Care in End-Stage Renal Disease.* 2nd ed. Chicago, Ill: American Dietetic Association; 1994.
4. American Medical Association Department of Foods and Nutrition. Multivitamin preparation for parenteral use: a statement by the Nutrition Advisory Group. *JPEN J Parenter Enteral Nutr.* 1979;3:258–262.
5. Parenteral multivitamin products; drugs for human use; drug efficacy study implementation amendment. 65 *Federal Register* 21200–21201 (2000) (codified at 21 CFR §5.70).
6. Wolk R. Nutrition in renal failure. In: Gottschlich MM, ed. *The Science and Practice of Nutrition Support: A Case-Based Core Curriculum.* Dubuque, Iowa: Kendall/Hunt Publishing; 2001: 575–599.
7. Expert Panel for Nutrition Advisory Group, American Medical Association Department of Foods and Nutrition. Guidelines for essential trace element preparations for parenteral use. *JAMA.* 1979;241:2051–2054.
8. Macias WL, Alaka KJ, Murphy MH, Miller ME, Clark WR, Mueller BA. Impact of the nutritional regiment on protein catabolism and nitrogen balance in patients with acute renal failure. *JPEN J Parenter Enteral Nutr.* 1996;20:56–62.
9. Miles J, Klein JA. Should protein be included in calorie calculations for a TPN prescription? Point-counterpoint. *Nutr Clin Pract.* 1996;11:204–206.
10. Van Way CW III. Total calories vs nonprotein calories. *Nutr Clin Pract.* 2001;16:271–273.
11. Feinstein EI, Blumenkrantz MJ, Healy M, Koffler A, Silberman H, Massey SG, Kopple JD. Clinical and metabolic response to parenteral nutrition in acute renal failure: a controlled double blind study. *Medicine.* 1981;60:124–137.
12. Piraino AJ, Firpo JJ, Powers DV. Prolonged hyperalimentation in catabolic chronic dialysis therapy patients. *JPEN J Parenter Enteral Nutr.* 1981;5:463–477.
13. Powers DV, Jackson A, Piraino AJ. Prolonged intradialysis hyperalimentation in chronic hemodialysis patients with an amino acid solution (RenAmin [amino acid] injection) formulated for renal failure. In: Kinney JM, Borum PR, eds. *Perspectives in Clinical Nutrition.* Baltimore, Md: Urban & Schwarzenberg; 1989:191–205.

14. Bartel LL, Hussey JL, Shrago E. Perturbation of serum carnitine levels in human adults by chronic renal disease and dialysis therapy. *Am J Clin Nutr*. 1981;34:1314–1320.
15. Evans AM, Faull R, Fornasini G, Lemanowicz EF, Longo A, Pace S, Nation RL. Pharmacokinetics of L-carnitine in patients with end-stage renal disease undergoing long-term hemodialysis. *Clin Pharmacol Ther*. 2000;68:238–249.
16. Hahn P, Allardyce DB, Frohlich J. Plasma carnitine levels during total parenteral nutrition of adult surgical patients. *Am J Clin Nutr*. 1982;36: 569–572.
17. Wanner W, Wackerle B, Boeckle H, Schollmeyer P, Horl WH. Plasma and red blood cell carnitine and carnitine esters during L-carnitine therapy in hemodialysis patients. *Am J Clin Nutr*. 1990;51: 407–410.
18. Golper TA, Wolfson M, Ahmad S, Hirschberg R, Kurtin P, Katz LA, Nicora R, Ashbrook D, Kopple JD. Multicenter trial of L-carnitine in maintenance hemodialysis patients, I. Carnitine concentrations and lipid effects. *Kidney Int*. 1990;38: 904–911.
19. Ahmad S, Robertson HT, Golper TA, Wolfson M, Kurtin P, Katz LA, Hirschberg R, Nicora R, Ashbrook DW, Kopple JD. Multicenter trial of L-carnitine in maintenance hemodialysis patients, II. Clinical and biochemical effects. *Kidney Int*. 1990;38:912–918.
20. Frankenfield DC, Reynolds HN, Badelino MM, Wiles CE III. Glucose dynamics during continuous hemodiafiltration and total parenteral nutrition. *Intensive Care Med*. 1995;21:1016–1022.
21. Bistrian BR. Hyperglycemia and infection: Which is the chicken and which is the egg? [editorial] *JPEN J Parenter Enteral Nutr*. 2001;25: 180–181.
22. van den Bergh G, Wouters PJ, Weekers F, Verwaest C, Bruyninckx F, Schetz M, Vlasselaers D, Ferdinande P, Lauwers P, Bouillion R. Intensive insulin therapy in critically ill patients. *N Engl J Med*. 2001;345:1359–1367.
23. van den Bergh G, Wouters PJ, Bouillion R, Weekers F, Verwaest C, Schetz M, Vlasselaers D, Ferdinande P, Lauwers P. Outcome benefit of intensive insulin therapy in the critically ill: insulin dose versus glycemic control. *Crit Care Med*. 2003;31:359–366.
24. Wolfe RR, O'Donnell TF Jr, Stone MD, Richmand DA, Burke JF. Investigation of factors determining the optimal glucose infusion rate in total parenteral nutrition. *Metabolism*. 1980;29: 892–900.
25. American Gastroenterological Association Clinical Practice and Practice Economics Committee. AGA technical review on parenteral nutrition. *Gastroenterol*. 2001;121:970–1001.
26. Gottschlich MM. Selection of optimal lipid sources in enteral and parenteral nutrition. *Nutr Clin Pract*. 1992;7:152–165.
27. Chambrier C, Leclercq M, Saudin F, Vignal B, Bryssine S, Guillaumont M, Bouletreau P. Is vitamin K supplementation necessary in long-term parenteral nutrition? *JPEN J Parenter Enteral Nutr*. 1998;22:87–90.
28. Matarese LE. Metabolic complications of parenteral nutrition therapy. In: Gottschlich MM, ed. *The Science and Practice of Nutrition Support: A Case-Based Core Curriculum*. Dubuque, Iowa: Kendall/Hunt Publishing; 2001:269–286.
29. Wolk R. Micronutrition in dialysis. *Nutr Clin Pract*. 1993;8:267–276.
30. National Advisory Group on Standards and Practice Guidelines for Parenteral Nutrition. Safe practices for parenteral nutrition formulations. *JPEN J Parenter Enteral Nutr.* 1998;22:49–66.
31. DeBiasse-Fortin MA. Minerals and trace elements. In: Matarese LE, Gottschlich MM, eds. *Contemporary Nutrition Support Practice: A Clinical Guide*. 2nd ed. Philadelphia, Pa: WB Saunders Co; 2003;164–172.
32. Burns DL, Mascioli EA, Bistrian BR. Parenteral iron dextran therapy: a review. *Nutrition*. 1995; 11:163–168.
33. Skipper A, Millikan KW. Parenteral nutrition implementation and management. In. American Society for Parenteral and Enteral Nutrition Board of Directors, ed. *ASPEN Nutrition Support Manual*. Silver Spring, Md: ASPEN; 1998:1–9.
34. Eisenberg PG, Gianino S, Clutter WE, Fleshman JW. Abrupt disconnection of cycled parenteral nutrition is safe. *Dis Colon Rectum*. 1995;38: 933–939.
35. Dudrick SJ, MacFadyn BV, Van Buren CT, Ruberg RL, Maynard AT. Parenteral hyperalimentation: metabolic problems and solutions. *Ann Surg*. 1972;176:259–264.

36. Wagman LD, Newsome HH, Miller KB, Thomas RB, Weir GC. The effect of acute discontinuation of total parenteral nutrition. *Ann Surg.* 1988;204: 524–530.
37. Krzywda EA, Andris DA, Whipple JK, Street CC, Ausman RK, Schulte WJ, Quebbeman EJ. Glucose response to abrupt initiation and discontinuation of total parenteral nutrition. *JPEN J Parenter Enteral Nutr.* 1993;17:64–67.
38. National Kidney Foundation. K/DOQI Clinical practice guidelines for nutrition in chronic renal failure. *Am J Kidney Dis.* 2000;35(suppl):S1–S104.
39. Buchman AL. Complications of long-term home total parenteral nutrition. *Dig Dis Sci.* 2001;46: 1–18.
40. Mulla H, Peek G, Upton D, Lin E, Loubani M. Plasma aluminum levels during sucralfate prophylaxis for stress ulceration in critically ill patients on continuous venovenous hemofiltration: A randomized, controlled trial. *Crit Care Med.* 2001;29:267–271.
41. Sacks G. Multivitamins for the millennium. *Nutr Clin Pract.* 2002;17:83–84.
42. Department of Health and Human Services. Food and Drug Administration. Aluminum in large and small volume parenterals used in total parenteral nutrition. 65 *Federal Register* 4103–4111 (2000) (codified at 21 CFR §201.323).
43. Department of Health and Human Services. Food and Drug Administration. Aluminum in large and small volume parenterals used in total parenteral nutrition; delay of effective date. 66 *Federal Register* 7864–7865 (2001) (codified at 21 CFR §201.323).
44. Department of Health and Human Services. Food and Drug Administration. Meeting Summary: HIMA/FDA; Discussion of the final rule provisions, LVP: Aluminum labeling. [Docket No. 90N-0056].
45. Benabe JE, Martinez-Maldonado M. The impact of malnutrition on kidney function. *Miner Electrolyte Metab.* 1998;24:20–26.
46. Fiaccadori E, Lombardi M, Leonardi S, Rotelli CF, Tortorella G, Borghetti A. Prevalence and clinical outcome associated with preexisting malnutrition in acute renal failure: A prospective cohort study. *J Am Soc Nephrol.* 1999;10:581–593.
47. Anderson RJ, Schrier RW. Acute renal failure. In: Schrier RW, Gottschalk CW, eds. *Diseases of the Kidney*. Boston, Mass: Little Brown and Co; 1997:1069–1113.
48. Maxvold NJ, Smoyer WE, Custer JR, Bunchman TE. Amino acid loss and nitrogen balance in critically ill children with acute renal failure: A prospective comparison between classic hemofiltration and hemofiltration with dialysis. *Crit Care Med.* 2000;28:1161–1165.
49. Brivet FG, Kleinknecht DJ, Loirat P, Landais PJM, Acute renal failure in intensive care units—causes, outcome, and prognostic factors of hospital mortality: a prospective, multicenter study. *Crit Care Med.* 1996;24:192–198.
50. Liano F, Junco E, Pascual J, Madero R, Verde E, Madrid Acute Renal Failure Study Group. The spectrum of acute renal failure in the intensive care unit compared with that seen in other settings. *Kidney Int.* 1998;53(Suppl 66):S16–S24.
51. Fiaccadori E, Lombardi M, Leonardi S, Fregonese O, Zambrelli P, Rotelli CF, Zinelli M, Minari M. Adequacy of nutrient stakes in patients with renal failure on artificial nutrition [abstract]. *J Am Soc Nephrol.* 1997;8(suppl):124A–125A.
52. Cachecho R, Millham FH, Wedel SK. Management of the trauma patient with pre-existing renal disease. *Crit Care Clin.* 1994;10:523–536.
53. Charney P, Charney D. Nutrition support in renal failure. *Nutr Clin Pract.* 2002;17:226–236.
54. Bellomo R, Farmer M, Parkin G, Wright, Boyce N. Severe acute renal failure: A comparison of acute continuous hemodiafiltration and conventional dialytic therapy. *Nephron.* 1995;71:59–64.
55. Goldstein-Fuchs DJ, McQuiston B. Renal failure. In: Matarese LE, Gottschlich MM, eds. *Contemporary Nutrition Support Practice: A Clinical Guide.* 2nd ed. Philadelphia, Pa: WB Saunders Co; 2003:460–483.
56. Navarro JF, Mora C, Leon C, Martin-del Rio R, Macia ML, Gallego E, Chahin J, Mendez ML, Rivero A, Garcia J. Amino acid losses during hemodialysis with polyacrylonitrile membranes: effect of intradialytic amino acid supplementation on plasma amino acid concentrations and nutritional variables in nondiabetic patients. *Am J Clin Nutr.* 2000;71:765–773.
57. Blumenkrantz MJ, Gahl GM, Kopple JD, Kamdar AV, Jones MR, Kessel M, Coburn JW. Protein losses during peritoneal dialysis. *Kidney Int.* 1981;19:593–602.

58. Davies SP, Reaveley DA, Brown EA, Kox, WJ. Amino acid clearances and daily losses in patients with acute renal failure treated by continuous arteriovenous hemodialysis. *Crit Care Med.* 1991;19:1510–1515.
59. Druml W. Protein metabolism in acute renal failure. *Miner Electrolyte Metab.* 1998;24:47–54.
60. May RC, Clark AS, Goheer A, Mitch WE. Specific defects in insulin-mediated muscle metabolism in acute uremia. *Kidney Int.* 1985;28:490–497.
61. Monaghan R, Watters JM, Clancey SM, Moulton SB, Rabin EZ. Uptake of glucose during continuous arteriovenous hemofiltration. *Crit Care Med.* 1993;21:1159–1163.
62. Kaufman DC, Haas CE, Spencer S, Veverbrants E. Adjustments of nutrition support with continuous hemodialfiltration in a critically ill patient. *Nutr Clin Pract.* 1994;14:120–123.
63. Monson P, Mehta RL, Fujioka K. Optimizing nutrition support in patients with acute renal failure (ARF) treated with CAVHD. Lecture presented at: ASPEN 17th Clinical Congress; January 16, 1993; San Diego, Calif.
64. Forni LG, Hilton PJ. Continuous hemofiltration in the treatment of acute renal failure. *N Engl J Med.* 1997;336:1303–1309.
65. Druml W, Fischer M, Sertl S, Schneeweiss B, Lenz K, Widhalm K. Fat elimination in acute renal failure: Long-chain vs medium-chain triglycerides. *Am J Clin Nutr.* 1992;55:468–472.
66. Basttistella FD, Widergren JT, Anderson JT, Siepler JK, Weber JC, MacColl K. A prospective, randomized trial of intravenous fat emulsion administration in trauma victims requiring total parenteral nutrition. *J Trauma.* 1997;43:52–60.
67. Klein CJ, Moser-Veillon PB, Schweitzer A, Douglass LW, Reynolds N, Patterson KY, Veillon C. Magnesium, calcium, zinc, and nitrogen loss in trauma patients during continuous renal replacement therapy. *JPEN J Parenter Enteral Nutr.* 2002;26:77–93.
68. Lim VS, Yarasheski KE, Flanigan MJ. The effect of uraemia, acidosis, and dialysis treatment on protein metabolism: a longitudinal leucine kinetic study. *Nephrol Dial Transplant.* 1998;13:1723–1730.
69. Price SR, Reaich D, Marinovic AC, England BK, Bailey JL, Caban R, Mitch WE, Maroni BJ. Mechanisms contributing to muscle wasting in acute uremia: activation of amino acid catabolism. *J Am Soc Nephrol.* 1998;9:439–443.
70. Fuhrman MP. Identifying your patient's risk for a vitamin deficiency. *Nutr Clin Pract.* 2001; 16(suppl):S8–S11.
71. Druml W, Schwarzenhofer M, Apsner R, Horl WH. Fat-soluble vitamins in patients with acute renal failure. *Miner Electrolyte Metab.* 1998;24: 220–226.
72. Story DA, Ronco C, Bellomo R. Trace element and vitamin concentrations and losses in critically ill patients treated with continuous venovenous hemofiltration. *Crit Care Med.* 1999;27:220–223.
73. Fuhrman MP. Overview of micronutrients and parenteral nutrition. *Support Line.* 2002;24(3): 8–12.
74. Mirtallo JM. Introduction to parenteral nutrition. In: Gottschlich MM, ed. *The Science and Practice of Nutrition Support: A Case-Based Core Curriculum.* Dubuque, Iowa: Kendall/Hunt Publishing; 2001:211–224.
75. Riella MC. Malnutrition in dialysis: malnourishment or uremic inflammatory response? *Kidney Int.* 2000;57:1211–1232.
76. Kaysen GA, Rathore V, Shearer GC, Depner TA. Mechanisms of hypoalbuminemia in hemodialysis patients. *Kidney Int.* 1995;48:510–516.
77. Malnutrition in chronic kidney disease. In: McCann L, ed. *Pocket Guide to Nutrition Assessment of the Patient With Chronic Kidney Disease.* 3rd ed. New York, NY: National Kidney Foundation; 2002:9–17.
78. Kopple JD, Foulks CJ, Piraino B, Beta JA, Goldstein DJ. National Kidney Foundation position paper on proposed Health Care Financing Administration guidelines for reimbursement of enteral and parenteral nutrition. *J Ren Nutr.* 1996; 6:45–47.
79. Rodriguez VO, Arem R, Adrogue HC. Hypoglycemia in dialysis patients. *Semin Dial.* 1995:8:95–101.
80. Foulks CJ, Goldstein J, Kelly MP, Hunt JM. Indications for the use of intradialytic parenteral nutrition in the malnourished hemodialysis patient. *J Ren Nutr.* 1991;1:23–33.
81. Chertow GMM, Ling J, Lew NL, Lazarus JM, Lowrie EG. The association of intradialytic parenteral nutrition administered with survival in hemodialysis patients. *Am J Kidney Dis.* 1994;24: 921–929.

82. Jones SA, Bushman M, Cohen R. Intradialytic parenteral nutrition after small bowel resection. *Nutr Clin Pract*. 1996;11:12–15.
83. Fuhrman MP, Charney P, Mueller C. Hepatic proteins and nutrition assessment. *J Am Diet Assoc.* 2004 (in press).
84. Foulks CJ. An evidence-based evaluation of intradialytic parenteral nutrition. *Am J Kidney Dis.* 1999;33:186–192.
85. *Regional Medical Policy on Parenteral Nutrition.* Columbia, SC: Palmetto Government Benefits Administrators; 1996.
86. Giordano C, Capodicosa G, DeSanto N. Artificial gut for total parenteral nutrition through the peritoneal cavity. *Int J Artif Organs.* 1980;3:326–330.
87. Wolfson, M, Jones MR. Nutrition impact of peritoneal dialysis solutions. *Miner Electrolyte Metab*. 1999;25:333–336.
88. Faller B, Aparicio M, Faict D, De Vos C, de Precigout V, Larroumet N, Guiberteau R, Jones M, Peluso F. Clinical evaluation of an optimized 1.1% amino-acid solution for peritoneal dialysis. *Nephrol Dial Transplant*. 1995;10:1432–1437.
89. Kopple JD, Bernard D, Messana J, Swartz R, Bergstrom J, Lindholm B, Lim V, Brunori G, Leiserowitz M, Bier DM, Stegnik LD, Martis L, Boyle CA, Serkes KD, Vonesh E, Jones MR. Treatment of malnourished PD patients with an amino acid based dialysate. *Kidney Int*. 1995;47: 1148–1157.
90. Bruno M, Bagnis C, Marangella M, Rovera L, Cantaluppi A, Linari F. CAPD with an amino acid dialysis solution: a long term cross-over study. *Kidney Int*. 1989;35:1189–1194.
91. Jones M, Hagen T, Boyle CA, Vonesh E, Hamburger R, Charytan C, Sandroni S, Bernard D, Piraino B, Schrieber M, Gehr T, Fein P, Friedlander M, Burkart J, Ross D, Zimmerman S, Swartz R, Knight R, Kraus A, McDonald L, Hartnett M, Weaver M, Martis L, Moran J. Treatment of malnutrition with 1.1% amino acid peritoneal dialysis solution: results of a multicenter outpatient study. *Am J Kidney Dis*. 1998;32:761–769.
92. Young GA, Dibble JB, Hobson SM, Tompkins L, Gibson J, Turney JH, Brownjohn AM. The use of an amino acid based CAPD fluid over 12 weeks. *Nephrol Dial Transplant*. 1989;4:285–292.
93. Arfeen S, Goodship THJ, Kirkwood A. The nutritional/metabolic and hormonal effects of 8 weeks of continuous ambulatory peritoneal dialysis with a 1% amino acid solution. *Clin Nephrol*. 1990;33: 192–199.
94. Jones MR, Gehr TW, Burkart JM, Hamburger RJ, Kraus AP, Piraino BM, Hagen T, Ogrinc FG, Wolfson M. Replacement of amino acid and protein losses with 1.1% amino acid peritoneal dialysis solution. *Perit Dial Int*. 1998;18:210–216.

Chapter 15

Medications Commonly Prescribed in Chronic Kidney Disease

Bruce Smith, MS, RD,
and Paul Garney, MS, RD

INTRODUCTION

A major challenge for the renal dietitian is determining the causes in compromised nutritional status. The patient on dialysis presents with the metabolic derangement of uremia, the effects of the dialysis treatment, comorbid conditions, and the consequences of polypharmacy.

This chapter is not intended to be a comprehensive list of medications or their side effects, but rather a reference for the more commonly prescribed medications used in chronic kidney disease (CKD) and end-stage renal disease (ESRD) patients. There is a focus on cardiac medications, especially antihypertensives. Prescription and dosage of these medications are routinely changed as physicians try to keep hypertension under control. Due to these frequent, and often unannounced, changes, it is easy to relate the side effects of these medications to other causes. Because of the prevalence of diabetes in CKD, the more common diabetic medications have also been included in this chapter.

Coronary artery disease continues to be a leading cause of morbidity and mortality in the United States (1). In response, the National Cholesterol Education Program Adult Treatment Panel III has established more aggressive lipid panel targets (refer to Chapter 10). This is leading to the use of combination therapies similar to those now seen with diabetes and hypertension, and the development of new medications such as ezetimibe and rosuvastatin. Therapies will likely include HMG-CoA reductase inhibitors (ie, statins) in combination with cholesterol-absorption inhibitors such as ezetimibe, or other medications including niacin, fibrates, or bile acid resins.

Studies are beginning to show the effectiveness of statins as inhibitors of inflammation (2,3). This may lead to increased use of these drugs for indications other than hyperlipidemia; dietitians should be cognizant of developments in research.

In recent years, soft-tissue calcification has begun receiving considerable attention for its role in cardiac disease (4,5). New recommendations and practice guidelines in this area will affect phosphorus binder and vitamin D prescriptions. Close attention should be paid to developments in this field.

The medications in this chapter are categorized by medical conditions. The side effects listed are limited to those affecting nutrition and gastrointestinal (GI) function. For a more complete picture of medical side effects and mechanisms, also consult other references, such as the *Physicians' Desk Reference,* reliable Internet resources, and textbooks of internal medicine. No attempt has been made to include alternative medications or their interactions in this chapter.

The following Web sites may be considered reliable resources:

- Drugs.com (http://www.drugs.com)
- Hypertension, Dialysis, and Clinical Nephrology (http://www.hdcn.com)
- Medscape (http://www.medscape.com)
- Merck Manual of Diagnostics and Therapies (http://www.merck.com/pubs/mmanual)
- National Library of Medicine Gateway Search (http://gateway.nlm.nih.gov/gw/cmd)
- PDRHealth (http://www.pdrhealth.com)
- RxList (http://www.rxlist.com)
- WebMD (http://www.webmd.com)

ANEMIA

Recombinant human erythropoietin

- Darbepoetin alfa (Aranesp, http://www.amgen.com)
- Epoetin alfa (Epogen, http://www.amgen.com)
- Epoetin alfa (Procrit [used in CKD], http://www.amgen.com)

These medications are used in the treatment of anemic patients with chronic renal failure (CRF) or ESRD who do not produce this hormone in adequate amounts for proper red blood cell production (6).

Possible GI Effects

GI effects from these medications may include GI distress.

Nutritional Implications and Other Side Effects

- Increased appetite.
- Increased blood pressure.
- May promote iron deficiency and low folate and vitamin B-12 stores.
- Polycythemia may occur if the hematocrit is not carefully monitored.

Dietary Management

- All hematologic parameters, as well as iron status, should be monitored regularly.
- Iron supplementation is frequently required in conjunction with this therapy.
- Vitamins containing folate and B-12 should be provided.
- As hematocrit increases, the viscosity of the blood increases, and blood pressure must therefore be monitored.

Oral Iron Preparations

- Ferrous fumarate
- Ferrous gluconate
- Ferrous sulfate
- Polysaccharide iron complex

These medications are used to treat iron-deficiency anemia caused by hemolysis, blood loss, lack of erythropoietin production, and inadequate iron intake; they are necessary to support erythropoiesis (7–9).

Possible GI Effects

Adverse effects can include constipation (which is common), as well as diarrhea, nausea, vomiting, altered taste, abdominal cramps, GI irritation, or dark stools.

Nutritional Implications and Other Side Effects

- Iron absorption is impaired if it is consumed at the same time as calcium, magnesium, fiber, phytates, tannins, certain sulfur-containing compounds, and cholesterol-lowering drugs.
- Geophagia (the practice of eating clay) also interferes with iron absorption.
- Iron absorption may be enhanced by ascorbic acid, fructose, sorbitol, vitamin E, and certain organic acids, including succinic, lactic, pyruvic, and citric acids.

Dietary and Medical Management

To minimize the risk of various substances in foods binding to iron and preventing absorption, iron supplements should not be taken with meals. However, if stomach upset occurs, iron may then be taken with some food.

Oral iron supplements should be taken 1 hour apart from antacids and phosphate binders. Some iron supplements also contain vitamin C or B-complex vitamins, which should be noted when considering vitamin recommendations for the renal population. Avoid slow-release iron preparations, which are not as well ab-

Table 15.1. Oral Iron Formulas

Iron Formula	*Elemental Iron (mg)*
Ferrous fumarate	
Chromagen	66
Ferro-Sequels	50
Hemocyte	106
Nephro-Fer	115
Ferrous sulfate	
Feosol	
Tablet	65
Capsule	50
Irospan	60
Polysaccharide iron complex	
Niferex	150
Niferex with vitamin C	150
Nu-Iron	
Capsule	150
Elixir	100

Source: Data are from references 7–9 and manufacturers—Chromagen: Savage Laboratories (Melville, NY 11747); Ferro-Sequels: Lederle Laboratories (Wayne, NJ 07470); Hemocyte: US Pharmaceutical Corp (Decatur, GA 30035); Nephro-Fer: R & D Laboratories Inc (Marina del Rey, CA 90292); Feosol: GlaxoSmithKline (http://www.gsk.com); Irospan: Fielding Pharmaceutical Co (Maryland Heights, MO 63043); Niferex and Niferex with vitamin C: Central Pharmaceuticals Inc (Seymour, IN 47274); Nu-Iron: Merz Pharmaceuticals (Greensboro, NC 27419; http://www.nuiron.com).

sorbed. See Table 15.1 for additional information on oral iron supplements (7).

Intravenous Iron Preparations

Intravenous (IV) iron preparations are indicated for the treatment of iron-deficiency anemia when oral iron supplements are not effective. In hemodialysis, oral iron supplements typically are not sufficient to replace iron stores, and therefore IV iron is given concomitantly with erythropoietin (7–9). Table 15.2 summarizes data on side effects and other concerns associated with these medications.

ANOREXIA

It is not uncommon for ESRD patients to experience periods of poor appetite and subsequent weight loss. These episodes can be caused by insufficient dialysis clearances, pain, depression, anxiety, and as a side effect of medications. To make matters more difficult, patients are often restricted from having many of the foods they enjoy.

When diet modification does not improve a patient's appetite or a patient is unable to eat enough to prevent weight loss, appetite-enhancing medications are often prescribed. These medications are indicated in the treatment of anorexia, cachexia, or unexplained significant weight loss, especially associated with both acquired immunodeficiency syndrome (AIDS) and cancer. They are also indicated as antiemetics. Although not specifically indicated for the above conditions associated with CKD, these medications (particularly Megace) are prescribed in the dialysis population (7–9). (See Table 15.3 for data on side effects and other concerns associated with these medications.)

CARDIAC MEDICATIONS

It is beyond the scope of this chapter and the knowledge of its authors to fully discuss the effect of medications on cardiac function (7–11). The reader is referred to textbooks of internal medicine or medical pathophysiology for an understanding of disorders of the cardiovascular system.

Antiarrhythmics

Generally, antiarrythmics are divided into four classes: Class I (A–C) drugs block inward sodium current, reducing depolarization; Class II drugs are antisympathetic agents; Class III drugs prolong action potential; and Class IV drugs are the calcium channel blockers, which decrease conduction velocity and increase refractoriness.

Amiodarone is a Class III medication and is used to treat acute ischemia. Quinidine is a Class I medication and is effective with tachycardia. (See Table 15.4 for more information on these medications.)

Antihypertensives

The heart and the kidney have been described as two parts of the same system. This conclusion can be readily

Table 15.2. Intravenous Iron Formulas

Drug	*Trade Name (Manufacturer)*	*Individual Side Effects and Comments*
Iron dextran	Infed (Schein Pharmaceuticals, Carmel, NY 10512) Dexferrum (Luitpold Pharmaceuticals Inc, Shirley, NY 11967)	Anaphylactic shock, chest pain, hypotension, hypertension, tachycardia, pruritits, rash, abdominal pain, nausea, vomiting, diarrhea.
Sodium ferric gluconate	Ferrlecit (Watson Pharmaceuticals, Morristown, NJ 07962)	Reactions are rare, but anaphylactic shock and hypotension are possible when intravenous iron is given.
Iron sucrose	Venofer (American Reagent, Shirley, NY 11967)	Reactions are rare, but anaphylactic shock and hypotension are possible when intravenous iron is given.

Table 15.3. Appetite Stimulants

Drug	*Trade Name (Manufacturer)*	*Individual Side Effects and Comments*
Megestrol	Megace (Bristol Myers Squibb, http://www.bms.com)	Constipation, diarrhea, dyspepsia, hyperglycemia, nausea and vomiting.
Dronabinol	Marinol (Unimed, http://www.solvaypharmaceuticals-us.com)	Tachycardia, central nervous system effects (amnesia, changes in mood, confusion, delusions, hallucinations, mental depression, nervousness or anxiety). Sleep disturbances may occur after discontinuation of therapy.

Source: Data are from references 7–9 and manufacturers.

Table 15.4. Antiarrythmics

Drug	*Trade Name (Manufacturer)*	*Individual Side Effects and Comments*
Amiodarone	Cordarone (Wyeth-Ayerst, http://www.wyeth.com)	Anorexia, abnormal taste, smell and salivation, nausea and vomiting, constipation, abdominal pain. Peripheral neuropathy and edema. Effects increased with hypokalemia.
Quinidine	Cardioquin (Purdue Frederick, http://www.pharma.com)	Diarrhea, loss of appetite, muscle weakness, nausea or vomiting. Take with food to decrease dyspepsia.

Source: Data are from references 7–9 and manufacturers.

observed in people with CKD or ESRD. Hypertension is a major cause of renal failure, and controlling blood pressure is an ongoing process for dialysis patients. In response to the widespread prevalence of hypertension, a wide array of medications has become available. In general, there are six classes of drugs: diuretics, antiadrenergic agents, vasodilators, calcium channel blockers, angiotensin-converting enzyme (ACE) inhibitors, and angiotensin receptor blockers. These classes may be used individually or in combination.

Because of the prevalence of these medications among renal patients, the renal dietitian should be familiar with their side effects. This is not to say that all the side effects are widespread, but when more common efforts are ineffective in resolving what seem to be nutritional metabolic problems, such as hyperkalemia, then these medications should be considered. Some side effects are specific, such as dry mouth, hyperglycemia, and fluid retention, whereas others are more subtle, such as depression, insomnia, and anorexia, and may be attributed to other causes.

Antihypertensive medications are generally prescribed in a stepwise fashion: a) oral diuretic; b) adrenergic inhibitor; c) vasodilator; and d) another sympathetic depressant. These are, of course, general guidelines and will vary with individual patients. By the time ESRD has occurred, most patients will already be at step c or d.

Diuretics

Thiazide Diuretics

These diuretics reduce the reabsorption of sodium and chloride in the first half of the distal convoluted tubule of the nephron. Water follows the unabsorbed sodium.

Thiazide diuretics may cause sensitivity to sunlight and may increase blood glucose levels. Side effects of particular concern include hyponatremia (confusion, convulsions, decreased mentation, fatigue, irritability, muscle cramps) and hypokalemia (dryness of mouth, increased thirst, irregular heartbeat, mood or mental changes, muscle cramps or pain, nausea or vomiting, unusual tiredness or weakness, weak pulse). There is also the possibility of developing metabolic alkalosis and hyperglycemia. (See Table 15.5 for other side effects.)

Loop Diuretics

These are powerful diuretics that block the reabsorption of sodium, potassium, and chloride in the ascending limb of the loop of Henle. These medications differ from other diuretics in their continued effectiveness even when extracellular fluid and blood volume have been depleted. (See Table 15.6 for side effects of loop diuretics.)

Aldosterone Antagonists (Potassium-Sparing Agents)

These agents block the exchange of sodium with potassium and hydrogen ions in the distal half of the convoluted tubule. They are often used in combination with thiazide diuretics to reduce the risk of potassium retention.

With aldosterone antagonists, hyperkalemia (confusion, irregular heartbeat, nervousness, numbness or

Table 15.5. Thiazide Diuretics

Drug	*Trade Name (Manufacturer)*	*Individual Side Effects*
Chlorthalidone	Hygroton (Aventis, http://www.aventis.com)	General effects discussed in text.
Hydrochlorthiazide	Hydrodiuril (Merck, http://www.merck.com) Microzide (Watson Labs, Inc, http://www.watsonutah.com) Esidrix (Novartis, http://www.novartis.com)	Nausea or decreased appetite, abdominal pain.
Indapamide	Lozol (Aventis, http://www.aventis.com)	Less or no hypercholesterolemia.
Metolazone	Zaroxolyn (Celltech Pharmaceuticals, http://www.celltechgroup.com)	General effects discussed in text.

Source: Data are from references 7–9 and manufacturers.

Table 15.6. Loop Diuretics

Drug	*Trade Name (Manufacturer)*	*Individual Side Effects*
Bumetanide	Bumex (Roche Pharmaceuticals, http://www.rocheusa.com)	Headache, dry mouth, hypokalemia, muscle cramps, thrombocytopenia; reduced phosphate reabsorption
Ethacrynic acid	Edecrin (Merck, http://www.merck.com)	Anorexia, diarrhea, dysphagia, gastrointestinal bleed, headache, nausea and vomiting
Furosemide	Lasix (Aventis Pharmaceuticals, http://www.aventis.com)	Dizziness, metabolic alkalosis, muscle cramps, nausea and vomiting
Torsemide	Demadex (Roche Pharmaceuticals, http://www.rocheusa.com)	Cough, diarrhea, dizziness, headache, hyperglycemia, nausea and vomiting

Source: Data are from references 7–9 and manufacturers.

tingling in hands, feet, or lips, shortness of breath or difficult breathing, unusual tiredness or weakness) is a particular concern. Excessive potassium intake should be avoided, including high-potassium substances such as salt substitutes that contain potassium. (See Table 15.7 for other side effects of potassium-sparing agents.)

Adrenergic Inhibitors

This class of medications acts on the nervous system, usually on the sympathetic system, but occasionally on the parasympathetic system as well. The primary action is the reduction of the movement of neurotransmitters that cause vasoconstriction, especially norepinephrine.

Central Agents

Central agents (see Table 15.8) stimulate a central alpha-adrenergic pathway, decreasing signal outflow to stimulate neurotransmitters.

Alpha Blockers

Adrenergic-receptor blocking agents are categorized by their site of action. Alpha blockers (see Table 15.9) act on postsynaptic ($alpha_1$) and/or presynaptic ($alpha_2$) nerve receptors. Again, the result is the blocking of norepinephrine action. Alpha-blockers are the only group of antihypertensives with a modest effect on reducing total cholesterol, especially low-density lipoprotein (LDL) cholesterol.

Beta Blockers

Beta blockers (see Table 15.10) block sympathetic effects on the heart, resulting in reduced arterial pressure and cardiac output. An added benefit of beta blockers is the decreased release of renin. Individuals with diabetes should use beta blockers with care because these medications inhibit the usual nervous response to hypoglycemia.

Table 15.7. Potassium-Sparing Agents

Drug	*Trade Name (Manufacturer)*	*Individual Side Effects*
Amiloride hydrochloride	Midamor (Merck, http://www.merck.com)	Dry mouth, nausea, vomiting, heartburn, diarrhea, constipation, dyspepsia
Spironolactone	Aldactone (Pfizer Inc, http://www.pfizer.com)	Dry mouth, nausea, vomiting, gastritis, diarrhea, cramps
Triamterene	Dyrenium (Wellspring Pharmaceutical Corp, http://www.wellspringpharm.com)	Dry mouth, nausea, vomiting, gastritis, diarrhea, cramps, decreased use of folate

Source: Data are from references 7–9 and manufacturers.

Table 15.8. Central Alpha-Agonists

Drug	*Trade Name (Manufacturer)*	*Individual Side Effects and Comments*
Clonidine hydrochloride	Catapres (Boehringer-Ingelheim, http://www.boehringer-ingelheim.com)	Fluid retention, constipation, dizziness, drowsiness dryness of mouth, unusual tiredness or weakness, loss of appetite, nausea or vomiting.
Guanabenz acetate	Wytensin (Wyeth-Ayerst, http://www.wyeth.com)	Drowsiness, dryness of mouth, weakness, nausea.
Guanfacine hydrochloride	Tenex (Esp Pharma Inc, Edison, NJ 08817)	Constipation, drowsiness, dryness of mouth, nausea or vomiting, unusual tiredness or weakness.
Methyldopa	Aldomet (Merck, http://www.merck.com)	Flatus, nausea, vomiting, constipation, diarrhea, distention, and/or weight gain. May cause sodium retention, edema, and/or anemia.

Source: Data are from references 7–9 and manufacturers.

Table 15.9. Alpha Blockers

Drug	*Trade Name (Manufacturer)*	*Individual Side Effects*
Doxazosin mesylate	Cardura (Pfizer Inc, http://www.pfizer.com)	Swelling of feet or lower legs, nausea, sleepiness or drowsiness
Prazosin hydrochloride	Minipress (Pfizer Inc, http://www.pfizer.com)	Swelling of feet or lower legs, lack of energy, dryness of mouth, unusual tiredness or weakness
Terazosin hydrochloride	Hytrin (Abbott Laboratories, http://www.abbott.com)	Swelling of feet or lower legs, unusual tiredness or weakness, drowsiness, nausea and vomiting, stuffy nose

Source: Data are from references 7–9 and manufacturers.

Table 15.10. Beta Blockers

Drug	*Trade Name (Manufacturer)*	*Side Effects Across Entire Class*
Acebutolol	Sectral (Esp Pharma Inc, Edison, NJ 08817)	Increased serum potassium, constipation, diarrhea, weakness, nausea or vomiting, stomach discomfort, stuffy nose, flatulence, heartburn. High incidence of central nervous system adverse effects: sleep disturbance, fatigue, lethargy. May mask insulin-induced hypoglycemia. Depressed HDL, increased TC, and TG except with drugs with intrinsic sympathomimetic activity, eg, acebutolol, carteolol, penbutolol, pindolol.
Atenolol	Tenormin (Astrazeneca, http://www.astrazeneca.com)	
Betaxolol	Kerlone (Sanofi-Synthelabo Inc, http://www.sanofi-synthelabous.com)	
Bisoprolol fumerate	Zebeta (Barr Laboratories, http://www.barrlabs.com/home.html)	
Carteolol hydrochloride	Cartrol (Abbott Laboratories, http://www.abbott.com)	
Metoprolol tartrate	Lopressor (Novartis, http://www.novartis.com)	
Metoprolol succinate	Toprol-XL (Astrazeneca, http://www.astrazeneca.com)	
Nadolol	Corgard (Apothecon Inc, Princeton, NJ 08543)	
Penbutolol sulfate	Levatol (Schwarz Pharma, http://www.schwarzpharma.com)	
Pindolol	Visken (Novartis, http://www.novartis.com)	
Propranolol hydrochloride	Inderal (Wyeth-Ayerst, http://www.wyeth.com) Inderal LA (Wyeth-Ayerst, http://www.wyeth.com)	
Timolol maleate	Blocadren (Merck, http://www.merck.com)	

Abbreviations: HDL, high-density lipoprotein cholesterol; TC, total cholesterol; TG, triglycerides.

Source: Data are from references 7–9 and manufacturers.

Vasodilators

Vasodilators cause the direct relaxation of vascular smooth muscle. These medications are indicated for both heart failure and hypertension. With heart failure, increased ventricular afterload may lead to increased pulmonary capillary pressures and pulmonary congestion/edema, a common problem in renal patients. Vasodilators improve cardiac output, thereby reducing the symptoms of cardiac failure. With hypertension, reduction in vasoconstriction leads directly to decreased blood pressure. (Table 15.11 identifies side effects of vasodilators.)

Calcium Channel Blockers

These medications act by binding to cellular voltage-dependent calcium channels, modifying calcium entry into the cells, resulting in vasodilation. (See Table 15.12 for more information on these drugs.)

ACE Inhibitors

ACE inhibitors inhibit the production of angiotensin, a vasoconstrictor, and slow the degradation of bradykinin, a vasodilator. They have been found to have a

Table 15.11. Vasodilators

Drug	*Trade Name (Manufacturer)*	*Individual Side Effects*
Hydralazine	Apresoline (Novartis, http://www.novartis.com)	Edema, nausea, vomiting, anorexia, diarrhea
Minoxidil	Rogaine (Pfizer Inc, http://www.pfizer.com) Loniten (Pfizer Inc, http://www.pfizer.com)	Marked edema
Nitroprusside	Nitropress (Abbott Laboratories, http://www.abbott.com)	Nausea, vomiting, weakness, apprehension

Source: Data are from references 7–9 and manufacturers.

Table 15.12. Calcium Channel Blockers

Drug	*Trade Name (Manufacturer)*	*Side Effects Across Class*
Benzothiazepine derivatives (diltiazem)	Cardizem (Aventis, http://www.aventis.com) Dilacor (Watson Pharmaceuticals, http://www.watsonpharm.com) Tiazac (Biovail Corp, http://www.biovail.com)	Possible side effects include dizziness, flushing, headache, weakness, nausea, pedal edema, constipation, diarrhea, dyspepsia, dryness of mouth. Caution with diabetic patients; may increase glucose and gastroparesis. Do not affect serum calcium concentrations.
Diphenylalkylamine derivatives (verapamil)	Calan (Pfizer Inc, http://www.pfizer.com) Isoptin (Abbott Laboratories, http://www.abbott.com) Covera (Pfizer, http://www.pfizer.com) Verelan (Elan Drug Co, http://www.elan.com)	
Dihydropyridines (amlodipine, felodipine, isradipine, nicardipine, nifedipine, nisoldipine)	Norvasc (Pfizer, http://www.pfizer.com) Plendil (www.astrazeneca.com) Dynacirc (Reliant Pharmaceuticals, http://www.reliantrx.com) Cardene (Roche Pharmaceuticals, http://rocheusa.com) Procardia (Pfizer Inc, http://www.pfizer.com) Sular (First Horizon, http://www.horizonpharm.com)	

Source: Data are from references 7–9 and manufacturers.

renal protective effect and are prescribed for CKD, independent of systemic hypertension.

Across the class, the most frequent adverse effect is a dry, irritating cough, possibly caused by a buildup of bradykinin. Other effects include swelling of face, mouth, hands, or feet; stomach pain, nausea, vomiting, diarrhea; loss of taste; unusual tiredness. They may cause increased blood urea nitrogen (BUN) and creatinine. An increase in serum potassium is possible; close monitoring is recommended. (For side effects associated with individual drugs in this category, see Table 15.13.)

Glycosides

The primary action of cardiac glycosides (eg, digoxin) is the increase of intracellular (myocardial) sodium, which in turn increases calcium intake and muscle contraction.

Side Effects

Side effects include diarrhea, loss of appetite (dose limiting), lower stomach pain, nausea, and vomiting.

Dietary Management

Hypokalemia and hypomagnesemia cause the myocardium to be sensitive to digoxin, and toxicity may occur. Hypercalcemia may increase the risk of digitalis toxicity. Toxicity is also possible with herbs that have digitalis-like effects: foxglove, dogbane, lily-of-the-valley, oleander. Absorption of digoxin occurs

Table 15.13. ACE Inhibitors

Drug	*Trade Name (Manufacturer)*	*Individual Side Effects and Comments*
Benazepril hydrochloride	Lotensin (Novartis, http://www.novartis.com)	General effects discussed in text.
Captopril	Capoten (Par Pharmaceuticals, http://www.parpharm.com/html/nf/Home.html)	May cause sodium retention; therefore, monitor fluid status.
Enalapril maleate	Vasotec (Biovail Corp, http://www.biovail.com)	May cause hyperglycemia in patients with diabetes.
Fosinopril sodium	Monopril (Bristol Myers Squibb, http://www.bms.com)	General effects as discussed in text.
Lisinopril	Prinivil (Merck, http://www.merck.com) Zestril (www.astrazeneca.com)	Nausea, vomiting, dyspepsia, diarrhea.
Moexipril	Univasc (Schwarz Pharma, http://www.schwarzpharma.com)	General effects as discussed in text.
Quinapril hydrochloride	Accupril (Pfizer Inc, http://www.pfizer.com)	High magnesium content.
Ramipril	Altace (Wyeth, http://www.wyeth.com)	May cause hyperglycemia in patients with diabetes.
Trandolapril	Mavik (Abbott Laboratories, http://www.abbott.com)	General effects as discussed in text.

Abbreviation: ACE, angiotensin-converting enzyme.

Source: Data are from references 7–9 and manufacturers.

by passive diffusion in the proximal part of the small intestine. Rate of absorption, but not amount of drug, is affected by concurrent food intake.

DIABETES

Inappropriate use of diabetic medications results in uncontrolled blood sugar—either increased or decreased (7–10,12).

- Low blood glucose: Symptoms can include anxiety, blurred vision, cold sweats, confusion, cool pale skin, difficulty in concentrating, drowsiness, drunken behavior, excessive hunger, fast heartbeat, headache, nausea, shakiness, slurred speech, and unusual tiredness or weakness.
- High blood glucose: Symptoms of high blood glucose appear more slowly than those of low blood glucose. Symptoms can include blurred vision; drowsiness; dry mouth; flushed and dry skin; fruit-like breath odor; increased urination; loss of appetite; stomachache, nausea, or vomiting; tiredness; troubled breathing (rapid and deep); and unusual thirst.
- Severe high blood glucose: Symptoms of severe high blood glucose (called ketoacidosis or diabetic coma) include flushed dry skin, fruit-like breath odor, ketones in urine, loss of consciousness, troubled breathing (rapid and deep).

Medications include oral hypoglycemic agents and insulin. Oral medications are grouped by action into three categories: a) stimulation of the beta cells of the pancreas to release more insulin; b) increase of receptor sites on cells or correction of post-receptor defect, and/or modification of production of glucose by the liver; c) slow breakdown of starches and certain sugars.

Sulfonylurea Agents

These medications stimulate beta cells. Onset of action of sulfonylureas is within 1.5 hours. All sulfonylureas have potential to cause hypoglycemia, so use with caution in older adults. Because sulfonylureas are metabolized by the liver, caution should be used with patients with hepatic dysfunction. (See Table 15.14 for more information about these medications.)

Meglitinides

Meglitinides are used to stimulate beta cells. These medications have a quick onset with short action time and should be taken at mealtime. They are effective on postprandial blood glucose and are effective for those

Table 15.14. Sulfonylurea Agents

Drug	*Duration of Action (hours)*	*Trade Name (Manufacturer)*	*Side Effects Across Class*
Chlorpropamide	60	Diabinese (Pfizer Inc, http://www.pfizer.com)	Changes in sense of taste, constipation, diarrhea, dizziness, heartburn, flatulence, dyspepsia vomiting, increased or decreased appetite, weight gain
Gliclazide	24	Diamicron (Servier, http://www.servier.com)	
Glimepiride	24	Amaryl (Aventis, http://www.aventis.com)	
Glipizide	12–24	Glucotrol (Pfizer Inc, http://www.pfizer.com)	
Glyburide	12–24	DiaBeta (Aventis, http://www.aventis.com) Glynase (Pfizer Inc, http://www.pfizer.com) Micronase (Pfizer Inc, http://www.pfizer.com)	
Tolazamide	12–24	Tolinase (Pfizer Inc, http://www.pfizer.com)	
Tolbutamide*	6–12	Orinase (Pfizer Inc, http://www.pfizer.com)	

*In patients with renal disease, tolbutamide is preferred because it is metabolized entirely by the liver.

Source: Data are from references 7–9 and manufacturers.

with irregular meal patterns. (See Table 15.15 for more information.)

Biguanides

Biguanides (ie, metformin [Glucophage, Bristol Myers Squibb, http://www.bms.com]) decrease hepatic glucose production and provide some increased peripheral sensitivity. This medication should *not* be given to patients with advanced renal disease. Other patients should start with a low dose at the evening meal and increase as tolerated. Adverse effects include bloating, diarrhea, and gas. Metformin can cause lactic acidosis.

Guidelines for CKD patients are as follows:

- Creatinine clearance (CrCl) > 60 L/min/1.73 m^2: maximum dose safe.
- CrCl < 60 L/min/1.73 m^2: limit to 1,000 to 1,500 mg/day.
- CrCl < 30 L/min/1.73 m^2: discontinue use.

Thiazoladinediones

These medications increase insulin sensitivity and are active only in the presence of insulin. They may be taken with or without food. (See Table 15.16 for more information.)

Alpha-Glucosidase Inhibitors

Table 15.17 presents information on these medications.

Insulin

Insulin is characterized by three components: a) onset: the length of time taken to begin reducing blood glucose; b) peak time: time of maximum strength in terms of reducing blood glucose; and c) duration: overall time of effect on blood glucose.

These three characteristics divide insulin into four categories:

1. *Rapid-acting:* Humalog (insulin lispro), NovoLog (insulin aspart). These begin working within 5 minutes, peak in 1 hour, and have a duration of 2 to 4 hours. These insulins should be injected immediately before a meal. They are effective in treating postprandial blood sugars; allow adjustment based on carbohydrate counting.

Table 15.15. Meglitinides

Drug	*Duration of Action (hours)*	*Trade Name (Manufacturer)*	*Selected Side Effects*
Nateglinide	3	Starlix (Novartis, http://www.novartis.com)	Diarrhea, dyspepsia, nausea
Repaglinide	3	Prandin (Novo Nordisk, http://www.novonordisk.com)	Cough, fever runny or stuffy nose, shortness of breath, sinus congestion with pain, sneezing, sore throat

Source: Data are from references 7–9 and manufacturers.

Table 15.16. Thiazoladinediones

Drug	*Trade Name (Manufacturer)*	*Individual Side Effects and Comments*
Pioglitazone	Actose (Eli Lilly and Co, http://www.lilly.com)	May decrease TG and increase HDL.
Rosiglitasone	Avandia (GlaxoSmithKline, http://www.gsk.com)	Fluid retention, congestive heart failure (CHF), liver disease. May increase LDL. May reduce hemoglobin in dose-related fashion (study mean: 1 g/dL).

Abbreviations: TG, triglycerides; HDL, high-density lipoprotein cholesterol; LDL, low-density lipoprotein cholesterol.
Source: Data are from references 7–9 and manufacturers.

Table 15.17. Alpha-Glucosidase Inhibitors

Drug	*Duration of Action (hours)*	*Trade Name (Manufacturer)*	*Selected Side Effects and Comments*
Miglitol	4	Glyset (Pfizer Inc, http://www.pfizer.com)	Abdominal pain, diarrhea, flatulence.
Acarbose	2–6	Precose (Bayer Healthcare, http://www.pharma.bayer.com)	Should *not* be used for individuals with kidney disease (creatinine > 2.0) due to poor renal clearance. Abdominal or stomach pain bloated feeling or passing of gas diarrhea.

Source: Data are from references 7–9 and manufacturers.

2. *Regular or short-acting:* Humalin R, Novolin R. These begin working within 30 minutes, peak from 2 to 3 hours, and have a duration of approximately 3 to 6 hours.
3. *Intermediate acting:* NPH, Lente classes. These begin working in approximately 2 to 4 hours, peak in 4 to 12 hours, and have a duration of approximately 12 to 18 hours. This class is often used in combination with short-acting insulin and should be injected within 15 minutes of eating.
4. *Long-acting:* Ultralente class, Lantus (insulin glargine). These begin working in 6 to 10 hours; continuous release is effective for 24 hours. (Note: Ultralente is now rarely used due to variable absorption. Lantus has continuous "peakless" action with 2- to 3-hour onset.) Usually given at bedtime; this class should not be mixed with other types of insulin in the same syringe.

GASTROPARESIS

Dopaminergic Blocking Agents

These medications (eg, metoclopramide) inhibit gastric smooth muscle relaxation, accelerate intestinal transit and gastric emptying, and relax the upper small intestine, decreasing reflux into the esophagus and improving acid clearance from the esophagus. Metocopramide is indicated primarily for diabetic gastroparesis and esophageal reflux.

Adverse effects include dry mouth, nausea, vomiting. Metoclopramide may alter insulin requirements.

HYPERKALEMIA

Potassium-Removing Resins

Sodium polystyrene sulfonate (Kayexalate; Sanofi Winthrop Pharmaceuticals, New York, NY 10016) is used for the reduction of serum potassium levels, resins' mechanism of removing potassium from the body is by exchange of sodium ions with potassium ions, primarily in the large intestine (7–10). The potassium-containing resin is then excreted in the feces.

Possible Gastrointestinal Effects

Diarrhea is the most common side effect. Gastric irritation, anorexia, nausea, vomiting, and constipation may occur, especially with high doses.

Nutritional Implications and Other Side Effects

Potassium-removing resins may cause sodium retention and should therefore be used with caution in those who cannot tolerate even a small increase in blood pressure. They may also cause hypocalcemia and hypomagnesemia.

Dietary and Medical Management

- Monitor serum potassium levels daily throughout treatment.
- Observe for clinical signs of hypokalemia.
- Consider further sodium restriction in diet during treatment.

HYPERLIPIDEMIA

Gemfibrozil

Indicated for the reduction of triglycerides (TG), gemfibrozil (Lopid, Pfizer, http://www.pfizer.com) may cause increased LDL cholesterol in type IV hyperlipidemia.

Gemfibrozil may increase effect of anticoagulants or worsen pre-existing renal insufficiency. There is an increased risk (rare) of rhabdomyolysis and myoglobinuria when gemfibrozil is used concurrently with lovastatin. With use of gemfibrozil, there is also an increased risk of cholelithiasis secondary to increased cholesterol secretion into the bile. Serum potassium may be decreased. Side effects include abdominal pain, diarrhea, fatigue, nausea, and vomiting.

HMG-CoA Reductase Inhibitors

Statins are a class of drugs that reduces the level of cholesterol in the blood by decreasing the liver's production of cholesterol. Statins reduce inflammation, which could be another mechanism that may beneficially affect atherosclerosis. This reduction of inflammation does not depend on statins' ability to reduce cholesterol. Further, these anti-inflammatory effects can be seen as early as 2 weeks after starting statins.

Grapefruit juice can increase the levels of simvastatin, lovastatin, fluvastatin, and atorvastatin (but not pravastatin) in the blood, increasing risk of rhabdomyolysis.

The most common side effects are headache, nausea, vomiting, constipation, diarrhea, headache, rash, weakness, and muscle pain. The most serious (but fortunately rare) side effects are liver failure and rhabdomyolysis. (See Table 15.18 for information about adverse effects associated with specific medications.)

Bile Acid Sequestrants

Bile acid sequestrants bind with cholesterol-containing bile acids in the intestines and are then eliminated in the stool. Bile acid sequestrants reduce LDL cholesterol by approximately 10% to 20%. Small dosages of sequestrants can produce beneficial reductions in LDL cholesterol. Bile acid sequestrants are sometimes prescribed with a statin to increase cholesterol reduction.

Folic acid supplementation is recommended for patients receiving sequestrants for prolonged periods; supplemental vitamin K may be required in some patients who develop bleeding tendencies or who take anticoagulants. Calcium absorption is decreased. Cholestyramine binds with intrinsic factor, preventing the formation of an intrinsic factor-vitamin complex needed for absorption of vitamin B-12; Schilling test may be abnormal. (See Table 15.19 for more information.)

Table 15.18. HMG-CoA Reductase Inhibitors

Drug	*Trade Name (Manufacturer)*	*Individual Side Effects*
Atorvastatin	Lipitor (Pfizer Inc, http://www.pfizer.com)	Abdominal pain, constipation, diarrhea, flatulence, muscle weakness, nausea
Fluvastatin	Lescol (Novartis, http://www.novartis.com)	Abdominal pain, constipation, diarrhea, flatulence, muscle weakness, nausea
Lovastatin	Mevacor (Merck, http://www.merck.com)	Abdominal pain, constipation, diarrhea, flatulence, muscle weakness, nausea
Pravastatin	Pravachol (Bristol Myer Squib Co, http://www.bms.com)	Abdominal pain, dizziness, headache, rash
Simvastatin	Zocor (Merck, http://www.merck.com)	Abdominal pain, constipation, diarrhea, flatulence, muscle weakness, nausea

Source: Data are from references 7–9 and manufacturers.

Table 15.19. Bile Acid Sequestrants

Drug	*Trade Name (Manufacturer)*	*Individual Side Effects and Comments*
Cholestyramine	Questran (Bristol Myer Squibb Co, http://www.bms.com) Questran Light (Bristol Myer Squibb Co, http://www.bms.com)	Constipation, heartburn or indigestion, nausea or vomiting, stomach pain. May increase (VLDL) production, increasing plasma concentration of triglycerides, especially in patients with hypertriglyceridemia. **Effects on laboratory values:** Alkaline phosphatase values and and phosphorous levels may be increased; potassium and sodium may be decreased.
Colestipol	Colestid (Pfizer Inc, http://www.pfizer.com)	Increased risk of developing hyperchloremic acidosis, causing renal function impairment. **Effects on laboratory values:** Alkaline phosphatase values and and phosphorous levels may be increased; potassium and sodium may be decreased.

Abbreviation: VLDL, very-low-density lipoprotein cholesterol.

Source: Data are from references 7–9 and manufacturers.

Ezetimibe

The mechanism of action of ezetimibe (Zetia Merck/ScheringPlough Pharmaceuticals, Wales, PA 19454) differs from other classes of cholesterol-lowering medications. It seems to act at the brush border of the small intestine and inhibits the absorption of cholesterol. This mechanism is complementary to that of HMG-CoA reductase inhibitors (decreased cholesterol production by the liver). Concurrent use with fibrates is contraindicated. Abdominal pain, diarrhea, rash, and tiredness are possible side effects.

Fibric Acids

Nutrition Management

Hypoglycemic effect of oral antidiabetic agents, especially tolbutamide, may be enhanced with concurrent use of clofibrate; glipizide, and glyburide may not be affected as much as the other oral agents.

Other Concerns

Because the potential benefits of combined therapy do not outweigh the risks of severe myopathy, rhabdomyolysis, and acute renal failure, concurrent use of fibrates with HMG-CoA reductase inhibitors is not recommended. (See Table 15.20 for more information on fibric acids.)

Niacin

Niacin reduces serum cholesterol and TG concentrations by inhibiting the synthesis of very-low-density lipoprotein cholesterol. Concurrent use of niacin with HMG-CoA reductase inhibitors may be associated with an increased risk of rhabdomyolysis and acute renal failure.

Pre-existing conditions should be considered before starting niacin therapy. Large oral doses may

- Exacerbate arterial bleeding, hemorrhage, or glaucoma
- Impair glucose tolerance in diabetes
- Exacerbate hypotension due to vasodilation
- Activate peptic ulcer

Initially, dosage should be 1 g three times per day, increased in increments of 500 mg per day every 2 to 4 weeks as needed. For maintenance, dosage should be 1 to 2 g taken orally three times per day.

OSTEODYSTROPHY

Calcium Replacements

Calcium replacements are used to treat hypocalcemia due to secondary hyperparathyroidism and renal osteodystrophy (7–9,13). They are often required after parathyroidectomies until calcium homeostasis is achieved. They may also be used to neutralize gastric acidity.

Possible GI Effects

Adverse effects include constipation, anorexia, nausea, belching, and flatulence.

Nutritional Implications and Other Side Effects

For optimal calcium absorption, active vitamin D is required. In ESRD, active vitamin D is given either orally or intravenously to compensate for the kidney's inability to provide adequate amounts of this necessary vitamin. (See section on Vitamin D Preparations in this chapter.)

Calcium absorption is impaired by the presence of iron salts, corticosteroids, and food sources of oxalic and phytic acids. Patients should be monitored for hypercalcemia. Calcium citrate increases aluminum absorption from other medications and sources.

Dietary and Medical Management

The recently published National Kidney Foundation Kidney Disease Outcomes Quality Initiative (K/DOQI) guidelines (14) indicate that serum calcium levels should be kept within "normal" laboratory ranges. When serum albumin levels are low (less than 4.0 g/dL), the corrected calcium formula should be used to determine a more accurate serum calcium status. Calcium supplements should be used only as needed. Serum calcium levels are not accurate indicators for assessment of soft tissue calcification. K/DOQI recommends intake of elemental calcium should not exceed 1,500 mg/day from phosphorous binders and no more than 2,000 mg/day total including dietary intake (14). The serum calcium level must be monitored, especially when active vitamin D is being given, to guard against

Table 15.20. Fibric Acids

Drug	*Trade Name (Manufacturer)*	*Individual Side Effects and Comments*
Clofibrate		More effective reducing TG (VLDL) than TC. Diarrhea and nausea most common side effects. **Note:** Flu-like syndrome or myositis occurs more frequently with existing renal disease.
Fenofibrate	Tricor (Abbott Laboratories, http://www.abbott.com)	Constipation, flatulence, flu-like symptoms, pruritis. Not removed by hemodialysis.

Abbreviations: TC, total cholesterol; TG, triglycerides; VLDL, very-low-density lipoprotein cholesterol.

Source: Data are from references 7–9 and manufacturers.

hypercalcemia. Calcium replacements should not be taken with food because phosphorus and other minerals within foods bind to calcium and inhibit its absorption. Oral iron should not be given at the same time as calcium. Calcium citrate should not be given if aluminum-containing phosphate binders are prescribed.

If constipation results from intake of calcium, a high-fiber diet or fiber supplement may be prescribed. (See Table 15.21 for more information on calcium replacements.)

Phosphate Binders

- Aluminum hydroxide (Amphojel, Wyeth-Ayerst Laboratories, Inc. St. Davids, PA 19087)
- Calcium salts (see Calcium Replacements section in this chapter)
- Magnesium carbonate (Magnebind, Nephro-Tech, Inc, Shawnee, KS 66203)
- Sevelamer hydrochloride (Renagel, Genzyme Corporation, Cambridge, MA 02139)

Phosphate binders are used to control hyperphosphatemia by binding the phosphorus from ingested foods in the GI tract, preventing absorption into the bloodstream. Calcium salts replaced aluminum as the phosphate binder of choice due to damage caused by aluminum toxicity and bone deposition. However, concerns of vascular calcification secondary to excessive intake of calcium are shifting current practice toward limiting calcium intake.

Dietary and Medical Management

- Acceptable serum levels of phosphorus are generally 2.6 to 5.5 mg/dL.
- Calcium × phosphorus product should ideally be less than 55; at this time, products less than 70 are commonly referenced in dialysis units.
- Although aluminum binders are not recommended for long-term use (more than 1 month), they may be helpful in getting phosphorus to manageable levels for other binders. Magnesium

Table 15.21. Calcium Replacements

Drug/Trade Name (Manufacturer)	*Elemental Calcium (mg)*
Calcium acetate	
Phoslo (Nabi Biopharmaceuticals, http://www.nabi.com, http://www.phoslo.com)	169
Calcium carbonate	
Calci-mix (R & D Laboratories, Marina del Rey, CA 90292)	500
Nephro-calci (R &D Laboratories, Marina del Rey, CA 90292)	600
Oscal 500 (GlaxoSmithKline, http://www.gsk.com)	500
Titralac (3M, http://www.3m.com/us)	
Tablet	168
Liquid (5 mL)	400
TUMS (GlaxoSmithKline, http://www.gsk.com)	
Regular	200
Extra strength	300
Ultra	400
Calcium citrate	
Citracal 950 (Mission Pharmacal, http://www.missionpharmacal.com)	200
Calcium glubionate	
Neo-Calglucon (Novartis, http://www.novartis.com)	115
Calcium gluconate	
1000 mg	93
485 mg	47
Calcium lactate	
325 mg	42
648 mg	84

Source: Data are from references 7–9 and manufacturers.

can be toxic at high levels; however, it is also removed by dialysis. Magnesium binders, used as directed, have not been shown to be a risk for the hemodialysis population. As a cautionary measure, when binders are started serum magnesium levels should be measured regularly.

Nutritional Implications and Other Side Effects

Calcium salts can cause constipation, anorexia, nausea, belching, and flatulence. Magnesium binders have the added benefit of acting as mild laxatives.

Phosphate binders should be taken with food, and the appropriate dose should be based on phosphorus content of meals and snacks. For obtaining acceptable serum phosphorus levels, dietary phosphorus should be restricted in conjunction with these drugs. Sevelamer hydrochloride may bind with other drugs and increase calcium absorption if used in conjunction with calcium binders.

Vitamin D Preparations

Oral Preparations

- Calcitriol (Rocaltrol, Hoffmann-La Roche Inc, Nutley, NJ 07110)
- Doxercalciferol (Hectorol, Bone Care International, Middleton, WI 53562)

Injectable Preparations

- Calcitriol (Calcijex, Abbott Laboratories, Abbott Park, IL 60064)
- Paricalcitol (Zemplar, Abbott Laboratories, Abbott Park, IL 60064)

Both of these types of preparations are used to provide the active form of vitamin D that CRF patients are typically unable to produce in adequate amounts. Active vitamin D is necessary for absorption of calcium from the GI tract and in the treatment of secondary hyperparathyroidism and resulting renal osteodystrophy.

Possible GI Effects

Nausea, vomiting, and constipation may be associated with vitamin D preparations.

Nutritional Implications and Other Side Effects

- Active vitamin D is necessary for absorption of calcium from the gut.
- These drugs should not be given if hypercalcemia and vitamin D toxicosis is evident.
- Mineral oil and cholestyramine impair the intestinal absorption of oral vitamin D preparations.

Dietary and Medical Management

Monitor serum calcium, phosphorus, and parathyroid hormone levels. K/DOQI recommendations for giving these drugs are as follows (14):

- Phosphorus within normal range: 3.5 to 5.5 mg/dL
- Calcium within normal range: 8.4 to 10.2 mg/dL (preferably within low end of range 8.4–9.5 mg/dL)
- Calcium × phosphorus product less than 55

The new trend in practice, however, is to keep calcium × phosphorus product less than 55 whenever possible to prevent metastatic calcification.

REFLUX/GI ULCERATION

Histamine H2–receptor Antagonists

These medications are indicated for the treatment of pathological gastric hypersecretion associated with Zollinger-Ellison syndrome, systemic mastocytosis, multiple endocrine adenoma, and gastroesophageal reflux disease (GERD) (7–9). (See Table 15.22 for information on side effects.)

Proton-Pump Inhibitors (PPIs)

PPIs are used for the prevention and treatment of acid-related conditions such as ulcers, GERD, and Zollinger-Ellison syndrome. They also are used in combination with antibiotics for eradicating *Helicobacter pylori*.

Oral iron efficacy will be diminished due to increased stomach pH. (See Table 15.23 for more information on PPIs.)

Table 15.22. Histamine H2–Receptor Antagonists

Drug	*Trade Name (Manufacturer)*	*Individual Side Effects*
Cimetidine	Tagamet (GlaxoSmithKline, http://www.gsk.com)	Alopecia, interstitial nephritis, polymyositis, urinary retention
Famotidine	Pepcid (Merck, http://www.merck.com)	Abdominal pain, alopecia, anorexia, constipation, dryness of mouth, nausea, vomiting
Nizatidine	Axid (Reliant Pharmaceuticals, http://www.reliantrx.com)	Abdominal pain, constipation, dryness of mouth, nausea, vomiting
Ranitidine	Zantac (GlaxoSmithKline, http://www.gsk.com)	Abdominal pain, alopecia, constipation, nausea, vomiting

Source: Data are from references 7–9 and manufacturers.

Table 15.23. Proton-Pump Inhibitors

Drug	*Trade Name (Manufacturer)*	*Individual Side Effects and Comments*
Rabeprazole	Aciphex (Janssen Pharmaceutica, http://janssen.com)	Diarrhea, headache
Esomeprazole	Nexium (AstraZeneca LP, http://www.astrazeneca.com)	Diarrhea, headache
Lansoprazole	Prevacid (TAP Pharmaceutical Products, http://www.tap.com)	Constipation, diarrhea, headache
Omeprazole	Prilosec (AstraZeneca LP, http://www.astrazeneca.com)	Diarrhea, headache; may increase risk of bleeding
Pantoprazole	Protonix (Wyeth, http://www.wyeth.com)	Diarrhea, headache

Source: Data are from references 7–9 and manufacturers.

OTHER MEDICATIONS WITH NUTRITIONAL IMPLICATIONS

Anabolic-Androgenic Hormones

These medications (eg, Oxymetholone [Unimed Pharmaceuticals, Inc, Marietta, GA 30062]) are used to promote lean body mass and weight gain, especially in AIDS wasting syndrome. The action of these medications is to reverse catabolic processes and negative nitrogen balance by promoting protein anabolism and by stimulating appetite. In the past, these medications have been used to treat anemia caused by damaged bone marrow, ineffective erythropoiesis, hemolytic anemia, or neutropenia. Now, however, these are now infrequently used to treat anemia due to the effectiveness of recombinant human erythropoietin.

Possible GI Effects

Anabolic-androgenic hormones may cause increased appetite, nausea, vomiting, diarrhea, or mild to moderate liver damage with abnormal liver function test values.

Nutritional Implications and Other Side Effects

Anabolic-androgenic hormones may cause dry weight gain (due to increased lean body mass); elevated creatinine and TG levels; retention of fluid, sodium, potassium, nitrogen, and phosphorus; and excretion of calcium. The use of anabolic steroids may increase the effects of anticoagulants by alteration of procoagulant factor synthesis (ie, prothrombin time may be increased).

Dietary and Medical Management

A diet adequate in energy, protein, vitamins, and minerals should be provided. Monitor serum levels of alanine aminotransferase (ALT), aspartate aminotransferase (AST), BUN, creatinine, electrolytes, calcium, and phosphorus, as well as fluid status.

Corticosteroids

Side Effects Across Class

Side effects include lower resistance to infections. Also, any infection may be harder to treat. Other possible effects include increased blood glucose, increased appetite, indigestion, gastric ulcer, loss of appetite (for triamcinolone only), nervousness or restlessness, and edema.

Side Effects That May Occur With Long-term Use

Long-term use may cause abdominal or stomach pain; bloody or black, tarry stools; filling or rounding out of the face; muscle cramps or pain; muscle weakness; nausea; unusual bruising; unusual increase in hair growth; unusual tiredness or weakness; vomiting; weight gain (rapid); or wounds that will not heal.

Nutritional Implications and Other Side Effects

Individuals taking corticosteroids may need increased intake of potassium, calcium, phosphorous, zinc, pyroxidine, folate, and vitamins A, C, and D. Serum changes may include increased TG and cholesterol.

RENAL VITAMINS

Vitamin uptake and use is altered in patients with renal impairment or failure (7,9,13). Differences in vitamin requirements for those on dialysis are largely due to impaired renal metabolism and altered urine losses. In general, the water-soluble B vitamins should be supplemented. In addition, some renal-specific formulas also offer minerals such as zinc, iron, and selenium along with vitamins C and E. (See Table 15.24 for data on specific brands.)

The following summarizes supplementation guidelines for other vitamins:

- Vitamin A concentration is usually elevated in the serum of patients both predialysis and on dialysis and should not be supplemented.
- Vitamin E requirements in kidney patients are not well defined, but supplementation with vitamin E is recognized as safe as no adverse effects have been reported.
- Vitamin K supplements are not recommended unless there is the risk of dietary deficiency due to poor dietary intake.
- Vitamin D is given in the active form when supplementation is required (see Vitamin D Preparations).

Table 15.24. Commonly Prescribed Renal-Specific Vitamins

	Trade Name (Manufacturer)						
Nutrient	*Dialyvite*	*Diatx*	*Nephplex Rx*	*Nephrocaps*	*Nephron FA*	*Nephrovite*	*Renax*
Vitamin C (mg)	60	60	60	100	40	60	50
Thiamin (vitamin B-1) (mg)	1.5	1.5	1.5	1.5	1.5	1.5	3.0
Riboflavin (vitamin B-2) (mg)	1.7	1.5	1.7	1.7	1.7	1.7	2.0
Pyridoxine (vitamin B-6) (mg)	10	50	10	10	10	10	15
Cyanocobalamin (vitamin B-12) (μg)	6	1	6	10	6	6	12
Niacin (vitamin B-3) (mg)	20	20	20	20	20	20	20
Biotin (μg)	300	300	300	300	300	300	300
Pantothenic acid (vitamin B-5) (mg)	10	10	10	10	10	10	10
Folic acid (mg)	0.8	5	1	1	1	1	2.5
Vitamin E (IU)	0	0	0	0	0	0	35

Source: Data are from references 7–9 and manufacturers—Dialyvite: Hillestad Pharmaceuticals (http://www.hillestadlabs.com); Diatx: Pam Labs, LLC (http://www.diatx.com); Nephplex Rx and Nephron FA: Nephro-Tech Inc (http://www.nephrotech.com); Nephrocaps: Fleming & Co Pharmaceuticals (http://www.flemingcompany.com); Nephrovite: R & D laboratories Inc (Marina del Rey, CA 90292); Renax: Everett Laboratories (www.everettlabs.com).

REFERENCES

1. National Institute of Diabetes and Digestive and Kidney Diseases. United States Renal Data System. Annual Data Report 2003: Patient Characteristics. Available at: htttp://www.usrds.org/2003/pdf/03_pt_chars_03.pdf. Accessed July 2, 2003.
2. Ridker PM, Rifai N, Pfeffer MA, Sacks F, Braunwald E; Cholesterol and Recurrent Events (CARE) Investigators. Long-term effects of pravastatin on plasma concentration of C-reactive protein. *Circulation.* 1999;100:230–235. Available at: http://circ.ahajournals.org/cgi/content/full/100/3/230. Accessed June 24, 2003.
3. Albert MA, Danielson E, Rifai N, Ridker PM. Effect of statin therapy on C-reactive protein levels. *JAMA*. 2001;286:64–70.
4. Giachelli CM. *Molecular Aspects of Vascular Calcification.* Presentation given at the ASN/ISN Satellite Symposium San Francisco, Calif, October 13, 2001. Available at: http://www.hdcn.com. Accessed July 2, 2003.
5. Salusky IB. *2001 Extraskeletal Calcification in Uremia: Cardiovascular Implications.* Presented at World Congress of Nephrology (ASN/ISN), San Francisco, Calif, October 2001. Available at: http://www.hdcn.com. Accessed July 3, 2003.
6. Anemia Management Institute. *Workshop 1 Independent Study: Basic Principles and Assessment Techniques.* Thousand Oaks, Calif: Amgen, Inc; 2002.
7. PDRhealth. Available at: http://www.pdrhealth.com. Accessed June 24, 2003.
8. Rxlist.com. Available at: http://www.rxlist.com. Accessed June 24, 2003.
9. Drugs.com. Available at: http://www.drugs.com. Accessed June 23–27, 2003.
10. Fauci AS, Braunwald E, Isselbacher KJ, eds. *Harrison's Principles of Internal Medicine.* New York, NY: McGraw-Hill; 1998.
11. Cardiovascular disorders. In: *The Merck Manual of Diagnostics and Therapies.* Available at: http://www.merck.com/mrkshared/mmanual/section16/sec16.jsp. Accessed July 3, 2003.
12. Diabetes mellitus. In: *The Merck Manual of Diagnostics and Therapies.* Available at: http://www.merck.com/mrkshared/mmanual/section2/chapter 13/13a.jsp. Accessed July 3, 2003.
13. Thompson Healthcare, ed. *Physicians' Desk Reference.* 56th ed. Des Moines, Iowa: Medical Economics; 2002.
14. Kasiske BL, ed. K/DOQI clinical guidelines for gone metabolism and disease in chronic kidney disease. *Am J Kidney Dis.* 2003;42(Suppl 3):S77–S84.

Chapter 16

Renal Osteodystrophy

Susan C. Knapp, MS, RD, CSR,
and Carol Liftman, MS, RD

Renal osteodystrophy is a generic term used to describe the wide spectrum of skeletal lesions that are associated with renal failure. Because of the kidney's crucial role in mineral homeostasis, metabolic bone diseases frequently develop in patients with chronic renal disease. The kidneys help maintain the body's balance of calcium, phosphorus, and magnesium. Additionally, the kidneys are responsible for the final step in the synthesis of calcitriol, the activated form of vitamin D, and, along with the liver, are involved in the degradation of parathyroid hormone (PTH). We now recognize that complications of disordered metabolism of calcium, phosphorus, calcitriol, and PTH are not limited to renal bone disease but are systemic. Other clinical consequences include cardiovascular, arterial, and valvular calcifications (1–4), arterial stiffening (5), metastatic calcification of other soft tissue (6), calciphylaxis (7,8), erythropoietin-resistant anemia (9), and increased morbidity and mortality (10–12). Renal bone disease develops in the early stages of renal insufficiency. The bone mineral density of patients beginning hemodialysis (HD) was found to be significantly lower than in healthy individuals (13).

CAUSES AND TYPES OF RENAL BONE DISEASE

Multiple factors are involved in the development of renal osteodystrophy. Causes of renal osteodystrophy include abnormal calcium and phosphorus metabolism, calcitriol deficiency, secondary hyperparathyroidism, resistance to PTH, and aluminum toxicity (14).

The histopathologic pattern of bones has been the basis for classification of the types of renal osteodystrophy. Typically, these classification groups are osteitis fibrosa, mild lesion, osteomalacia, mixed uremic osteodystrophy, and adynamic bone disease. A simpler classification into three groups has been suggested. These groups are a) predominant hyperparathyroid bone disease, b) low-turnover bone disease (including osteomalacia and adynamic bone disease), and c) mixed uremic osteodystrophy (15,16). Transformation between types and severity may occur (16). The dietitian can be influential in modifying some of these factors, potentially altering patients' development of renal bone disease.

Predominant Hyperparathyroid Bone Disease

Predominant hyperparathyroid bone disease (PHBD) is a disorder of increased bone turnover, characterized by elevated bone formation and resorption, along with an increased osteoid volume (15,16). In addition to the greater number of bone cells, many are shaped and arranged irregularly. This classification includes both osteitis fibrosa and mild disease. The severity of this disorder ranges from mild to severe, with mild having a smaller increase in osteoclastic activity and lacking fibrosis. In addition to high levels of PTH, PHBD is associated with metabolic acidosis and hyperphosphatemia (17). A range of from 5% to 50% of dialysis patients have been reported in various bone histology series to have osteitis fibrosa and the occurrence seems to be decreasing (15,17). The prevalence is higher in HD patients than in peritoneal dialysis (PD) patients (17,18). Because mineralization of the bone is deficient and haphazard, the bone is prone to fracture (17).

Several factors are believed to lead to an excessive secretion of PTH, causing high serum PTH levels and resulting in high-turnover renal osteodystrophy. These factors include altered vitamin D metabolism, hypocalcemia, phosphorus retention, skeletal resistance to PTH, reduced degradation of PTH, and metabolic acidosis.

Altered Vitamin D Metabolism

The kidneys are the major site for the production of the active form of vitamin D, 1,25-dihydroxyvitamin D (calcitriol). Calcitriol binds to vitamin D receptors in the parathyroid glands and causes a decrease in PTH gene transcription. This reduces PTH synthesis and secretion. Calcitriol and PTH are both involved with regulation of calcium homeostasis in the body. The synthesis of calcitriol and the secretion of PTH are affected by changes in the calcium concentration of extracellular fluid. Calcitriol and PTH cause an increase in serum calcium. Calcitriol increases intestinal calcium absorption. PTH directly stimulates the renal tubules to increase calcitriol production. Calcitriol increases the expression of the vitamin D-3 receptor genes (VDR) in the parathyroid gland, resulting in increased VDR protein synthesis and an increased binding of calcitriol (19,20). A decreased density of VDR was found to be associated with severe parathyroid hyperplasia, with the density less in nodular hyperplasia than diffuse hyperplasia (20).

As kidney function fails and levels of calcitriol fall, active transport of calcium from the intestine is hampered, leaving only primarily passive absorption of calcium, thus contributing to hypocalcemia. Decreased phosphorus excretion adds to the hypocalcemia by stimulating PTH production and inhibiting the action of calcitriol. The result is hyperphosphatemia, hypocalcemia, and calcitriol deficiency, which leads to parathyroid cell hyperplasia.

Recent research has also shown a role for vitamin D in the function of immunity, bone marrow, vasculature, reproduction, and the growth and differentiation of many cell types. Target cells for vitamin D have been found in the intestines, kidneys, bone, bone marrow, parathyroid glands, skin, liver, and muscle, among others, illustrating the diverse biological roles of vitamin D. Secondary hyperparathyroidism may impair red blood cell production despite the use of erythropoietin in HD patients (9).

Calcium

Serum calcium concentration is the most important factor regulating PTH secretion (21). Consequently, hypocalcemia is a powerful stimulant of PTH secretion. One reason for increased PTH levels in high-turnover bone disease may be a shift in the "set-point" for calcium; that is, requiring a higher calcium level in the blood to decrease the production of PTH. One study of 20 patients found that those with hyperparathyroidism had a significantly higher set-point for calcium than those with mild disease or adynamic bone disease; meaning a higher calcium level in the blood was required to decrease the production of PTH (21).

Phosphorus Retention

As renal function deteriorates, the excretion of phosphorus and calcitriol production per nephron increases in response to an increased secretion of PTH. Therefore, phosphorus levels in the blood usually remain near normal, especially in Stages 2 and 3 of chronic kidney disease (CKD). When the glomerular filtration rate (GFR) decreases to approximately 25% of normal (Stages 4 and 5), changes in phosphorus excretion and calcitriol production can no longer be maintained by the reduced renal mass (17).

Research indicates that the synthesis and secretion of PTH are directly stimulated by phosphate, independent of serum calcium or calcitriol (22). In addition, phosphate stimulates parathyroid gland hyperplasia. Studies with uremic rats found that an increase in dietary phosphorus increased parathyroid gland hyperplasia. When the rats were changed from a high- to low-phosphorus diet, although the serum phosphorus and PTH decreased, the parathyroid glands remained enlarged (22,23). Another study using uremic rats found that a high-phosphorus diet enhanced parathyroid cell proliferation whereas a low-phosphorus diet led to a decreased PTH and the total absence of parathyroid cell proliferation (24). A high-phosphorus diet seems to rapidly increase parathyroid cell growth. In a study by Dendra et al, uremic rats fed a high-phosphorus diet showed a significant increase in parathyroid gland weight within 2 days (25). This rapid growth continued for 1 week prior to leveling off and then plateaued in 2 weeks.

Nodular parathyroid hyperplasia has been shown to be associated with reduced levels of vitamin D receptors and calcium-sensing receptors (22,26). Parathyroid growth can progress to the nodular stage, resulting in severe hyperparathyroidism, phosphate efflux from bone, and calcitriol resistance. A parathyroidectomy may be required at this stage (17).

In addition to worsening secondary hyperparathyroidism, an elevated phosphorus level can limit the use of calcitriol and cause resistance to calcitriol therapy. An increased serum phosphorus level may result not only from dietary phosphate intake, but also from enhanced bone breakdown due to secondary hyperparathyroidism (17).

Skeletal Resistance

It is generally accepted that two to three times the normal circulatory levels of PTH are needed to maintain normal bone turnover in uremic patients. Uremia seems to interfere with at least one step of the bone remodeling cycle, osteoclastic bone resorption. This is referred to as skeletal resistance (27,28).

Reduced Degradation of PTH

The major factor responsible for the high plasma levels of PTH in patients with renal insufficiency is the increased secretion of PTH. A contributing factor could be decreased catabolism of PTH because the kidneys play an important role in the degradation of PTH. Intact PTH contains a sequence of 84 amino acids, including amino N terminal and carboxyl C terminal regions. The active part of the PTH is within the first 34 amino acids, whereas the carboxy-terminal fragment seems to be inactive. Because the kidneys are the only organs responsible for the removal of carboxy-terminal fragments, these fragments can accumulate in renal failure patients (29).

Metabolic Acidosis

Chronic metabolic acidosis is another possible factor involved in the development of osteodystrophy in individuals with chronic kidney disease. Metabolic acidosis, indicated by a low serum CO_2 (generally considered less than 22 mmol/L), is increasingly present in patients from Stage 3 through initiation of dialysis. Chronic metabolic acidosis causes dissolution of bone minerals. Evidence is limited that a correction of metabolic acidosis alone leads to an improvement or correction of osteodystrophy (30). However, in a small study of chronic HD patients with secondary hyperparathyroidism, correction of acidosis was found to reduce the intact parathyroid hormone (iPTH) concentrations (31). Another mechanism whereby acidosis can impact osteodystrophy is that vitamin D analog therapy seems to be more effective in the absence of acidosis (30).

Low-Turnover Renal Osteodystrophy

Low-turnover renal osteodystrophy includes two subclassifications. These are osteomalacia (LTOM) and adynamic (or aplastic) bone disease (ABD).

Low-Turnover Osteomalacia

Osteomalacia is defined by decreased bone turnover, defective bone mineralization, and an accumulation of unmineralized bone matrix (17). LTOM is associated with severe vitamin D deficiency, aluminum and/or iron toxicity, and profound hyperphosphatemia. Because aluminum binders are used much less frequently now compared with the past, the prevalence of LTOM is decreasing and is found in only 4% to 8% of patients in ESRD (15).

Adynamic Bone Disease

ABD refers to bone histologic findings that show very low rates of bone formation and resorption (decreased numbers of osteoblasts and osteoclasts) (17, 27). Total bone volume is usually reduced (16). Although low blood levels of PTH (< 100 pg/mL) suggest adynamic bone, a high PTH level does not necessarily exclude it because PTH levels greater than 400 pg/mL have been found in patients with ABD (30). In chronic renal failure, suppression of PTH levels to "normal range" is not desirable and may lead to adynamic bone disease. The prevalence of adynamic bone disease without evidence of aluminum toxicity has been increasing, and has been found to be between 25% and 60% in dialysis patients (15). Bone biopsies of adults on HD and PD indicated adynamic renal osteodystrophy in more than 40% and 50%, respectively (32).

Factors that are associated with development of ABD include PD, males on continuous ambulatory peritoneal dialysis, diabetes, advanced age, aluminum toxicity, low albumin level, immobilization, steroid-induced osteopenia, estrogen deficiency, hypermagnesemia, and total parathyroidectomy. Other modifiable factors include a chronic positive calcium balance due to high-dose calcium salts for phosphate binders or use of a high-calcium dialysate (such as 3.5 mEq/L), and more frequent and aggressive calcitriol therapy (30). An increased risk of ABD in malnourished patients may be related to a decreased protein intake, leading to hypophosphatemia (27). Hypophosphatemia can reduce PTH secretion and therefore be involved in the development of low bone turnover (6). The suppression of PTH in individuals with diabetes mellitus may be due to hyperglycemia and advanced glycation end product (27). In addition to its direct effect on suppressing PTH secretion, calcitriol may enhance the onset of ABD by reducing bone metabolism (27).

Serum calcium concentrations tend to be higher in patients with ABD than those with other types of renal osteodystrophy (32). Adynamic bone is essentially inert and does not modulate calcium and phosphate levels properly (30). Thus, a small amount of additional calcium can lead to hypercalcemia. Because adynamic bones cannot amass calcium, other tissues become susceptible to the accumulation of calcium, leading to metastatic calcification, with calciphylaxis as the most formidable result (30). Additionally, hypercalcemia caused by immobilization and decreased ability of the bone to buffer calcium can further suppress PTH and bone remodeling (27). In addition to abnormal calcium homeostasis, patients with ABD have been found to have higher incidences of fractures, more bone pain, delayed healing, and higher morbidity and mortality than patients with other renal osteodystrophy diseases (16).

Mixed Renal Osteodystrophy or Mixed Uremic Osteodystrophy

Mixed uremic osteodystrophy (MUO) is identified by the coexistence of areas of bone that have a variety of remodeling activities, including both high and low turnover, with or without mineralization defect. Thus, overall activity of the bone can be normal or elevated. Contributing factors to MUO include hyperphosphatemia, hyperparathyroidism, calcium and calcitriol deficiency, acidosis, and aluminum ingestion (17).

The reported prevalence of MUO in dialysis patients ranges from 11% to 80% (15). In a study of dialysis patients between 1983 and 1995, 52.9% of those with renal bone diseases were found to have mixed renal osteodystrophy (17).

DIAGNOSIS OF RENAL OSTEODYSTROPHY

Histomorphometry (bone biopsy) is considered the "gold standard" for diagnosis (33). In addition to identifying the types of renal osteodystrophy, a bone biopsy can provide information about the severity of the bone lesions and the presence and amount of deposition of aluminum in the bones (16).

Because the treatment will vary depending on the type of osteodystrophy, it is important to know what type is present, especially in those patients with intermediate PTH levels (100 to 400 pg/mL) (15). It is recognized that patients may transform from one type of bone lesion to another (15). Variables that may alter histology include the phosphate content of the diet, type and amount of phosphate binders used, vitamin D analog therapy, dialysate calcium concentration, and parathyroidectomy. Adynamic bone disease is especially difficult to diagnose using traditional indicators of bone turnover, such as PTH (33). Monier-Faugere et al found that patients with PTH levels less than or equal to 100 pg/mL had low bone turnover, whereas 89.4% of patients with PTH levels greater than or equal to 500 pg/mL had high or normal bone turnover (34). However, of the patients with PTH levels between 100 and 500 pg/mL, 59% had low bone turnover and 41% had high or normal bone turnover (34). In another study, Qi et al found that serum PTH levels between 65 and 450 pg/mL are not predictive of the underlying bone disease (35). Thus, serum PTH levels greater than 500 pg/mL are reasonably predictive of hyperparathyroid bone disease and levels less than 100 are reasonably predictive of low-turnover bone disease.

Several methods may be utilized for the differentiation and diagnosis of renal osteodystrophy. These may include clinical symptoms (such as muscle weakness, joint pain, bone pain, pruritus); biochemical indicators such as calcium, phosphorus, alkaline phosphatase, serum bone alkaline phosphatase (BAP), and PTH concentration; bone x-rays; bone mineral density (BMD); ultrasonography of the parathyroid; and bone histomorphometry. These methods range from relatively noninvasive to the invasive bone biopsy for histomorphometry. Balon and Bren found that a combination of several noninvasive parameters (iPTH, densitometry, radiology, alkaline phosphatase, phosphorus, and patient age) provided accurate diagnosis in 73.3% of the patients in their study (36). A study by Fletcher et al found that the measurement of serum PTH is a useful screening tool for detection of hyperparathyroid bone disease, confirmed by an increased BAP or parathyroid enlargement (33).

Measurement of PTH

The blood level of PTH that accurately predicts low vs high bone turnover has not been clearly established, but it is often used for assessment of bone turnover. The PTH molecule consists of 84 amino acids and thus is referred to as 1–84 PTH. Various amino-terminal and carboxy-terminal fragments (non-1–84 PTH) result from the metabolism of PTH in the liver and kidneys. Carboxy-terminal fragments are primarily inactive. Because the kidneys normally excrete them, circulating levels of these inactive non-1–84 PTH fragments tend to increase with renal failure.

In the 1970s, PTH was measured by competitive radioimmuno assay (RIA), now known as first-generation PTH assays. Second-generation "intact" PTH immunoassays, also known as sandwich assays, provided a more accurate assessment. These assays rely on two detection antibodies to avoid measurement of inactive PTH fragments. It is now recognized that the "intact" parathyroid hormone assay measures a non-1–84 PTH truncated fragment, likely 7–84, in addition to 1–84 PTH. New third-generation "whole" PTH assays measure only the biologically active 1–84 PTH molecule (37). One method also provides a ratio of the 1–84 PTH to the 7–84 PTH (18,38,39). These new assays may improve the accuracy of the interpretation of PTH to renal osteodystrophy.

The target value for PTH depends on the analytical method used. Close monitoring of PTH levels is important, particularly with vitamin D analog therapy to both optimize vitamin D analog therapy and to avoid low bone turnover (17).

TREATMENT AND PREVENTION

When considering the best option for preventing or treating renal osteodystrophy in a renal patient, it is important to evaluate various parameters, including PTH, calcium, and phosphorus levels; bone status; and clinical symptoms such as severe pruritus. Available options for controlling phosphorus, calcium, and PTH levels and the possible use of vitamin D analogues can then be reviewed. The benefit vs risk of each treatment option should be considered on an individual patient basis.

Risks of Hyperphosphatemia

Hyperphosphatemia is an independent risk factor for cardiovascular mortality in dialysis patients (10,40). The cardiovascular mortality rate is 20 to 40 times higher for adults on HD than for the general population for a variety of reasons (41). In a group of dialysis patients, 20 to 30 years old and on dialysis for at least 5 years, coronary artery calcification was found in 88% compared with normal subjects in the same age group, where it is quite uncommon. Patients with calcification had a higher phosphorus level, higher calcium × phosphorus products, and took a higher dose of calcium-containing binders (1).

Two large studies, using US Renal Data System data found that 39% of dialysis patients had a serum phosphorus level greater than 6.5 mg/dL (10,40). These hyperphosphatemic patients had a relative risk of mortality 27% higher than those with a phosphorus level between 2.4 and 6.5 mg/dL. Approximately 20% of the patients studied had a calcium × phosphorus product greater than 72. These patients had a 34% higher relative risk of mortality than patients with a calcium × phosphorus product of 42 to 52. The relative risk from cardiac death was 41% higher in the patients with a serum phosphorus greater than 6.5 mg/dL. All patients had been on dialysis for more than 1 year. The increase in cardiac deaths was thought to be a result of vascular calcification, including plaque calcification, leading to the accelerated atherosclerosis seen in dialysis patients. Patients with elevated phosphorus were also found to have an increased risk of death from infection. It is unclear whether serum phosphorus impairs the immune system or contributes to poor wound healing through abnormalities in the circulation. In these studies, serum calcium was not found to be an independent risk factor (10,40).

Phosphorus Control

The cornerstone for the treatment and prevention of secondary hyperparathyroidism, renal osteodystrophy, and soft tissue calcification is phosphorus control (42).

Table 16.1. Summary of Select K/DOQI Clinical Practice Guidelines on Bone Metabolism and Disease in Chronic Kidney Disease (CKD)

	CKD Stage 3	*CKD Stage 4*	*CKD Stage 5*
GFR range (mL/min/1.73m^2)	30–59	15–29	< 15 or Dialysis
Frequency of measurement of PTH*	Every 12 mo	Every 3 mo	Every 3 mo
Frequency of measurement of calcium/phosphorus*	Every 12 mo	Every 3 mo	Every mo
iPTH goal (pg/mL)	35–70	70–110	150–300
Serum phosphorus goal (mg/dL)	2.7–4.6	2.7–4.6	3.5–5.5
Serum calcium goal	"Normal" range for laboratory	"Normal" range for laboratory	"Normal" range for laboratory, preferably toward lower end (8.4–9.5 mg/dL)
Serum calcium × phosphorus goal	< 55	< 55	< 55
Dietary restriction of phosphorus (mg/d) (initiated when phosphorus or PTH > goal)	800–1000	800–1000	800–1000
Total elemental calcium intake (dietary + calcium-based binders) (mg/d)	< 2000	< 2000	< 2000 (< 1500 total dose elemental calcium-based phosphate binders)

Abbreviations: GFR, glomerular filtration rate; PTH, parathyroid hormone; iPTH, intact parathyroid hormone.

*Frequency of measurements may need to be increased if the patient is restricting dietary phosphorus, receiving vitamin D or analog therapy, or after kidney transplant.

Source: Data are from reference 30.

See Table 16.1 for a summary of select National Kidney Foundation Kidney Disease Outcome Quality Initiatives (K/DOQI) Clinical Practice Guidelines (30). The interventions to achieve and maintain serum phosphorus levels in the target range include a low-phosphorus diet, phosphate binders, and dialysis.

Dialysis

During HD, a limited amount of phosphorus is removed from the blood compartments; the slow movement of phosphorus from the intracellular to the extracellular compartments limits the amount removed in a 3– to 4–hour treatment. The rate-limiting step in phosphorus removal seems to be the movement from intracellular to extracellular compartments and not the dialyzer clearance. Intracellular phosphorus is 50 times higher than extracellular phosphorus (43). There is no agreement about whether different dialyzers increase clearance (43). The average phosphorus removal with PD is 300 to 315 mg per day. HD removes, on average, 800 mg of phosphorus per treatment. Thus, the phosphorus removed per week with HD is approximately 2,400 mg or a mean of 343 mg per day. This is similar to the phosphorus removal with daily PD (30). Longer dialysis times and more frequent dialysis, as in nocturnal dialysis, have been shown to be more efficient at phosphorus removal by allowing a slower equilibration of phosphorus between body compartments. HD six times per week or 8 hours three times per week has been shown to normalize serum phosphorus without the use of binders. Phosphorus supplementation may be needed for those patients doing daily nocturnal dialysis (43–45).

Diet

The K/DOQI nutrition guidelines for optimal protein intake are at least 1.2 g/kg/day for HD patients and 1.3 g/kg/day for PD patients (30). The recommended phosphorus allowance is 10 to 12 mg/g of protein per day, or 800 to 1,000 mg/day adjusted for protein needs (30). All foods high in protein (such as meat, fish, eggs, poultry, milk, and dried beans) are high in phosphorus.

The average absorption of phosphorus from the gastrointestinal (GI) tract is 60% to 70%. Even with the use of a phosphate binder (a compound which binds phosphorus in the gut and prevents absorption), phosphorus absorption can still be 30% to 40%. The use of calcitriol can increase phosphorus absorption from the GI tract up to 86% (11).

The average amount of phosphorus per gram of protein is 10 to 16 mg (30). For a patient weighing 80 kg, requiring 96 grams of protein, the phosphorus content of the diet would be in the range of 1,152 to 1,536 mg, depending on the protein sources

For dialysis patients, the amount of phosphorus in the diet can be reduced without greatly affecting the protein content by excluding those foods highest in phosphorus. A diet that avoids milk and milk products (such as yogurt and cheese), liver, dried beans, and dried peas while relying on meats, eggs, fish, and poultry can provide adequate protein. Liquid nondairy creamers or nondairy milk substitutes containing lower levels of phosphorus can be used in place of milk. Other high-phosphorus foods to avoid or limit include beer; nuts; chocolate; quick breads; whole-grain or bran products; and carbonated beverages, canned ice tea, or juice drinks containing phosphoric acid. Peanut butter and cheese, although somewhat high in phosphorus, may be included in the patient's diet if other protein sources are not tolerated. Individuals on a low-phosphorus diet should avoid enhanced meat, which is fresh meat marinated in a solution of sodium, phosphate, and water. This process, used to increase shelf life and improve tenderness in packaged meats, increases the phosphorus content.

A detailed diet history can help the dietitian individualize each patient's diet to maintain adequate nutrients while minimizing phosphorus intake. Ethnic or cultural food habits need to be considered when restricting the diet. For patients following a vegetarian diet, it can be a challenge to maintain an adequate protein intake with an acceptable phosphorus intake. It may be necessary to include milk products in the vegetarian diet for their protein content. A plant-based diet will need to rely on beans, legumes, and lentils, which are high in phosphorus, for dietary protein. (See Appendix C for more information about renal vegetarian diets.)

Phosphate Binders

The third method for controlling serum phosphorus levels is the use of phosphate binders. Historically, aluminum hydroxide was used as a phosphate binder. Although these medications are very efficient at binding phosphorus, it was discovered that aluminum was being absorbed and patients developed aluminum overload (30). Because of serious side effects such as osteomalacia, dementia, and myopathy, the use of aluminum-based binders are limited (30). Magnesium-based products such as antacids have also been used as phosphate binders, but their use is also limited because of the potential for absorption and accumulation of magnesium in the body. Magnesium is removed during dialysis, but overload can occur and lead to inhibition of bone mineralization and suppression of the central nervous system (46). Monitoring the patient's magnesium levels and adjusting the magnesium in the dialysate may be necessary for those patients taking magnesium-based binders (47,48). Additionally, diarrhea can be a limiting side effect of magnesium binders (48). With no long-term studies on the safety and efficacy of magnesium-based binders, K/DOQI recommends their use only if all other compounds have failed (30).

Calcium-based binders, such as calcium carbonate and calcium acetate, largely replaced aluminum-based binders in the last decade. Calcium salts are effective in binding phosphorus in the GI tract. However, these too have some negative side effects. Large amounts of calcium salt are often needed to control serum phosphorus, and unbound calcium is absorbed from the gut. This can lead to hypercalcemia, especially when the patient is also receiving the active form of vitamin D (49). There is evidence that hypercalcemia can lead to oversuppression of PTH and ABD. Excessive calcium absorption can also lead to deposition in the soft tissue, especially when the phosphorus and calcium × phosphorus product are elevated. Other risks of excessive calcium intake include calciphylaxis, cardiovascular calcification, and metastatic calcification (49).

The serum calcium may or may not reflect total body calcium and bone status because only approximately 0.1% of the total body calcium is found in the extracellular fluid (50). In other words, a normal serum calcium does not guarantee a normal body calcium. K/DOQI guidelines recommend a standard calcium dialysate of 2.5 mEq/L (30). Dialysate concentrations of 1.5 to 2.0 mEq/L, or even lower, can be used to treat hypercalcemia. However, these low calcium dialysate levels can lead to marked bone demineralization and are not recommended for long-term use. Negative calcium balance may aggravate secondary hyperparathyroidism (49).

Calcium acetate and calcium carbonate are both effective phosphate binders. Calcium acetate, a more efficient phosphate binder, allows the use of a smaller dose of elemental calcium, compared with calcium carbonate, to bind an equal amount of phosphorus. The use of calcium acetate may therefore reduce the total calcium load to the patient (41,51).

Calcium citrate should be avoided because citrate enhances absorption of aluminum (52). Even if the patient is not taking any aluminum-based phosphate binders, other medications may contain aluminum. Calcium supplements inhibit the absorption of iron from supplements and foods when taken simultaneously. Oral iron supplements, if indicated, should be taken between meals because calcium-based binders must be taken with meals to be effective.

Sevelamer hydrochloride is a phosphate binder that does not contain aluminum, calcium or magnesium. Sevelamer has been shown to have comparable efficacy to calcium acetate in controlling hyperphosphatemia, but with less hypercalcemia (53). A study by Chertow et al (54) followed 200 maintenance HD patients from 15 participating units for 52 weeks. Patients were randomized to either sevelamer or calcium-based binders after a washout period. Both binders controlled serum phosphorus within the range of 3.0 to 5.0 mg/dL. Subjects on the calcium-based binders experienced significantly more hypercalcemia (defined as a calcium greater than 10.5 mg/dL when corrected for serum albumin) and intact PTH levels were below the target range of 150 to 300 pg/mL. Both coronary artery and aortic calcification progressed significantly with calcium-based binders, but not with sevelamer. This difference was seen as early as 6 months into the study. The sevelamer subjects ingested on average 6.5 grams of the polymer, or about eight (800 mg) tablets. The subjects in the calcium group ingested 4.3 to 4.6 g of calcium per day. Other studies have also shown sevelamer to be a safe and effective phosphate binder. Doses of two to four (800 mg) capsules with each meal have been shown to control serum phosphorus (55).

A study by Chertow et al (56) observed an increase in serum calcium, although still in the normal range, in patients on sevelamer even without a change in vitamin D dosage. They theorized that sevelamer competes for phosphate binding with dietary calcium, allowing more free calcium to be absorbed. Alternatively, with a reduction in serum phosphorus on sevelamer, and a lower calcium × phosphorus product, they speculated that fewer calcium-phosphate crystals were deposited in the tissue, therefore increasing the serum calcium. Other research comparing calcium acetate to sevelamer has shown a reduction in the incidence of hypercalcemia (defined as a serum calcium > 11.0 mg/dL) with sevelamer, from 22% to 5% (11,53).

Sevelamer also acts as a bile acid sequestrant and is therefore capable of reducing low-density lipoprotein (LDL) cholesterol levels. Short-term studies have shown a 20% to 30% reduction in LDL cholesterol and a 5% to 15% increase in high-density lipoprotein cholesterol (55). Other calcium-free, non-aluminum phosphate binders, such as lanthanum carbonate, are under investigation (49,57).

Adherence

Poor adherence to diet and medication recommendations is a common problem in dialysis patients. This seems to be especially true with phosphorus control. Patient compliance to phosphate binders has reported to range from 30% to 100% (30). Aggressive education and encouragement of the patient need to be provided by the dietitian and other health care team members for the treatment to be successful. Phosphate binders must be taken with food to be effective. Remembering to take several fairly large pills with all meals and snacks can be a difficult task. The need to limit fluids for swallowing these pills as well as other medications can also be a deterrent to adherence. GI side effects such as bloating, constipation, or diarrhea may also decrease adherence. Phosphate binders are often prescribed in equally divided doses such as "3 TID"; however, patients rarely eat three meals of equal size per day. The phosphate binder dosage must be customized to match the phosphorus content of the meal or snack. The dietitian can be instrumental in instructing the patient to match binder dosage with the phosphorus content of foods consumed.

The choice of a phosphate binder must consider other factors in addition to clinical efficacy. Cost to the patient, comorbid illnesses, patient's ability to swallow the pills, and any GI side effects must be evaluated before recommending a specific phosphate binder. The following are suggestions on binder usage based on the K/DOQI guidelines:

1. Both calcium-based and non–calcium-, non–aluminum-, non–magnesium-based binders (such

as sevelamer) are effective in reducing serum phosphorus (30).

2. For patients with a serum phosphorus greater than 5.5 mg/dL despite the use of calcium-based or non–calcium-, non–aluminum-, non–magnesium-based binders, a combination should be used (30).

Overview of Phosphorus Control

To control phosphorus, pursue the following steps:

1. Work with patient to reduce dietary phosphorus.
2. Evaluate the phosphorus content of meals and snacks.
3. Match the number of binders to the phosphate content of the meals and snacks. The general consensus is that binders should be taken 10 to 15 minutes before or during the meal for optimal effect (30).
4. Monitor calcium (corrected calcium) and phosphorus at least monthly (30).
5. Maintain serum phosphorus between 3.5 and 5.5 mg/dL. (30)
6. Reduce binder dosage if phosphorus drops to less than 3.0 mg/dL.
7. Consider increasing binder dosage if phosphorus is greater than 5.5 mg/dL, patient is compliant with diet and binders, and the maximum recommended binder dosage has not been reached.
8. Try to keep corrected calcium × phosphorus product at less than 55 (30,41,47).
9. For non-calcium-based binders, keep in mind the following:
   - Sevelamer is an excellent phosphate binder because it does not add to the calcium load and has the extra benefit of reducing LDL cholesterol (53).
   - The manufacturer recommends a starting dose of sevelamer (Renagel, Genzyme Corporation, Cambridge, MA 02193) of 800 to 1,600 mg with each meal, depending on the severity of hyperphosphatemia. An average of eight Renagel tablets per day have been required to control serum phosphorus (54).
   - If GI complaints occur with sevelamer, try a lower dose and assess tolerance.
   - If a lower dose is tolerated, but phosphorus is elevated, try adding another binder.
   - Because of cost, it may be necessary to use sevelamer at a lower dose in combination with a calcium-based binder.
10. For calcium-based binders, keep in mind the following:
    - Calcium-based binders are effective and may be used as the primary binder (30).
    - Total calcium from binders should be limited to 1,500 mg/day and the total calcium including dietary calcium should not exceed 2,000 mg/day (30).
    - Calcium acetate is preferred over calcium carbonate because a lower dose of elemental calcium will bind the same amount of phosphorus (41,51). The recommended initial dosage of calcium acetate is two tablets (667 mg each) with each meal.
    - Calcium carbonate can be used if the patient cannot obtain or tolerate calcium acetate.
    - If corrected calcium becomes greater than 10.2 mg/dL, try reducing the dosage of calcium-based binders (30). Sevelamer may be added if phosphate is not controlled on the reduced dosage of calcium-based binders.
    - An aluminum- or magnesium-based binder may be used (for up to 4 weeks) alone or in combination with a calcium-based binder if phosphorus is not controlled on the reduced dosage of calcium alone (30).
    - When hypercalcemia persists, consider reducing the dialysate calcium.
11. Based on the K/DOQI guidelines (30), calcium-based binders should be avoided by the following individuals:
    - Patients who have hypercalcemia (corrected calcium > 10.2 mg/dL).
    - Patients whose plasma PTH levels are less than 100 pg/mL, or less than 150 pg/mL on two consecutive measurements.
    - Patients with severe vascular or other soft-tissue calcification.
12. For magnesium-based binders, keep in mind the following:
    - Magnesium-based or combination calcium/magnesium-based binders can be effective. If they are used, magnesium levels in the patient should be checked monthly.
    - The magnesium level in the dialysate may need to be reduced (48).

13. For aluminum-based binders, keep in mind the following:
    - Aluminum-based binders may be appropriate for a patient with a phosphorus level greater than 7.0 mg/dL and inability to obtain or tolerate sevelamer.
    - The use of aluminum binders should be limited to 1 month. The patient should then be switched to another binder (30,50).

(Refer to Chapter 15 for more information about medications.)

Vitamin D

As previously mentioned, the primary action of vitamin D is the regulation of PTH by the parathyroid glands. Active vitamin D is generated from the precursor vitamin D-3 (cholecalciferol) from animal sources and vitamin D-2 (ergocalciferol) from plant sources. Vitamin D-3 is also generated from provitamin D-3 in the skin upon exposure to ultraviolet light. The liver and kidneys convert the precursors to the biologically active form in the body. In the liver, vitamin D is hydroxylated to form 25–hydroxyvitamin D. In the kidney a second hydroxyl group is added to form 1,25–dihydroxyvitamin D (calcitriol). Calcitriol binds with high affinity to vitamin D receptors.

The replacement of vitamin D has become a major tool for the treatment of secondary hyperparathyroidism. These medications can be given orally or intravenously (IV). When administered orally they can be given intermittently (2 to 3 times per week) or continuously (daily). IV versions can be given three times per week at HD treatments. Intermittent IV calcitriol has been shown to be more effective than daily oral calcitriol (30). IV dosing has the advantage of not relying on patient compliance with oral medication. The important issue is not just whether PTH is suppressed, but to what extent is there is regression of parathyroid gland hyperplasia (49). One study showed IV calcitriol to have a superior effect on bone remodeling over oral pulse or oral intermittent calcitriol therapy, despite similar changes in PTH levels, after 6 months (58).

For patients on PD, evidence suggests that intraperitoneal (IP) calcitriol is at least as effective as oral calcitriol in reducing PTH levels and slowing the progression of renal osteodystrophy (59). IP calcitriol is associated with a lower incidence of hyperphosphatemia and elevated calcium × phosphorus products (59).

Calcitriol has been shown to successfully suppress PTH levels and improve bone histology, but its use is limited by its stimulation of intestinal absorption of both calcium and phosphorus, resulting in the occurrence of hypercalcemia, hyperphosphatemia, and elevated calcium × phosphorus product. The risk of hypercalcemia is greatest when the patient is on calcium-based phosphate binders. Any calcium × phosphorus product greater than 55 increases the risk of metastatic calcification (47,60,61).

Vitamin D analogs were developed to retain the high affinity for vitamin D receptors, with less calcemic activity, while suppressing PTH secretion (61). Paricalcitriol, 19-nor $1,25(OH)_2D_2$ (19–NOR) (Zemplar, Abbott Laboratories, North Chicago, IL 60064) is a vitamin D analog developed to overcome some of calcitriol's shortcomings. Paricalcitriol has shown long-term efficacy in reducing PTH levels by 60% (62). This is accomplished with only slight increases in serum calcium, while phosphorus and calcium × phosphorus product remain within an acceptable range. Patients with baseline hypocalcemia were found to have more normalized calcium while PTH was suppressed (63). Although hypercalcemia has occurred in some patients, it occurs more often in patients with relatively lower PTH levels (< 150 pg/mL) (62–64).

Doxercalciferol, ($1 \times (OH)D_2$) (Hectorol, Bone Care International, Madison, WI 53711), another vitamin D analog, is a pro-vitamin and must be converted in the liver to the active form. Both oral and IV preparations of doxercalciferol have been shown to be effective in controlling secondary hyperparathyroidism (65). Intermittent oral doxercalciferol suppressed PTH with acceptable mild increases in serum calcium, even when calcium-based binders were used (66). In a study of 99 HD patients with hyperparathyroidism, 80% of the patients had a 70% decrease in PTH when treated with doxercalciferol (67). Research continues on new vitamin D analogs. Two currently under investigation are 22-oxacalcitriol (OCT) and falecitriol (64).

K/DOQI guidelines (30) recommend that patients with an intact PTH greater than 300 pg/mL should be evaluated for vitamin D therapy. The target range for an intact PTH is 150 to 300 pg/mL. When initiating or titrating the dose of vitamin D, calcium and phosphorus should be monitored at least every 2 weeks.

Success with any vitamin D therapy depends on appropriate timing for initiation of therapy, adequate dosing, and careful monitoring for side effects. Individual dialysis facilities may have protocols for vitamin

D analog usage and doses. (Refer also to Chapter 15 on medications.)

Calcimimetics

In secondary hyperparathyroidism, there is a decrease in the calcium-sensing receptor, which regulates PTH release. This receptor becomes an ideal target for the development of compounds that enhance the affinity of the receptor for calcium and reduce PTH secretion. Compounds that mimic calcium at the receptor site are called calcimimetic agents (68).

Cinacalcet HCL (Sensipar TM, Amgen, Inc, Thousand Oaks, CA 91320–1799) is a new calcimimetic agent, which has been shown to directly lower PTH levels by increasing the sensitivity of the calcium-sensing receptor sites to extracellular calcium. The reduction in PTH is associated with a concomitant decrease in serum calcium levels. In a study of 75 patients with PTH greater than 350 pg/mL, a decrease in PTH, calcium × phosphorus product, and phosphorus occurred with cinacalcet HCL compared to a placebo. The drug was well tolerated (69).

The manufacturer recommends starting with an oral dose of 30 mg once a day. It is recommended that serum calcium and phosphorus be measured within 1 week, and PTH 1 to 4 weeks after initiation or dose adjustment. Cinacalcet HCL should be titrated no more frequently than every 2 to 4 weeks through sequential doses of 60, 90, 120, and 180 mg once daily until target PTH is reached. Because cinacalcet HCL lowers calcium, a calcium level less than 8.4 mg/dL is a contraindication. Cinacalcet HCL can be used alone or in combination with vitamin D sterols and/or phosphate binders. There is no pharmacokinetic interaction with cinacalcet HCL and calcium carbonate or sevelamer HCL (70).

Early Intervention

Evidence is compelling that in early renal disease the use of calcitriol is beneficial for retarding or preventing metabolic bone disease with minimal risk to the patient (71). Calcium, phosphorus, and PTH levels should be monitored closely. K/DOQI (30) recommends the initiation of an oral vitamin D sterol when the serum level of 25(OH)-vitamin D is less than 30 ng/mL and the plasma levels of iPTH are above the target range for the CKD stage. (See Table 16.1. Also refer to Chapter 3 for more information about early renal disease.)

Parathyroidectomy

A normal parathyroid gland weighs 30 to 40 mg. In comparison, a hyperplastic gland in secondary hyperparathyroidism may weigh 2 to 3 g. Four glands are typical, but more glands may be present in up to 13% of subjects. K/DOQI guidelines recommend considering parathyroidectomy in patients with intact PTH persistently more than 800 mg/dL, and hypercalcemia and/or hyperphosphatemia that are refractory to medical treatment (30). Another indication would be calciphylaxis with PTH levels more than 500 pg/mL (30).

Conflicting evidence exists for performing parathyroidectomy for severe hyperparathyroidism prior to transplant. However, a total parathyroidectomy is not recommended because control of calcium levels may be difficult to manage after transplant (30).

In addition to the effects of excess PTH on bone, calcium, and phosphorus regulation, PTH has been shown to affect the function of many organs and tissues such as the brain, heart, smooth muscles, lungs, erythrocytes, lymphocytes, pancreas, adrenal glands, and testes (72). One would therefore expect a parathyroidectomy to have a positive impact on nutritional status and humoral and cellular immunity.

Surgical Procedures for Parathyroidectomy

The following three surgical procedures are available:

- *Subtotal parathyroidectomy*—involves removal of all identifiable parathyroid tissue except for 40 to 60 mg of the least hyperplastic gland. Drawbacks include the risk of persistent or recurrent disease, with repeated neck surgery needed.
- *Total parathyroidectomy with autotransplantation*—total parathyroidectomy with small amount of tissue transplanted, usually in the forearm. A main advantage of this procedure is the remaining gland can easily be removed from the implantation site if repeat surgery is necessary.
- *Total parathyroidectomy*—minimizes the chances of recurrent disease. Disadvantages of this procedure include development of ABD and osteomalacia, permanent hypoparathyroidism, impaired bone healing, and need for long-term calcium and vitamin D therapy.

At this time there is no consensus as to which procedure is the best. Effective surgical treatment can be accomplished with subtotal, total, or total with autotransplantation (36).

Nonsurgical Parathyroidectomy

Ethanol injection under ultrasonographic guidance has been suggested as a safe and simple approach to refractory hyperparathyroidism (73,74). Ethanol is injected into the largest gland. The plasma PTH is measured in 1 week, and if it is still more than 200 pg/mL, ethanol is injected into the same or the next largest gland, with PTH again measured in 1 week. This process continues until the PTH is less than 200 pg/mL. Currently this procedure remains experimental until its efficacy and safety are established in a large number of patients (75). Another experimental treatment that seems encouraging is injecting calcitriol directly into the parathyroid gland (76).

Hungry Bone Syndrome

Hypocalcemia following parathyroidectomy can be mild or severe. "Hungry bone" syndrome occurs from a sudden reduction in PTH that upsets the exchange of calcium to and from the bone that is necessary for normal remodeling. The result is hypocalcemia. Severe hypocalcemia postoperatively may be treated with IV calcium. Careful monitoring of calcium and phosphorus is essential. Once the patient can tolerate oral medications, calcium supplements should be given between meals for maximum absorption. A calcium dosage of up to 12 g per day may be required. Phosphorus may also need supplementation. Calcitriol, up to 6 μg/day, is normally given to stimulate calcium and phosphorus absorption (49).

CONCLUSION

Renal osteodystrophy is a challenging problem that has evolved to encompass much more than bone health. It can have a tremendous impact on the morbidity and mortality of individuals with kidney disease. Many of the factors that impact renal osteodystrophy are modifiable, including phosphorus intake and binders, calcium, and vitamin D analog therapy. Because of this, the dietitian has the opportunity to positively impact renal osteodystrophy of patients.

REFERENCES

1. Goodman WG, Goldin J, Kuizon BD, Yoon C, Gales B, Sider D, Wang Y, Chung J, Emerick A, Greaser L, Elashoff R, Salusky IB. Coronary-artery calcification in young adults with end-stage renal disease who are undergoing dialysis. *N Engl J Med.* 2000;342:1478–1483.
2. Ribeiro S, Ramos A, Brandao A, Rebelo JR, Guerra A, Resina C, Vila-Lobos A, Carvalho F, Remedio F, Ribeiro F. Cardiac valve calcification in haemodialysis patients: role of calcium-phosphate metabolism. *Nephrol Dial Transplant.* 1998;13:2037–2040.
3. London GM, Pannier B, Marchais S, Guerin AP. Calcification of the aortic valve in the dialyzed patient. *J Am Soc Nephrol.* 2000;11:778–783.
4. Rostand SG, Drueke TB. Parathyroid hormone, vitamin D, and cardiovascular disease in chronic renal failure. *Kidney Int.* 1999;56:383–392.
5. Guerin A, London GM, Marchais S, Metivier F. Arterial stiffening and vascular calcifications in end-stage renal disease. *Nephrol Dial Transplant.* 2000;15:1014–1021.
6. Cannata Andia JB. Adynamic bone and chronic renal failure: an overview. *Am J Med Sci.* 2000; 320:81–84.
7. Llach F. Hyperphosphatemia in end-stage renal disease patients: pathophysiological consequences. *Kidney Int.* 1999;56(Suppl 73):S31–S37.
8. Llach F. The evolving pattern of calciphylaxis: therapeutic considerations. *Nephrol Dial Transplant.* 2001;16:448–451.
9. Drueke TB, Eckardt K. Role of secondary hyperparathyroidism in erythropoietin resistance of chronic renal failure patients. *Nephrol Dial Transplant.* 2002;17(Suppl 5):28–31.
10. Block GA, Hulbert-Shearon TE, Levin NW, Port FK. Association of serum phosphorus and calcium (phosphate product with mortality risk in chronic hemodialysis patients: a national study. *Am J Kidney Dis.* 1998;31:607–617.
11. Block GA, Port FK. Re-evaluation of risks associated with hyperphosphatemia and hyperparathyroidism in dialysis patients: recommendations for a change in management. *Am J Kidney Dis.* 2000; 35:1226–1237.
12. Block GA. Prevalence and clinical consequences of elevated Ca × P product in hemodialysis patients. *Clin Nephrol.* 2000;54:318–324.
13. Balon BP, Radovan H, Zavratnik A, Kos M. Bone mineral density in patients beginning hemodialysis treatment. *Am J Nephrol.* 2002;22:14–17.

14. Hruska K. New concepts in renal osteodystrophy. *Nephrol Dial Transplant.* 1998;13:2755–2760.
15. Ho LT, Sprague SM. Percutaneous bone biopsy in the diagnosis of renal osteodystrophy. *Semin Nephrol.* 2002;22:268–275.
16. Malluche HH, Langub MC, Monier-Faugere M-C. The role of bone biopsy in clinical practice and research. *Kidney Int.* 1999;56(Suppl 73): S20–S25.
17. Malluche HH, Monier-Faugere MC. Understanding and managing hyperphosphatemia in patients with chronic renal disease. *Clin Nephrol.* 1999; 52:267–277.
18. Monier-Faugere M-CM, Langub MC, Malluche HH. Mineralized bone histology in normal and uremic states. In: Bushinsky D, ed. *Renal Osteodystrophy*. Philadelphia, Pa: Lippincott-Raven; 1998:81.
19. Beckerman P, Silver J. Vitamin D and the parathyroid. *Am J Med Sci.* 1999;317:363–375.
20. Fukuda N, Tanaka H, Tominaga Y, Fukagawa M, Kurokawa K, Seino Y. Decreased 1,25-dihydroxyvitamin D3 receptor density is associated with a more severe form of parathyroid hyperplasia in chronic uremic patients. *J Clin Invest.* 1993;92: 1436–1443.
21. Olaizola I, Aznarez A, Jorgetti V, Petraglia A, Caorsi H, Acuna G, Fajardo L, Ambrosoni P, Mazzuchi N. Are there any differences in the parathyroid response in the different types of renal osteodystrophy? *Nephrol Dial Transplant.* 1998;13(Suppl 3):15–18.
22. Slatopolsky E, Dusso A, Brown AJ. The role of phosphorus in the development of secondary hyperparathyroidism and parathyroid cell proliferation in chronic renal failure. *Am J Med Sci.* 1999; 317:370–376.
23. Slatopolsky E, Finch J, Denda M. Phosphate restriction prevents parathyroid cell growth in uremic rats: High phosphate directly stimulates PTH secretion in vitro. *J Clin Invest.* 1996;97:2534–2540.
24. Naveh-Many T, Rahamimov R, Livni N, Silver J. Parathyroid cell proliferation in normal and chronic renal failure rats: The effects of calcium, phosphate, and vitamin D. *J Clin Invest.* 1995;96: 1786–1793.
25. Dendra M, Finch J, Slatopolsky E. Phosphorus accelerates the development of parathyroid hyperplasia and secondary hyperparathyroidism in rats with renal failure. *Am J Kidney Dis.* 1996;38: 596–602.
26. Arnold, A, Brown MF, Urena P, Gaz RD, Sarfati E, Drueke TB. Monoclonality of parathyroid tumors in chronic renal failure and in primary parathyroid hyperplasia. *J Clin Invest.* 1995;95: 2047–2053.
27. Fukagawa M, Akizawa T, Kurokawa K. Is aplastic osteodystrophy a disease of malnutrition? *Curr Opin Nephrol Hypertens.* 2000;9:363–367.
28. Disthabanchong S, Gonzalez E. Regulation of bone cell development and function: implication for renal osteodystrophy. *J Investig Med.* 2001;49:240–249.
29. Divieti P, John MR, Juppner H, Bringhurst FR. Human PTH-(7–84) Inhibits bone resorption in vitro via actions independent of the type 1 PTH/PTHrP receptor. *Endocrinology.* 2002;143: 171–176.
30. K/DOQI clinical practice guidelines for bone metabolism and disease in chronic kidney disease. *Am J Kidney Dis.* 2003;42(suppl):S7–S169.
31. Movilli E, Zani R, Carli O, Sangalli L, Pola A, Camerini C, Scolari F, Cancarini G, Maiorca R. Direct effect of the correction of acidosis on plasma parathyroid hormone concentrations, calcium and phosphate in hemodialysis patients: a prospective study. *Nephron.* 2001;87:257–262.
32. Salusky IB, Goodman WG, Adynamic renal osteodystrophy: is there a problem? *J Am Soc Nephrol.* 2001;12:1978–1985.
33. Fletcher S, Jones RG, Rayner HC, Harnden P, Hordon LD, Aaron JE, Oldroyd B, Brownjohn AM, Turney JH, Smith MA. Assessment of renal osteodystrophy in dialysis patients: use of bone alkaline phosphatase, bone mineral density and parathyroid ultrasound in comparison with bone histology. *Nephron.* 1997;75:412–419.
34. Monier-Faugere M-C, Geng Z, Mawad H, Friedler RM, Gao P, Cantor TL, Malluche HH. Improved assessment of bone turnover by the PTH-(1–84)/large C-PTH fragments ratio in ESRD patients. *Kidney Int.* 2001;60:1460–1468.
35. Qi Q, Monier-Faugere MC, Geng Z, Malluche HH. Predictive value of serum parathyroid hormone levels for bone turnover in patients on chronic maintenance dialysis. *Am J Kidney Dis.* 1995;26:622–631.
36. Balon BP, Bren A. Bone histomorphometry is still the golden standard for diagnosing renal osteodystrophy. *Clin Nephrol.* 2000;54:463–469.

37. Coen G, Bonucci E, Ballanti P, Balducci A, Calabria S, Nicolai GA, Fischer MS, Lifrieri F, Manni M, Morosetti M, Moscaritolo E, Sardella D. PTH 1–84 and PTH "7–84" in the noninvasive diagnosis of renal bone disease. *Am J Kidney Dis.* 2002;40:348–354.
38. Slatopolsky E, Finch J, Clay P, Martin D, Sicard G, Singer G, Gao P, Cantor T, Dusso A. A novel mechanism for skeletal resistance in uremia. *Kidney Int.* 2000;58:753–761.
39. Gao P, Scheibel S, D'Amour P, John MR, Rao SD, Schmidt-Gayk H, Cantor T. Development of a novel immunoradiometric assay exclusively for biologically active whole parathyroid hormone 1–84: implications for improvement of accurate assessment of parathyroid function. *J Bone Min Res.* 2001;16:605–614.
40. Ganesh SK, Stack AG, Levin NW, Hulbert-Shearon T, Port FK. Association of elevated serum PO4, Ca (PO4 product, and parathyroid hormone with cardiac mortality risk in chronic hemodialysis patients. *J Am Soc Nephrol.* 2001; 12:2131–2138.
41. Fatica RA, Dennis VW. Cardiovascular mortality in chronic renal failure: Hyperphosphatemia, coronary calcification, and the role of phosphate binders. *Cleveland Clin J Med.* 2002;69(Suppl): S21–S27.
42. Hsu CH. Are we mismanaging calcium and phosphate metabolism in renal failure? *Am J Kidney Dis.* 1997;29:641–649.
43. Pohlmeier R, Vienken J. Phosphate removal and hemodialysis conditions. *Kidney Int.* 2001; 59(Suppl 78):S190–S194.
44. Mucsi I, Hercz G, Uldall R, Ouwendyk M, Francoeur R, Pierratos A. Control of serum phosphorus without any phosphate binders inpatients treated with nocturnal hemodialysis. *Kidney Int.* 1998;53:1399–1401.
45. Drueke TB. Renal osteodystrophy: management of hyperphosphatemia. *Nephrol Dial Transplant.* 2000;15(Suppl 5):32–33.
46. Delmez JA, Slatopolsky E. Hyperphosphatemia: its consequences and treatment in patients with chronic kidney disease. *Am J Kidney Dis.* 1992; 19:303–317.
47. Malluche HH, Monier-Faugere MC. Hyperphosphatemia: pharmacologic intervention yesterday, today, and tomorrow. *Clin Nephrol.* 2000;54: 309–317.
48. Chertow GM, Martin KJ. Current and future therapies for the medical management of secondary hyperparathyroidism. *Semin Dial.* 1998;11:267–270.
49. Locatelli F, Cannata-Andia JB, Drueke TB, Horl WH, Fouque D, Heimburger O, Ritz E. Management of disturbances of calcium and phosphate metabolism in chronic renal insufficiency, with emphasis on the control of hyperphosphatemia. *Nephrol Dial Transplant.* 2002;17:723–731.
50. Krieger N. Calcium and phosphorus. In: Bushinsky D, ed. *Renal Osteodystrophy*. Philadelphia, Pa: Lippincott-Raven; 1998:91.
51. Mai ML, Emmett M, Sheikh MS, Santa Ana CA, Schiller L, Fordtran JS. Calcium acetate, as effective phosphate binder in patients with renal failure. *Kidney Int.* 1989;36:690–695.
52. Nolan CR, Califano JR, Butzin CA. Influence of calcium acetate or calcium citrate on intestinal aluminum absorption. *Kidney Int.* 1990;38:937–941.
53. Bleyer AJ, Burke SK, Dillon M, Garrett B, Kant KS, Lynch D, Rahman SN, Schoenfeld P, Teitelbaum I, Zeig S, Slatopolsky E. A comparison of calcium-free phosphate binder sevelamer hydrochloride with calcium acetate in the treatment of hyperphosphatemia in hemodialysis patients. *Am J Kidney Dis.* 1999;33:694–701.
54. Chertow GM, Burke SK, Paggi P. Sevelamer attenuates the progression of coronary and aortic calcification in hemodialysis patients. *Kidney Int.* 2002;62:245–252.
55. Slatopolsky EA, Burke SK, Dillon MA. Renagel, a nonabsorbed calcium- and aluminum-free phosphate binder, lowers serum phosphorus and parathyroid hormone. *Kidney Int.* 1999;55:299–307.
56. Chertow GM, Burke SK, Dillon MA, Slatopolsky E. Long- term effects of sevelamer hydrochloride on the calcium × phosphate product and lipid profile of hemodialysis patients. *Nephrol Dial Transplant.* 1999;14:2907–2914.
57. Hutchinson AJ. Calcitriol, lanthanum carbonate, and other new phosphate binders in the management of renal osteodystrophy. *Perit Dial Int.* 1999;19(Suppl 2):S408–S412.
58. Turk AM, Yildiz A, Gurbilek M. Comparative effect of oral pulse and intravenous calcitriol treatment in hemodialysis patients: the effect of serum

IL-1 and IL-6 levels and bone mineral density. *Nephron.* 2002;90:188–94.

59. Gadallah MF, Arora N, Torres C, Ramdeen G, Schaeffer-Pautz A, Moles K. Pulse oral verses pulse intraperitoneal calcitriol: a comparison of efficacy in treatment of hyperparathyroidism and renal osteodystrophy in PD patients. *Adv Perit Dial.* 2002;16:303–307.
60. Malluche HH, Mawad H, Koszewski NJ. Update on vitamin D and its newer analogues: actions and rationale for treatment in chronic renal failure. *Kidney Int.* 2002;62:367–374.
61. Slatopolsky EA, Dusso A, Brown AJ. New analogs of vitamin D3. *Kidney Int.* 1999;56(suppl): S46–S51.
62. Martin KJ, Gonzalez EA, Gellens M, Hamm LL, Abboud H, Lindberg J. 19-Nor-1-alpha-25-dihydroxyvitamin D2 (paricalcitol) safely and effectively reduces the levels of intact parathyroid hormone in patients on hemodialysis. *J Am Soc Nephrol.* 1998;9:1427–1432.
63. Lindberg J, Martin KJ, Gonzalez EA, Acchiardo SR, Valdin JR, Soltanek C. A long-term, multicenter study of the efficacy and safety of paricalcitol in end-stage renal disease. *Clin Nephrol.* 2001;56:315–323.
64. Slatopolsky E, Dusso A, Brown AJ. Control of uremic bone disease: role of vitamin D analogs. *Kidney Int.* 2002;61(suppl):S143–S148.
65. Maung HM, Elangovan L, Frazao JM, Bower JD, Kelley BJ, Acchiardo SR, Rodriguez HJ, Norris KC, Sigala JF, Rutkowski M, Robertson JA, Goodman WG, Levine BS, Chesney RW, Mazess RB, Kyllo DM, Douglass LL, Bishop CW, Coburn JW. Efficacy and side effects of intermittent intravenous and oral doxercalciferol (1alpha-hydroxyvitamin D2) in dialysis patients with secondary hyperparathyroidism: a sequential comparison. *Am J Kidney Dis.* 2001;37: 532–543.
66. Tan AU, Levine BS, Mazess RB, Kyllo DM, Bishop CW, Knutson JC, Kleinman KS, Coburn JW. Effective suppression of parathyroid hormone by 1 alpha-hydroxy-vitamin D2 in hemodialysis patients with moderate to severe secondary hyperparathyroidism. *Kidney Int.* 1997; 51:317–323.
67. Frazao JM, Elangovan L, Maung HM, Chesney RW, Acchiardo SR, Bower JD, Kelley BJ, Rodriguez HJ, Norris KC, Robertson JA, Levine BS, Goodman WG, Gentile D, Mazess RB, Kyllo DM, Douglass LL, Bishop CW, Coburn JW. Intermittent doxercalciferal (1 alpha-hydroxyvitamin D2) therapy for secondary hyperparathyroidism. *Am J Kidney Dis.* 2000;36:550–561.
68. Frazao JM, Martins P, Coburn JW. The calcimimetic agents: perspectives for treatment. *Kidney Int.* 2002;61(suppl):S149–S154.
69. Drueke TB. The place of calcium and calcimimetics in the treatment of secondary hyperparathyroidism. *Nephrol Dial Transplant.* 2001; 16(Suppl 6):15–17.
70. Sensipar. Amgen Web site. Available at: http://www.amgen.com. Accessed March 24, 2004.
71. Coburn JW, Elangovan L. Prevention of metabolic bone disease in the pre-end-stage renal disease setting. *J Am Soc Nephrol.* 1998;9(Suppl 12):S71–S77.
72. Bro S, Olgaard K. Effects of excess PTH on nonclassical target organs. *Am J Kidney Dis.* 1997; 30:606–620.
73. Kitaoka M, Fukagawa M, Ogata E, Kurokawa K. Reduction of functioning parathyroid cell mass by ethanol injection in chronic dialysis patients. *Kidney Int.* 1994:46:1110–1117.
74. Giangrande A, Castiflioni A, Solbiati L, Allaria P. Ultrasound-guided percutaneous fine-needle ethanol injection into parathyroid glands in secondary hyperparathyroidism. *Nephrol Dial Transplant.* 1992;7:412–421.
75. de Francisco A, Fresnedo GF, Rodrigo E, Pinera C, Amado JA, Arias M. Parathyroidectomy in dialysis patients. *Kidney Int.* 2002;61(suppl): S161–S166.
76. Fukagawa M, Tominaga Y, Kitaoka M, Kakuta T, Kurokawa K. Medical and surgical aspects of parathryoidectomy. *Kidney Int.* 1999;73(suppl): S65–S69.

Chapter 17

Management of Anemia in Chronic Kidney Disease

Paula J. Frost, RD, CSR

PATHOPHYSIOLOGY

Anemia is one of the major clinical pathologic conditions associated with chronic kidney disease (CKD). The specific type of anemia associated with CKD is hypoproliferative anemia, in which the number of red blood cells (RBCs) produced is less than normal. These RBCs are normocytic (healthy and normal in size) and normochromic (normal color and quantity of hemoglobin), although some irregularly shaped cells have been documented (1–5). Symptoms attributed to hypoproliferative anemia include the following (2–4,6):

- Changes in brain function with decreased cognition and ability to concentrate, decreased intellectual functions
- Left ventricular hypertrophy (LVH)
- Decreased delivery of oxygen to the tissues
- Increased cardiac output
- Decreased sexual function
- Menstrual cycle dysfunction
- Cardiomegaly
- Chronic fatigue
- Malnutrition
- Changes in pulmonary diffusion capacity
- Decreased humeral and cellular immunity
- Congestive heart failure
- Angina
- Decreased overall quality of life
- Increased hospitalization
- Higher mortality rates

Anemia associated with CKD results from insufficient production and release of erythropoietin (EPO) due to impaired kidney function (2–4,7). EPO, a glycoprotein hormone produced primarily in the kidney, regulates the process of erythropoiesis (2–4,7) by monitoring the division and differentiation of committed erythroid progenitor cells in the bone marrow. In CKD there is a loss of nephrons, which are the basic functional units of the kidney. These nephrons are replaced by fibrous connective tissue that lacks the capability to produce EPO. As a result, EPO production in the kidney diminishes. Because the kidney produces approximately 90% of EPO in the body, the deficiency of this hormone is a major cause of anemia in the CKD patient (4). Red blood cell transfusions have decreased significantly since EPO therapy was initiated. They are recommended by the National Kidney Foundation (NKF) Kidney Disease Outcome Quality Initiative (K/DOQI) only for patients who are severely anemic as a result of acute blood loss and EPO resistance (3).

Iron is essential for erythropoiesis; consequently, an insufficient supply of iron in the bone marrow is another major factor contributing to anemia (8). Additional contributing conditions include the following (2, 3,6–9):

- Blood loss through frequent laboratory testing
- Blood residue left in the blood lines and dialyzers
- Inflammation
- Gastrointestinal bleeding
- Menstrual bleeding
- Oozing from hemodialysis (HD) venipuncture sites
- Aluminum toxicity
- Inadequate nutrient intake
- Inadequate absorption of iron
- Folic acid deficiency
- Vitamin B-12 deficiency
- Hyperparathyroidism
- Decrease in RBC survival time
- Neoplasia

EPO THERAPY

The development of recombinant human erythropoietin (rHuEPO) and darbepoetin alfa through genetic engineering has been a major breakthrough in treating anemia in CKD. The most recent literature documents the benefits of EPO treatment. Many of the physiologic symptoms associated with anemia have improved markedly, and the quality of life has been enhanced for these patients. The benefits include lower rates of patient hospitalizations (10,11), improved nutritional status (4,9), improved brain function (12), better physical performance (13), regression of LVH (14), and improvement in patient survival with a hemoglobin (HGB) more than 11g/dL (10,15–17).

Professionals working with CKD patients recognized a need to provide comprehensive standards of practice to improve the outcomes of CKD patients. In 1995 the NKF formed an interdisciplinary work group to address ways to improve patient outcomes and survival. The NKF Dialysis Outcomes Quality Initiative (NKF-DOQI) guidelines were developed and published in 1997. These guidelines were updated in 2000 and are now called Kidney Disease Outcome Quality Initiative (K/DOQI). The goal of these evidence- and opinion-based guidelines is to improve the outcomes of CKD patients with anemia. The 27 guidelines chart a course of action that covers the following (2,3):

- Anemia workup
- Target ranges for HGB and hematocrit (HCT)
- Iron support
- Administration of EPO
- What to do when there is an inadequate EPO response
- Role of RBC transfusions
- Possible adverse effects of EPO therapy

The K/DOQI anemia guidelines recommend the range of HGB to be 11 to 12 g/dL and the range of HCT to be 33% to 36%. EPO is routinely being initiated via subcutaneous administration for predialysis, peritoneal dialysis, and transplanted kidney patients who have been diagnosed with anemia. Historically, most HD patients have been given intravenous (IV) EPO. EPO injections can produce a burning or stinging sensation, whereas IV administration eliminates this discomfort. K/DOQI guidelines continue to recommend the subcutaneous route of administration for HD patients because the EPO is used more efficiently and cost savings are estimated to be considerable (2,3,18).

Medicare is the major insurer for the coverage of EPO and currently sets the guidelines for reimbursement. The target range is a HGB of 11 to 12 g/dL or a HCT of 33% to 36%. The Centers for Medicare and Medicaid Services (CMS) requires medical justification for maintaining a HCT more than 36% (19).

The dosing of EPO should be individualized according to the physician's orders in conjunction with the manufacturer's guidelines. Each dialysis unit usually has a written protocol, approved by the medical director, for dosing EPO to achieve the target HGB. The K/DOQI Anemia Work Group includes in its guidelines how often to test HGB and how to dose and titrate EPO (2,3).

The updated guidelines now recommend using HGB as the measurement of anemia instead of HCT, based on the rationale that HCT is affected by temperature, the amount of time after the sample has been drawn until it is analyzed, hyperglycemia, and excess fluid. The HGB remains stable under these same conditions and is therefore more accurate (3).

Prior to the initiation of treatment with EPO it is important to rule out other potential causes of anemia using specific blood tests. These tests should include HGB iron parameters (total iron-binding capacity [TIBC], serum iron, percent transferrin saturation and serum ferritin), a reticulocyte count, and a test for occult blood in the stool. This workup will help determine whether the patient has sufficient iron stores for RBC synthesis (2,3).

If, as reflected in the HGB and HCT, there is an inadequate response after EPO has been initiated, this could indicate resistance to the drug. If a patient continues to demonstrate an unexplained resistance to EPO, the K/DOQI guidelines recommend that a hematology consult be considered (2). Documented causes for EPO resistance include the following (2–4,14,20–22):

- Iron deficiency (the most common cause of EPO resistance)
- Malnutrition (low serum albumin)
- Aluminum toxicity (historically caused by aluminum-based phosphate binders)
- Osteitis fibrosa (active bone marrow erythroid elements are replaced with fibrosis caused by hyperparathyroidism)
- Folate and vitamin B-12 deficiency
- Infection/inflammation (including rheumatologic disease, access infections, peritonitis, old graft inflammations, elevated C-reactive protein, HIV/AIDS)
- Hemoglobinopathies (including sickle cell anemia)
- Chronic blood loss
- Hemolysis
- Underlying hematologic disease
- Multiple myeloma
- Dialysis-related carnitine disorder

IRON

Because iron is essential for the formation of hemoglobin, it is important to make sure that there is enough iron available to meet the demand of erythropoiesis. In the normal healthy kidney, iron is incorporated into the RBC and then is salvaged when the RBC is broken down during catabolism. The iron is then stored in a stable iron pool. The RBCs carry 65% of the total body iron, and 15% of the iron is stored as serum ferritin and 1% is in the transit form of transferrin. One milligram of iron is incorporated into each molecule of hemoglobin (23). The best laboratory indicators presently available to measure adequate iron include: serum iron, TIBC, and serum ferritin (2,3). The percent of transferrin saturation (TSAT) can be calculated from these laboratory tests. It is recommended that the TSAT be at least 20% and no more than 50%. Serum ferritin levels should be between 100 and 800 ng/mL. Serum ferritin is an acute-phase reactant and may be elevated by chronic or acute inflammation, sometimes making it an inaccurate marker of iron status (2,3). If ferritin is greater than 800 ng/mL, the physician will evaluate the patient to determine whether they should still receive iron therapy.

There is an increased demand for iron during the production of RBCs. If sufficient iron is not available, red cell production can be inhibited and the improvement of HGB and HCT will be adversely affected. To maximize the benefits of EPO therapy and to avoid the development of iron-deficiency anemia, assessing and maintaining adequate availability of iron is critical (24–27). Also, the administration of higher doses of EPO may not improve HGB and HCT levels if iron deficiency is present. The K/DOQI Anemia Work Group mentions some important concerns that need to be addressed in treating iron deficiency in the CKD patient. These include the high incidence of blood loss during hemodialysis, gastrointestinal bleeding, frequent blood testing, and inadequate oral iron therapy in replacing or sustaining a sufficient level of iron stores in these patients. All of these factors put patients at additional risk for iron-deficiency anemia. By giving EPO, the uptake of iron can lead to "functional iron deficiency," which is defined by K/DOQI as a deficiency that is caused during the production of RBCs because the iron is used more rapidly than it can be released from the iron stores. The recommendation for prevention of this type of deficiency is to give a smaller amount of IV iron as a weekly maintenance dose (3).

When there is "absolute iron deficiency" (defined by K/DOQI in the CKD population as serum ferritin levels < 100 ng/mL and TSAT levels < 20%), K/DOQI guidelines recommend giving a series of IV iron doses to replenish iron stores. After giving a series of IV iron, TSAT and ferritin should be tested, and if the results are still in the "absolute iron deficiency" range, another series of IV iron can be given (3).

The types of IV iron available in the United States have increased in the past few years. Iron dextran was the only IV iron available before 1999, when the Food and Drug Administration approved iron gluconate and iron sucrose. The main benefit of these two new iron compounds is that the hypersensitivity reactions are reported to be very rare (28–30).

In the predialysis, peritoneal dialysis (PD), and posttransplant patient populations, oral iron is generally used to treat iron-deficiency anemia. When these patients do not respond to oral iron therapy, IV iron may be given. The most common oral iron compounds are ferrous gluconate, ferrous sulfate, ferrous fumarate, and a polysaccharide-iron complex. K/DOQI recommends a dosage of 200 mg elemental iron per day for adults, divided into two to three doses. Compliance with taking oral iron is a major concern along with inadequate absorption. Various side effects have been reported with oral iron intake, including bloating, gastric irritation, cramping, and constipation. (2,3,24–27). Some of these side effects may be dose-related: the higher the dose, the more side effects. When patients have an increase in the number of medications prescribed, their compliance rate usually decreases. Therefore, oral iron administration must be evaluated on an individual basis. Some patients may tolerate smaller, more frequent doses whereas others may need iron increased at a slower rate to reach the target dosage. Some patients may tolerate a larger dose at bedtime (31,32).

In addition, medications commonly used for CKD may adversely affect iron absorption and should be considered when oral iron is prescribed (2,3). Some of these medications include phosphate binders, antacids, antibiotics, and cholesterol-reducing resins. Although it is recognized that ascorbic acid (vitamin C) enhances iron absorption, the amount needed to enhance iron absorption is more than presently recommended for CKD patients. Ascorbic acid should be used with caution because excessive amounts can lead to oxalosis. Further studies need to be done to evaluate ascorbic acid supplementation. Ascorbic acid may be used for predialysis, PD, and posttransplant patients after being evaluated on an individual basis (33,34). (Refer to Chapter 15 for additional information.)

CONCLUSION

The successful treatment of CKD-induced anemia is one of the important advances in treating CKD. This success is contingent on continual individual patient assessments and consistent and effective administration of EPO and iron therapy. Such treatment has improved the outcomes for these patients and has increased overall quality of life, including improved nutritional status. Other significant benefits that have been documented include decreased mortality, fewer number of hospitalizations, regression of LVH, improved exercise tolerance, improved cognitive function, decreased depression, and less fatigue.

REFERENCES

1. *PDR Medical Dictionary.* Montvale, NJ: Medical Economics Co; 1995.
2. National Kidney Foundation. *Clinical Practice Guidelines for the Treatment of Anemia of Chronic Renal Failure.* New York, NY: National Kidney Foundation; 1997.
3. National Kidney Foundation. K/DOQI clinical proactive guidelines for anemia of chronic kidney disease, 2002. *Am J Kidney Dis.* 2001;37(suppl 1):S182–S238.
4. Besarb A. Treatment of anemia in dialysis subjects. In: Henrich WL, ed. *Principles and Practice of Dialysis.* 3rd ed. Baltimore, Md: William & Wilkins; 2003:464–501.
5. Wilkins KG. Nutritional care in renal disease. In: Mahan KL, Escott-Stump S, eds. *Krause's Food Nutrition & Diet Therapy.* 9th ed. Philadelphia, Pa: WB Saunders Co; 1996:771–773.
6. Burke JR. Low-dose subcutaneous recombinant erythropoietin in children with chronic renal failure. *Pediatr Nephrol.* 1995;9:558–561.
7. Briglia A, Paganini EP. The use of intravenous iron in the anemia of end-stage renal disease (ESRD). *Contemp Dial Nephrol.* 1998;19: 21–25.
8. Schaefer RM, Schaefer L. Iron monitoring and supplementation: how do we achieve the best results? *Nephrol Dial Transplant.* 1998;13(Suppl 2):9–12.
9. Evans RW, Rader B, Manninen DL. Cooperative Multicenter EPO clinical trial group: the quality of life of hemodialysis recipients treated with recombinant human erythropoietin. *JAMA.* 1990; 263:825–830.
10. Foley RN, Parfrey PS, Harnett JD, Kent GM, Murray DC, Barre PE. The impact of anemia on cardiomyopathy, morbidity, and mortality in end stage renal disease. *Am J Kidney Dis.* 1996;28: 53–61.
11. Xia H, Ebben J, Ma JZ, Collins AJ. Hematocrit levels and hospitalization risks in hemodialysis patients. *J Am Soc Nephrol.* 1999;10:1309–1316.
12. Pickett JL, Theberge DC, Brown WS, Schweitzer SU, Nessenson AR. Normalizing hematocrit in dialysis patients improves brain function. *Am J Kidney Dis.* 1999;33:1122–1130.
13. McMahon LP, McKenna JF, Sangkaburtra T, Mason K, Sostaric S, Skinner SL, Burge C, Murphy B, Crankshaw D. Physical performance and associated electrolyte changes after haemoglobin normalization: A comparative study in haemodialysis patients. *Nephrol Dial Transplant.* 1999; 14:1182–1187.
14. Sikole A, Polenakovic M, Spiroska V, Polenakovic B, Klinkmann H, Scigalla P. Recurrence of left ventricular hypertrophy following cessation of erythropoietin therapy. *Artif Organs.* 2002;26:98–102.

15. Ifudu O, Feldman J, Friedman EA. The intensity of hemodialysis and the response to erythropoietin in patients with end-stage renal disease. *New Engl J Med.* 1996;12:420–425.
16. Locatelli F, Conte F, Marcelli D. The impact of haematocrit levels and erythropoietin treatment on overall and cardiovascular mortality and morbidity: the experience of the Lombardy Dialysis Registry (news). *Nephrol Dial Transplant.* 1998; 13:1642–1644.
17. Xia H, Ebbens J, Ma JZ, Collins AJ. Hematocrit level and associated mortality in hemodialysis patients. *J Am Soc Nephrol.* 1999;10:610–619.
18. Besarb A, Reyes CM, Hornberger J. Meta-analysis of subcutaneous versus intravenous epoetin in maintenance treatment of anemia in hemodialysis patients. *Am J Kidney Dis.* 2002;40:439–446.
19. Collins AJ, Roberts TL, St Peter WL, Chen S-C, Ebbens J, Constantini E. United States renal data system assessment of the impact of the National Kidney Foundation-Dialysis Outcomes Quality Initiative guidelines. *Am J Kidney Dis.* 2002;39: 784–795.
20. Muller-Wiefel DE, Sinn H, Gilli G, Scharer K. Hemodialysis and blood loss in children with chronic renal failure. *Clin Nephrol.* 1977;8:481–486.
21. Barany P, Divino Filho JC, Bergstrom J. High C-reactive protein is a strong predictor of resistance to erythropoietin in hemodialysis patients. *Am J Kidney Dis.* 1997;29:565–568.
22. Eknoyan G, Latos DL, Lindberg J. Practice recommendations for the use of l-carnitine in dialysis-related carnitine disorder, National Kidney Foundation, carnitine consensus conference. *Am J Kidney Dis.* 2003;4:868–876.
23. Fishbane S, Paganini EP. Hemalogic abnormalities. In: Daugirdas JD, Blake P, Ing T, eds. *Handbook of Dialysis.* 3rd ed. Philadelphia, Pa: Lippincott Williams and Wilkins; 2001:477–494.
24. Fishbane S, Frei GL, Masesaka J. Reduction in recombinant human erythropoietin doses by the use of chronic intravenous iron supplementation. *Am J Kidney Dis.* 1995;26:41–46.
25. Macdougall IC, Tucker B, Thompson J, Tomson CRV, Baker LR, Raine AE. A randomized controlled study of iron supplementation in patients treated with erythropoietin. *Kidney Int.* 1996;50: 1694–1699.
26. Taylor JE, Peat N, Porter C, Morgan AG. Regular lose-dose intravenous iron therapy improves response to erythropoietin in haemodialysis patients. *Nephrol Dial Transplant.* 1996;11:1079–1083.
27. Sepandj F, Jindal K, West M, Hirsch D. Economic appraisal of maintenance parenteral iron administration in treatment of the anaemia in chronic haemodialysis patients. *Nephrol Dial Transplant.* 1996;11:319–322.
28. Van Wyck DB, Cavallo G, Spinowiz BS, Adhikarla R, Gagnon S, Charytan C, Levin N. Safety and efficacy of iron sucrose in patients sensitive to iron dextran: North American clinical trial. *Am J Kidney Dis.* 2000;36:88–97.
29. Charytan C, Levin N, Al-Saloum M, Hafeez T, Gagnon S, Van Wyck DB. Efficacy and safety of iron sucrose for iron deficiency in patients with dialysis-associated anemia: North American Clinical Trial. *Am J Kidney Dis.* 2001;37:300–307.
30. Sinverberg DS, Blum M, Peer G, Kaplan E, Iaina A. Intravenous ferric saccharate as an iron supplement in dialysis patients. *Nephron.* 1996;72: 413–417.
31. Wingard RL, Parker RA, Ismail L, Hakim RM. Efficacy of oral iron therapy in patients receiving recombinant human erythropoietin. *Am J Kidney Dis.* 1995;25:433–439.
32. Moore LW, Sergio A, Sargent JA, Burk L. Causes and treatment of iron deficiency in hemodialysis patients. *J Ren Nutr.* 1992;2:105–112.
33. Chazot C, Kopple JD, Vitamin metabolism and requirements in renal disease and renal failure. In: Kopple KD, Massry SG, eds. *Nutritional Management of Renal Disease.* Baltimore, Md: William & Wilkins; 1997:448–469.
34. Makoff R. Water-soluble vitamin status in patients with renal disease treated with hemodialysis or peritoneal dialysis. *J Ren Nutr.* 1991;1: 56–73.

Appendix A

Practice Guidelines, Reimbursement, and Continuous Quality Improvement in Chronic Kidney Disease

Jessie Pavlinac, MS, RD, CSR

DEFINITION OF MEDICAL NUTRITION THERAPY

The American Dietetic Association (ADA) defines medical nutrition therapy (MNT) as

> The assessment of the nutritional status of patients with a condition, illness, or injury that puts them at risk. This includes the nutrition assessment where practitioners obtain and analyze medical and diet histories and anthropometric measurements, and review laboratory values. Based on the assessment, the nutrition diagnosis is made and the nutrition intervention(s) most appropriate to manage the condition or treat the illness or injury are chosen. Nutrition interventions can include:
>
> - Diet modification and counseling leading to the development of a personal diet plan to achieve nutritional goals and desired health outcomes.
> - Specialized nutrition therapies including supplementation with medical foods for those unable to obtain adequate nutrients through food intake only; enteral nutrition delivered via tube feeding into the gastrointestinal tract for those unable to ingest or digest food; and parenteral nutrition delivered via intravenous infusion for those unable to absorb nutrients (1).

Nutrition evaluation and monitoring is another step in the nutrition care process of providing MNT. The purpose of this step is to determine the degree to which progress is being made and goals or desired outcomes of nutrition care are being met (2).

When Congress added reimbursement for MNT for type 1, type 2, and gestational diabetes and nondialysis kidney disease with the passage of section 105 of the Medicare, Medicaid, and State Children's Health Insurance Program (SCHIP) Benefits Improvement and Protection Act (BIPA) in 2000, MNT was defined as "nutritional diagnostic, therapy, and counseling services for the purpose of disease management which are furnished by a registered dietitian or nutrition professional" (3,4).

MEDICAL NUTRITION THERAPY PROTOCOLS AND EVIDENCE-BASED GUIDES TO PRACTICE

To standardize the process dietetics professionals use to provide nutrition services, MNT protocols were developed and published in 1998 in *Medical Nutrition Therapy Across the Continuum of Care* (5). This publication represented a partnership between the ADA Quality Management Team, the ADA Dietetic Practice Groups (DPGs), and Morrison Health Care (6). This publication included a pre–end-stage renal disease (pre-ESRD) protocol for adult patients 18 years and older as well as other disease-specific protocols. The initial protocols or practice guidelines were developed using experts in the fields of nutrition care and quality assurance reaching a consensus about the number of recommended nutrition interventions; length for each of these interventions; key clinical, behavioral, functional outcome assessment factors to be measured; as well as expected outcomes.

With the advent of MNT provider status by the Centers for Medicare and Medicaid Services (CMS), nutrition guides for practice must reflect the best clinical evidence (7–10). In 2000 the ADA House of Delegates approved an evidence grading system for use in the production of future ADA guides for practice. This standardized grading system of the evidence would help practitioners determine the strength of the particular nutrition intervention on patient nutrition goals and outcomes. The ADA Quality Management Committee adopted the Institute for Clinical Systems Improvement (ICSI) Methodology to grade research evidence (5). Several guides for practice have been published for renal and transplant patients (7,8,11). The third edition of the *Guidelines for Nutrition Care of Renal Patients* has incorporated the National Kidney Foundation Kidney Disease Outcomes Quality Initiatives (K/DOQI) clinical practice guidelines that were developed using an evidence rating system (11). These practice guides include the following patients/conditions: adult pre-ESRD, adult dialysis, enteral/parenteral nutrition support for adult dialysis, adult hospitalized dialysis, adult acute renal failure, adult transplant, and adult pregnant ESRD. The adult pre-ESRD practice guidelines have undergone rigorous evidence grading and were published separately as the *American Dietetic Association Medical Nutrition Therapy Evidence-Based Guides for Practice: Chronic Kidney Disease (Non-dialysis) Medical Nutrition Therapy Protocol* (7). The details of this protocol are found in Figure A.1.

In addition, many organizations and dialysis companies have developed their own set of protocols/guidelines for nutrition care that outline standards and expectations for appropriate MNT, timeframes for initial and follow-up care, expected outcomes, and documentation criteria.

REIMBURSEMENT FOR MNT

Payment for MNT by third-party payers—Medicare, health maintenance organizations, standard health insurance companies, and state Medicaid programs—has been limited by the lack of recognition of registered dietitians as providers. With the passage of BIPA 2000, registered dietitians and nutrition professionals have been granted status as Medicare providers of MNT. This act provides reimbursement for MNT to all qualifying Medicare Part B beneficiaries with non-dialysis kidney disease (GFR of 13 to 50 mL/min/1.73 m^2), inclusive of post-kidney transplantation for up to 36 months, and diabetes (type 1, type 2, and gestational). Prior to such recognition, in 2001 the ADA established the first three MNT procedure codes through the American Medical Association code proposal process. The codes defined initial, follow-up, and group MNT. The three procedure codes for MNT are 97802 (initial assessment), 97803 (follow-up assessment), and 97804 (group MNT). With a physician's referral, Medicare Part B patients who have these conditions are eligible for 3 hours of MNT the first year and 2 hours each subsequent year. The patient's physician can authorize additional hours of MNT based on medical necessity, such as when there is a change in the patient's medical condition. In 2003 CMS added two additional codes for assessment and reassessment of individuals (G0270) and groups (G0271). These codes are used when additional MNT, based on the physician referral, is needed within the same calendar year. Dialysis patients are excluded from this benefit because they already receive MNT as part of the overall conditions of coverage for dialysis units as established by Congress in 1976 and implemented as part of the ESRD program by Medicare (8).

Medicare requires any qualified registered dietitian or nutrition professional who wishes to provide MNT to Medicare Part B beneficiaries to become a Medicare provider (3). The steps to become a Medicare provider and provide Medicare MNT are

- Complete an application to become a Medicare provider (CMS855I), and if you work for an organization complete the Medicare reassignment of benefit form (CMS855R). If you are a member

Figure A.1. *(See facing page.)* Summary page, Chronic Kidney Disease (Non-dialysis) Medical Nutrition Therapy Protocol. *Medical Nutrition Therapy Evidence Based Guides For Practice. Chronic Kidney Disease (Non dialysis) Medical Nutrition Therapy Protocol* [CD-ROM]. Chicago, Ill: American Dietetic Association. © 2002. American Dietetic Association.

Summary Page
Chronic Kidney Disease (non-dialysis)
Medical Nutrition Therapy Protocol

Setting: Ambulatory Care or adapted for other healthcare settings (Adult 18+ years old) **Number of encounters: 3 to 6**

No. of Encounters	Length of encounters	*Time between encounters*
1	60-90 minutes	3-4 weeks
2	45-60 minutes	3-4 weeks
3	30-45 minutes	3-4 weeks
4,5,6	30-45 minutes	6- 8 weeks or as identified by reassessment

Expected Outcomes of Medical Nutrition Therapy

Baseline Evaluation of Outcomes

Outcomes **Assessment Factors**	1	2	3	4*	**Expected Outcomes**	**Ideal/goal Value**
Clinical Assessment						
Laboratory Values:						
• Serum albumin	X		X	X	• Maintain normal range	• Serum Albumin: > 4.0 g/dL **(Grade II)**
• Serum CO_2	X			X	• Maintain normal range	• Serum CO_2: 24-32 mEq/L **(Grade II)**
• Serum potassium	X	X	X	X	• Maintain normal range	• Serum Potassium: 3.5-5.5 mmol/L **(Grade II)**
• Serum calcium	X	X	X	X	• Progress toward goal	• Serum Calcium: 8.5- 10.2 mg/dL (corrected)
• Serum phosphorus	X	X	X	X	• Progress toward goal	• Serum Phosphorus:3.4-5.5 mg/dL**(Grade II)**
• PTH	X			X	• Progress toward goal	• Intact PTH: 100-300 pg/ml **(Grade II)**
• Serum glucose (if diabetic)	X			X	• ↓ 10% or at goal	• Random glucose:<140-160 mg/dL(blood); <160-180 mg/dL (plasma); A1C: <7% **(Grade I)**
• A1C (if diabetic)	X			X		
• Serum lipids	X		X	X	• Within normal range or △ by 10% to 20% if abnormal	• Cholesterol:>160 to <200 mg/dL • LDL-chol:<100 mg/dL;TG:<150 mg/dL • HDL-chol: >45 mg/dL (M) >55 (F)
• Serum Creatinine/GFR	X	X	X	X	• Stabilize creatinine, GFR and urinary albumin excretion	• Serum creatinine/GFR: stabilizes
• Urine albumin	X	X	X	X		• Urine albumin:<30 mg/d or <3 mg/dL
• Hemoglobin	X			X	• Adequate iron, folate for erythropoiesis when rHuEPO is administered	• Hgb: 12 g/L (M); 11 g/L (F) **(Grade II)**
• Ferritin	X			X		• Ferritin: >100 ng/mL,
• Transferrin saturation	X			X		• Transferrin saturation: >20%
• RBC folate	X			X		• RBC folate: >200 ng/ml
<u>Nutrition/Physical:</u>					• Maintains height, skeletal muscle, weight, fat stores (Weight should be edema free)	• Height: Yearly heights to monitor spinal osteoporosis/bone loss
• Height	X					
• Weight/BMI	X	X	X	X		• BMI: ≥24
• Body composition/SGA	X	X	X	X		
• Blood pressure	X	X	X	X	• Achieves blood pressure goal	• Blood pressure: <125/75: >1 g proteinuria or diabetic nephropathy; <130/85 without proteinuria **(Grade II)**
<u>Functional Status:</u>					• Improves/maintains functional status	• Optimum functional status
• ADLs, IADLs	X	X	X	X		
Therapeutic Lifestyle Changes						**MNT Goal: Maintain kidney function, ↓ progression; maintain nutritional status**
• Food/Meal Plan	X	X	X	X	• Chooses appropriate kinds and amounts of food	• <u>Kcal</u>: BEE (consider stress, dietary protein, weight goals) **(Grade I)**
	X	X	X	X	• Chooses 50% high biological animal or plant sources of protein	• <u>Protein:</u> 0.6 to 1.0 g/kg/IBW based on GFR, urinary protein excretion, degree of malnutrition, stress, motivation **(Grade I)**
	X	X	X	X	• Limits total fat, SF, cholesterol to meet serum lipid goals	• <u>Fat</u>: 25-30%, <7% SFA, <200 mg cholesterol
	X	X	X	X	• Eats at consistent times if diabetic	• <u>Carbohydrate:</u> 50 to 60% kcal
	X	X	X	X	• Limits high sodium foods	• <u>Sodium:</u> individualized, 1-3 g/d
	X	X	X	X	• Consumes potassium per labs	• <u>Potassium:</u> Individualized based on labs
	X	X	X	X	• Limits phosphorus per labs	• <u>Phosphorus</u>: 8-12 mg/kg IBW; phosphate binders/vitamin D analogues may be needed
	X	X	X	X	• Consumes calcium supplements if prescribed, based on labs	• <u>Calcium</u>: Individualized: ~800 to 1200 mg/d
• Food/supplement intake	X	X	X	X	• Maintains adequate appetite	• Consumes >80% meals/supplements • Adequate to maintain weight, body composition
• Food label reading		X	X	X	• Accurately reads food labels	
• Recipe modification	X	X	X	X	• Modifies recipes as needed	
• Food preparation	X	X	X	X	• Uses methods to ↓ sodium	
• Self-monitoring	X	X	X	X	• Records daily food intake	• Dietary intake = prescription >80% of time
• Eating away from home			X	X	• Selects food appropriately	
• Potential food/nutrient/drug interaction	X	X	X	X	• Follows protocols for medications	• Consumes >80% phosphate binders with meals/snacks if prescribed
• Smoking/use of alcohol	X	X	X	X	• Participates in smoking cessation program; limits use of alcohol	
• Physical activity	X	X	X	X	• Participates in physical activity	• Maintains muscle stores/strength

- Print additional copies of this form for additional encounters.

of a group practice you will need to fill out form CMS855B. Access the Medicare enrollment forms from CMS's Web site (http://www.cms.gov/providers/enrollment/forms); from the Medicare carrier's Web site, or from ADA's Web site (http://www.eatright.org/gov).

- Provide proof of qualifications—for registered dietitians, proof of the credential from the Commission on Dietetic Registration; for nutrition professionals, proof of completion of a bachelor of science degree or higher, completion of the nutrition academic requirements, and completion of at least 900 hours of supervised professional practice. In states with licensure or certification, RDs and nutrition professionals must show proof of state licensure or certification (3,4).
- Receive a unique provider identification number (PIN) number from CMS that will be used for billing.
- Receive a referral from a physician for MNT (3,4).
- Use specific billing forms—CMS1500. However, hospital outpatient nutrition clinics may use the UB92 form if the CMS1500 is not available in the hospital's billing system.
- Codes—RDs must use the MNT CPT Codes 97802, 97803, 97804 (3) (or, if appropriate, G0270, G0271) when billing for these services. Medicare MNT services cannot be billed incident to physician's services.
- Provide MNT using nationally recognized protocol for diabetes, chronic kidney disease, and kidney transplantation, such as ADA's *MNT Evidence-Based Guides for Practice* (7,8,11).
- Maintain documentation in the medical record that supports the necessity for MNT.
- Track outcomes data for each Medicare patient who receives MNT services.

Achieving recognition and coverage for Medicare MNT is just the first step in the reimbursement challenge. Registered dietitians should continue to work with their state Medicaid offices and private insurance carriers to be recognized as providers to expand coverage for MNT services.

CONTINUOUS QUALITY IMPROVEMENT IN CHRONIC KIDNEY DISEASE

All of the previously mentioned guidelines for nutrition care and ADA's *MNT Evidence-Based Guides for Practice* incorporate the K/DOQI Clinical Practice Guidelines for Nutrition in Chronic Renal Failure. The K/DOQI guidelines provide a framework to establish a continuous quality improvement (CQI) or performance improvement (PI) program to assure quality nutrition care for adult and pediatric patients with chronic kidney disease. There are 22 nutrition care guidelines for the adult dialysis patient, five guidelines for the adult chronic renal failure without dialysis patient, and 10 guidelines for the pediatric patient (9). These guidelines provide the framework for establishing a CQI program to provide quality nutrition care to chronic renal patients.

STEPS IN DEVELOPING A CQI PROGRAM

Evidence-based practice indicates that it is a responsibility of practitioners and organizations to utilize practices with the best available evidence when providing care. The guidelines just referenced will have evidence of specific assessment factors and interventions that are proven to be effective. The way to introduce these best practices is through CQI. For example, using the Plan Do Study Act (PDSA) methodology of CQI, you would complete the following steps when integrating evidence-based recommendations of nationally developed guidelines into practice. Implementing evidence-based practice is a process rather than a static event. This process involves a cycle of continuous improvement of care considering evidence-based recommendations.

Plan—The Improvement

Select an improvement topic. Review the evidence-based guidelines and compare these to what you are currently doing in practice. Collect data on how your process currently operates. The challenge is not just to identify inadequate care, but also to change clinical practice to improve patient care. To this end, a plan will focus on the changes that have the greatest potential for improvement based on good science, linking process to improved outcomes.

Do—Implement the Change

Changing clinical practice requires a systematic approach and strategic planning. In CQI, tools such as flow sheets, reminder systems, and order forms are aids in initiating process change and assuring consistent care for all patients. This requires diagnostic analysis, development of dissemination and implementation strategy, and a plan to monitor and evaluate the impact of any changes made. In the analysis of the available information, identify

- All groups affected by or influencing the proposed change
- Potential internal and external barriers to change, including whether practitioners are willing to change
- Enabling factors for change, such as resources and skills

Study—Monitor and Evaluate

Collect follow-up data (indicators) to evaluate the effectiveness of the change and degree of compliance and to develop strategies to maintain and reinforce change.

Act—To Hold the Gain and Standardize the Improvement

Act on the modifications by repeating the quality cycle to minimize the chance of the change going back to preimprovement state. At this step you should have full implementation of actions taken to integrate the best practice. If new information or job instructions are to be used, indicate what they are and where they are located. This can be accomplished through changes in policy and procedures. Educate, communicate, and follow-up with training for any practice of coaching that may be required. Be sure to establish a process for training new employees. A systems approach to CQI is an ongoing process that aids in the continual evaluation and improvement on the delivery of health care to patients.

Perhaps the greatest benefit that clinical practice guidelines/MNT protocols offer to the health care system is improved outcomes for service users through consistent and effective treatment. By promoting interventions with proven benefit, they can reduce morbidity and mortality and improve quality of life for some conditions, thereby increasing the cost-effectiveness of care provided.

POSSIBLE CQI TOPICS

Possible CQI projects might include the following:

1. Adult dialysis: evaluation of protein-energy nutritional status
   - Panels of nutritional measures—predialysis or stabilized albumin, percent of usual body weight, percent of standard body weight, subjective global assessment, dietary interviews and diaries, normalized protein nitrogen appearance (nPNA), prealbumin, serum creatinine and the creatinine index, and serum cholesterol
   - Management of acid-base status—measurement and treatment of serum bicarbonate
   - Management of protein and energy intake—dietary protein intake and daily energy intake
   - Nutritional intervention, initial and follow-up—intensive nutrition counseling, indications for nutrition support, protein intake during acute illness, and energy intake during acute illness
2. Advanced chronic renal failure without dialysis
   - Panels of nutritional measures for nondialyzed patients
   - Dietary protein intake for nondialyzed patients
   - Dietary energy intake for nondialyzed patients
   - Intensive nutritional intervention/counseling for chronic renal failure
3. Pediatric Guidelines
   - Evaluation of protein-energy nutritional status
   - Management of acid-base status
   - Urea kinetic modeling
   - Interval measurements of growth and nutritional parameters
   - Energy intake for children treated with maintenance dialysis
   - Protein intake for children treated with maintenance dialysis
   - Vitamin and mineral requirements
   - Nutrition management
   - Nutritional supplementation for children treated with maintenance dialysis

REFERENCES

1. Position of the American Dietetic Association: cost-effectiveness of medical nutrition therapy. *J Am Diet Assoc*. 1995;95:88–91.
2. Nutrition care process and model: ADA adopts road map to quality care and outcomes management. *J Am Diet Assoc*. 2003;103:1061–1072.
3. Medicare Program; Revisions to Payment Policies and Five-Year Review of and Adjustments to the Relative Values Units Under the Physician

Fee Schedule for Calendar Year 2002: Final Rule. 66 *Federal Register* 55275–55281 (2001) (codified at 42 CFR §405, 410, 411, 414, 415).
4. Williams ME, Chianchiano D. Medicare medical nutrition therapy: legislative process and product. *J Ren Nutr*. 2002;12:1–7.
5. The American Dietetic Association and Morrison Health Care. *Medical Nutrition Therapy Across the Continuum of Care*. Chicago, Ill: American Dietetic Association; 1998.
6. Myers ES, Pritchett E, Johnson EQ. Evidence-based practice guides vs protocols: what's the difference? *J Am Diet Assoc*. 2001;101:1085–1090.
7. American Dietetic Association. *The American Dietetic Association Medical Nutrition Therapy Evidence-Based Guides for Practice: Chronic Kidney Disease (Non-dialysis) Medical Nutrition Therapy Protocol* [CD-ROM]. Chicago, Ill: American Dietetic Association; 2002.
8. Wiggins KL. *Guidelines for Nutrition Care of Renal Patients*. 3rd ed. Chicago, Ill: American Dietetic Association; 2001.
9. Wiggins KL, Harvey KS. A review of guidelines for nutrition care of renal patients. *J Ren Nutr*. 2002;12:190–196.
10. Conditions for Coverage of Suppliers of End-Stage Renal Disease (ESRD) Services. Revised 2000. Codified at 42 CFR §405.2102.
11. National Kidney Foundation. Kidney Disease Outcomes Quality Initiative (K/DOQI) clinical practice guidelines for nutrition in chronic renal failure. *Am J Kidney Dis*. 2000;35(Suppl 2):S1–S140.

ADDITIONAL RESOURCES

To learn more about the ADA *MNT Evidence-Based Guides for Practice*, reimbursement, or CQI, consult the following Web sites.

American Dietetic Association

http://www.eatright.org
Key words: MNT, medical nutrition therapy, reimbursement, quality management

Centers for Medicare and Medicaid Services

http://www.cms.hhs.gov
Key words: MNT, medical nutrition therapy, ESRD

Appendix B

Counseling Skills for the Renal Dietitian: From Past Myths to New Practices

Kathleen Hunt, RD

Renal dietitians are acutely aware that proper nutrition improves the lives of people with kidney disease. Yet they are also aware that simply passing on nutritional knowledge to clients or patients does not change eating behaviors. Thanks to several major nutritional and medical intervention studies, new and well-tested techniques are available to help dietitians improve patient adherence (1–6). Grasping these new counseling philosophies and techniques first requires eliminating past ways of thinking. Here are some common myths of the past along with some skills to master.

MYTH: The Health Care Worker Knows What Is Best for the Patient

It's all about choices, independence, and who is in control. Effective teaching designates the *patient* as the primary decision-maker. Health care professionals no longer dole out advice or tell patients what needs to be changed. Instead, they initiate two-way conversations and actively listen to the patient. Then, knowing what is important to that individual, they offer choices to the patient. "You should," "you must," and scare tactics are replaced with restating a patient's own goal and then offering to educate and facilitate the important change. Here are some examples:

Possible patient goals	**Possible choices**
Because you . . .	*Then decide . . .*
Want to stay active and strong	Is the diet something you are ready to work on?
Want to stay as healthy as possible	Would you like to problem solve this together?

MYTH: Patients Who Fail to Follow the Diet for Kidney Disease Are Noncompliant, Apathetic, or Lazy

Before patients ever enter a facility, they bring issues that we alone cannot change. For them, the diet that we are eager to offer may not be a high priority in their lives. They may have little hope for a long, satisfying life. They may be faced with other adjustments, changes, or problems in their lives that distract them. They may still be in denial of their disease. Or, their definition of "quality of life" may not include changing their food habits!

For others, the diet may be too difficult to understand and apply. Many have cognitive impairment from uremia, dementia, medications, or advanced age. Issues with finances, lack of social support, culture, or depression may reduce their ability to make changes.

MYTH: Dietitians Should Not Waste Time on Patients Who Do Not Follow the Diet or Take Diet-Related Medications

People are ready to make changes at different times in their lives. The renal dietitian who is flexible and open-minded provides a sense of hope for future improvements. With new philosophies, labels like "noncompliant" and "hopeless" are replaced with "lack of readiness."

Patients may become more motivated as they adapt to their new lives. Dietitians can be a part of that change by

- Providing recognition or praise for any small achievements
- Including laughter/fun/lightheartedness in communications
- Writing upbeat newsletter articles
- Organizing "buddy visits" with encouraging patients
- Sending a card to an individual in the mail

MYTH: Poor Dietary Compliance Means the Dietitian Is Not Doing a Good Job

The dietitian alone cannot reach everyone. Do not get trapped in unwarranted guilt, frustration, and burnout. Changing a diet involves the support of many people other than the dietitian. Studies show that the nephrologist's involvement is critical (7,8). For some patients, active participation of their family and friends may be the link to success. Other health care workers can also contribute to patient acceptance or understanding of the renal diet. When dietitians are good facilitators, they incorporate a wide circle of influences to bring lifestyle changes for the patient with kidney disease.

MYTH: Verbal Instruction Is the Best Method to Teach Diet-Related Skills

For years it has been said that people learn only 10% of what they read and 20% of what they hear (9), but dietitians continue to rely heavily on written and verbal diet instructions. Much has been studied about how people learn (10). Consider these ideas for teaching dietary skills:

- Do your methods incorporate a variety of learning styles?
  - *Visual techniques:* graphics, pictures, videos, food models
  - *Audio techniques:* two-way discussions, tapes, compact discs
  - *Hands-on techniques:* activities that manipulate food cards, food pictures or food models, workbook activities, simple sketching activities
- Do you keep your teaching short and simple? You can increase cognitive retention by
  - Selecting several, small sessions to interact
  - Keeping diet changes to a few at a time
  - Presenting information simply, clearly, and concisely (a fifth grade level is often recommended)
- Does your teaching include practice and feedback?
  - Asking questions
  - Providing interactive workbooks
  - Role modeling situations
  - Sorting of food pictures or food models
  - Solving problems
  - Sharing experiences
- Do you provide *ongoing* patient education? The initial one-on-one consultations may not reach everyone. Here are some ideas that dietitians have successfully employed to continue the learning process:
  - Group activities: bulletin boards, contests that recognize participation or improved outcomes, guest presentations (in waiting rooms, at support groups), newsletters including patient testimonies or physician interviews
  - Teaching videos
  - Modeling desirable dietary behaviors: food samplings, cooking demonstrations (in person or on video), innovative and up-to-date meal planning, displays of cookbooks, cooking magazines, recipes

CONCLUSION

The information in this appendix is just a sampling of the motivational techniques and behavior-based, patient-centered education methods available to the renal dietitian. Further resources to master new skills are listed after the references.

REFERENCES

1. Gillis BP, Caggiula AW, Chiavacci AT, Coye T, Doroshenko L, Milas NC, Nowalk MP, Scherch

LK. Nutrition intervention program of the Modification of Diet in Renal Disease Study: a self-management approach. *J Am Diet Assoc.* 1995; 95:1288–1294.

2. Benfari RC. The Multiple Risk Factor Intervention Trial (MRFIT) III: the model for intervention. *Prev Med.* 1981;10:426–442.
3. Bowen D, Henderson MM, Iverson D, Burrows ER, Henry HJ, Foreyt J. Reducing dietary fat: understanding the success of the Women's Health Trial. *Cancer Prev.* 1994;1:21–30.
4. Lipid Research Clinics Program. The Coronary Primary Prevention Trial: design and implementation. *J Chronic Dis.* 1983; 36:451–465.
5. Jeffery RW, Tonascia S, Bjornson-Benson W, Schlundt DG, Sugars C, for the Hypertension Prevention Trial Research Group. Treatment in the Hypertension Prevention Trial. *Control Clin Trials.* 1989;10(3 Suppl):65S-83S.
6. Mojonnier ML, Hall Y, Berkson DM, Robinson E, Wether B, Pannbacker B, Moss D, Pardo E, Stamler J, Shekelle RB, Raynor W. Experience in changing food habits of hyperlipidemic men and women. *J Am Diet Assoc.* 1980;77:140–148.
7. Samir S, Shah VS, Peterson RA, Kimmel PL. Psychosocial variables, quality of life, and religious beliefs in ESRD patients treated with hemodialysis. *Am J Kidney Dis.* 2002;40;5.
8. Julie A, Patel SS, Peterson RA, Kimmel PL. Patient satisfaction with care and behavioral compliance in end-stage renal disease patients treated with hemodialysis. *Am J Kidney Dis.* 2002; 39;6.
9. Heinz A. Power of multisensory approach. *Slingerland Institute for Literacy Newsletter.* Fall 2000.
10. Armstrong T. *Seven Kinds of Smart; Identifying and Developing Your Multiple Intelligences.* New York, NY: Plume Books; 1999.

ADDITIONAL RESOURCES

DeSouza DM. *Handbook of Creative Approaches to Patient Compliance.* Pembroke Pines, Fla: Professional Nutrition Services; 2001.

Eitington JE. *The Winning Trainer: Winning Ways to Involve People in Learning.* Houston, Tex: Golf Publishing Company; 1996.

Franz MJ, ed. *A CORE Curriculum for Diabetes Education, Diabetes Education and Program Management.* 4th ed. Chicago, Ill: American Association of Diabetes Educators; 2001.

Mid-Atlantic Renal Coalition. Patient-Centeredness CEU Opportunity. Available at: http://www.esrdnet5.org under "Education" menu. Accessed September 6, 2003.

Miller WR, Rollnick S. *Motivational Interviewing: Preparing People for Change.* 2nd ed. New York, NY: Guilford Press; 2002.

Miller WR, Rollnick S. *What is MI?* Available at: http://www.motivationalinterview.org. Accessed September 6, 2003.

Appendix C

Helpful Hints for Common Problems

Sharon R. Schatz, MS, RD, CSR, CDE

This appendix addresses some of the common problems that a dialysis patient may encounter while trying to achieve or maintain a well-nourished state. Practical suggestions are provided regarding taste changes, nausea and vomiting, constipation, excessive interdialytic weight gains, and options for patients following a vegetarian diet. Individualized solutions are encouraged. Tips for combating early satiety are discussed in Chapter 6.

LOSS OF APPETITE, TASTE CHANGES, AND EATING PROBLEMS

A drop in blood urea nitrogen (BUN) may indicate a diminished intake and predict a subsequent reduction in serum albumin. Poor appetite and/or altered taste sensation may exist due to inadequate dialysis, an overly restrictive diet, side effects from medications, anxiety, weakness, and/or depression. Fluid restriction might also negatively impact hunger through a physiological feedback mechanism (1). Careful monitoring of dialysis adequacy through kinetics with an adjustment in the dialysis prescription may prove useful when appetite and intake decline. Additionally, changes in the prescribed medications and/or liberalizing the diet might stimulate better oral intake. The diet history should include what the patient says about the taste of food because it may be possible to improve nutrient intake by manipulating flavors (2). If depression or anxiety persists for a long period, referral to appropriate health care professionals may be indicated.

Physical factors that can affect intake include dry mouth; mouth sores; and the patient's ability to chew, swallow, and self-feed. Texture changes and artificial saliva preparations may be beneficial. Keeping foods moist by using gravies, melted margarine or butter, and the addition of sour cream are helpful, especially when fluid is restricted in the diet. Use of mouthwash with low alcohol content can lessen drying of the mouth. Limiting acidic and spicy foods will minimize irritation to the mouth. For severe swallowing problems, diagnostic follow-up may be indicated, and the renal diet may require alterations for dysphagia.

Being on hemodialysis can interfere with food consumption. The dialysis unit's schedule may conflict with the person's usual mealtimes. Sometimes a patient is too exhausted posttreatment to eat. Blood pressure changes during the hemodialysis session can result in nausea and/or vomiting. Consequently, fewer meals may be eaten on dialysis days. Use of nutrition supplements or blenderized high-protein/high-calorie shakes may be of assistance on these days.

The elderly often have reduced sense of taste and smell that cause decreased pleasure with eating. Incidentally, they consume higher concentrations of sugar and salt than younger patients, making glycemic and fluid control challenging in some patients. Older persons regard taste and flavor perception as the strongest determinants of food choices, and intake can become more monotonous due to generalized reduction in these senses (3).

The following suggestions may help improve altered taste or loss of appetite:

- Appetite is a learned response triggered by food intake, and lack of food can deter necessary physiological feedback mechanisms. Small, frequent meals may increase the total daily intake and be easier to consume than less frequent, larger ones. Established mealtimes may reinforce the need to eat.
- Food odors should be minimized. Cold foods might be more appetizing.
- Patients should be encouraged to eat in a calm atmosphere.
- The pleasurable physical aspects of dining may entice the appetite. The setting and presentation of food contribute to the eating experience.
- A bad taste in the mouth can be reduced by using mouthwash, brushing the teeth and tongue, chewing gum, or sucking lemon wedges or hard candy before the meal. Good mouth hygiene is essential.
- Patients' food preferences should be encouraged within the limitations of the diet. Liberalization may be required when intake is extremely poor.
- The addition of seasonings, herbs, and spices can improve the aroma and taste of foods.

NAUSEA AND VOMITING

Nausea and vomiting may be transient or persistent. Causes are variable and include uremia, concurrent medical problems, side effects from medications or other medical treatments such as chemotherapy or radiation. The following tips may be useful when counseling patients about how to overcome the effects of nausea and vomiting:

- While still in bed before rising in the morning, the person can eat unsalted crackers, hard candy, or other dry carbohydrate foods.
- Suggest the patient have small, frequent feedings, taking fluid feedings only if previous dry feedings have been tolerated. Patient should avoid highly seasoned foods and fried and other high-fat foods. As tolerance for food increases, fats and fluids may be gradually added and time between meals increased until three to four meal per day are reestablished.
- Patient should avoid cooking odors.
- Nausea and vomiting during a hemodialysis treatment may be lessened by eating a light meal 2 hours before or waiting to eat until after the treatment. Food intake just prior to the treatment is not recommended.
- If nausea and vomiting persist, medications can be initiated. The patient may need referral to the nephrologist.

CONSTIPATION

Factors contributing to constipation include phosphate-binding medications, fluid restriction, a reduced dietary fiber intake, lack of exercise, medication side effects, and surgery. Commercially available fiber supplements may be indicated, with special attention given to phosphorus content. Even small amounts of high-fiber items with potassium and/or phosphorus may be beneficial and could be integrated into the total diet. The incorporation of small amounts of several high-fiber foods may be easier to ingest than trying to eat a large portion of a single high-fiber item. Examples are the addition of shredded cabbage to salads, homemade applesauce from unpeeled fruit, or dried cranberries for snacking or in hot cereal or cookies. Usable high-fiber foods include the following:

- Grain and cereal products (< 26 mg phosphorus/g fiber and < 33 mg potassium/g fiber): cooked pearl barley, cooked roasted buckwheat groats, crude corn bran, roasted cooked kasha, and spinach egg noodles
- Fruits (< 75 mg potassium/g fiber): dried and fresh pears, dried and fresh figs, tangerines, applesauce, dried and fresh apples, Asian pear, kumquat, and berries (strawberries, loganberries, blackberries, boysenberries, blueberries, raspberries, and dried and fresh cranberries)
- Vegetables (< 100mg potassium/g fiber): boiled green peas, cooked green beans, raw or cooked shredded cabbage, cooked cauliflower, cooked corn, cooked carrots, cooked chopped collard or turnip greens, or raw green pepper

EXCESSIVE INTERDIALYTIC FLUID WEIGHT GAINS

The dialysis patient needs to understand the relationship of fluid intake and weight gains, and be able to identify the physical signs of fluid overload. Those on peritoneal dialysis need to comprehend the relationship of sodium and fluid control with the adjustment of dialysate solution as well as its impact on subsequent absorption of sugar and excess calories. Thirst has been associated with high BUN levels (4). Blood sugar control will influence fluid consumption because hyperglycemia contributes to thirst. Patients diagnosed with diabetes, especially those with neuropathy, may be more prone to symptoms of dry mouth, decreased salivary flow rates, and the effects of xerogenic drugs (5–9). Consider the following ideas for controlling fluid gains.

Controlling Thirst

- Sodium control: Many patients may not use salt but are unaware of hidden sodium sources in foods. Teach methods that simplify food label reading.
- Encourage patients to minimize dry mouth and lips. Rinsing the mouth with cold water, keeping lips moist with lip balms or moisturized lipsticks, and using mouthwash with low alcohol content will help. Good mouth hygiene is essential. Patients should brush teeth often.
- Snacking on hard candies, especially sour ones, and chewing sugar-free gum or special thirst-quencher gum eases thirst.
- Very cold items will quench thirst better. Advise patients to drink beverages that are less sweet.

Staying Cool

- When away from home in hot weather, patients should carry pre-moistened towelettes or diaper wipes and apply to back of neck or forehead to cool down. When home, applying a cold, damp washcloth to back of neck or forehead will help the individual cool down.
- Patients should limit outdoor exposure when the sun is hottest.
- Encourage patients to suck on a frozen fruit pop (such as a Popsicle); this takes longer to consume than drinking larger amounts of fluid.
- Suggest patients keep a small freezer chest in the car with small containers of liquids, frozen fruit pops, or frozen grapes.

Portion Awareness and Control

- Educate the patient about the measurement of fluid. Use handouts or create a bulletin board display with actual containers that indicate their amounts of fluid. Encourage use of smaller glasses and cups. Regular use of the same-size beverage container makes measurement easier.
- Use handouts with pictures of foods that need to be counted as fluid. Foods such as grapefruit, watermelon, lettuce, or cucumbers may need to be counted.
- Individuals on dialysis need to be able to equate the amount of fluid ingested to the amount of weight that is gained. Ask patients to weigh themselves every morning to track gains.
- Patients who are home most of the day can fill a container with water for the day's fluid allowance. Every time a liquid is used, they should pour out an equal amount of water from the container and discard it. Some patients find it helpful to record what they drink on a small index card to track their fluid consumption.
- Suggest that patients use applesauce or baby fruit to help swallow pills.
- Encourage patients to drain liquids from canned fruits and cooked vegetables.
- Patients may want to ration fluid throughout the day to spread it out and minimize feelings of deprivation. If going out to eat, they should budget fluid to prepare for this. In the restaurant, they should decline water or other beverage refills.
- Advise patients against drinking while doing another activity such as watching television or reading the newspaper.

VEGETARIAN RENAL DIETS

It is the position of the American Dietetic Association and Dietitians of Canada that appropriately planned vegetarian diets are healthful, nutritionally adequate, and provide health benefits in the prevention and treatment of certain diseases (10). In-depth nutrition assessment is needed to determine what the vegetarian practices are including, what foods are avoided, the nutritional adequacy of the intake, and what modifications may be indicated. The following aspects may need to be considered for the successful coordination of vegetarianism with nutrient goals for dialysis.

Reasons That the Patient Is a Vegetarian

Among end-stage renal disease (ESRD) patients, the three most important reasons for following vegetarian diets were religious, ethnic/cultural, and health (11). Concern for the environment, animal welfare factors, economic considerations, and world hunger issues may also play a role (10). The belief system may influence acceptance of food recommendations.

Type of Vegetarian Diet

Vegetarian diets include the following types (12,13):

- Vegan (total vegetarian): excludes all meat, fish, poultry, eggs, dairy, and their derivatives
- Lacto-ovo vegetarian: excludes animal flesh but permits use of eggs and dairy
- Lacto-vegetarian: vegan diet plus dairy
- Ovo-vegetarian: vegan diet plus eggs
- Pesco-vegetarian or pescetarian: lacto-ovo vegetarian diet plus fish
- Semi-vegetarian: excludes only red meat or includes less meat than average person's diet
- Fruitarian: diet based on fruits and vegetables that are botanically considered fruits or can be harvested without killing the plant

Other Foods Excluded From Diet

Some foods may be excluded due to processing or derivation. This will vary depending on the type of vegetarianism and food manufacturing employed. It is important to determine this on an individualized basis. Examples of foods that may be excluded include honey (bees may be killed in processing), sugar (bone charcoal may be used as decolorant), chocolate (milk products and sugar as ingredient), maple syrup (environmental concerns and/or use of animal-derived defoaming agent), cheese (if rennin in processing is animal-derived), gelatin (including Kosher gelatin), some red dyes (from cochineal beetle), and possibly items with additives sodium stearoyl lactylate, mono- and diglycerides, stearic acid, and glycerine (13,14).

Adequacy of Protein Intake

Instead of emphasizing complete sources of protein as in an animal-based diet, the vegetarian diet is based on the complete intake of amino acids throughout the day. Plant sources of protein alone can provide adequate amounts of essential amino acids if a variety of plant foods are consumed daily and energy needs are met (15). It was previously believed that protein sources needed to be complemented at each meal, but this is no longer the accepted practice. Evaluation of protein quality by the protein efficiency ratio has been replaced by the protein digestibility corrected amino acid score.

Vegetarian Meal Planning

Key vegan protein sources include soy products (tofu, tempeh, textured vegetable protein, and soy milk), pulses (peas, beans, lentils, and peanuts), nuts, and seeds. Whey protein is acceptable for vegetarian diets that allow dairy. A wide array of grains may be employed including barley, rye, corn, oats, millet, buckwheat, triticale, amaranth, quinoa, rice, and wheat.

Vegetarian food guide pyramids are available (16–18), but none were found with modification for the renal diet. Due to their higher protein requirement, the patients on dialysis may need different numbers of daily servings than those listed in these guides. Serving sizes for major protein foods are $^1/_2$ cup cooked dried peas, beans, or lentils; 2 tablespoons nuts, seeds, or peanut butter; 1 cup soy milk; 1$^1/_2$ ounces soy cheese; 1 egg or 2 egg whites; or 3 ounces meat substitute (16). Caloric adequacy is imperative to promote positive nitrogen balance. Commercially available liquid nutrition supplements, protein powders, and protein-energy bars made from soy or whey could augment the food intake. Nutrient data can vary for similar types of processed foods due to their formulation or additive profile, making some brands more usable.

Concerns About Vegetarianism in the Renal Diet

The renal diet emphasizes adequate phosphorus control. Egg whites have the lowest quantity of phosphorus relative to the quantity and quality of protein; animal flesh has the next lowest amount of phosphorus relative to protein. About 50% to 70% of phosphorus is absorbed in a mixed diet. Due to the phosphate form of phytic acid (inositol phosphate) in grains and legumes, their phosphorus absorption is reduced to 50% (15). Diet recommendations are for total milligrams of phosphorus, and food values and intake records are not adjusted for actual bioavailability. It is possible that total dietary intake of phosphorus could be higher, but there is a lack of research on the impact of a plant-based diet on actual phosphorus control. Therefore, it would be wise to advise use of foods with the least amount of phosphorus per gram of protein and limit low-protein foods with a high phosphorus load. Close monitoring of phosphorus control with possible increase in prescribed binder therapy would be indicated.

Potassium content can also be higher in some plant-based protein sources, especially those from soy. If potassium restriction is needed, foods with the least amount of potassium per gram of protein would be emphasized as well as intake of lower potassium fruits, vegetables, and grains. If hyperkalemia is a problem, the potassium bath in hemodialysis might need reduction; or potassium-binding resins such as sodium polystryrene sulfonate could additionally be prescribed.

Other Nutrient Concerns

The nutrient concerns of the vegetarian diet regarding adequacy of iron, calcium, riboflavin, vitamin D, and vitamin B-12 may be less prevalent in those on dialysis because of the specially formulated renal vitamins typically prescribed as well as the close monitoring of anemia and renal osteodystrophy.

SUMMARY

This appendix provided an overview for some common problems encountered by dialysis patients. It does not represent an all-inclusive list of remedies but should afford the renal dietitian with techniques to combat some of the frequent concerns among this unique patient population.

REFERENCES

1. Schoorlemmer GH, Evered MD. Reduced feeding during water deprivation depends on hydration of the gut. *Am J Physiol Regul Integr Comp Physiol.* 2002;283:R1061–R1069.
2. van der Eijk I, Farinelli MA. Taste testing in renal patients. *J Ren Nutr.* 1997;7:3–9.
3. Schatz SR. Malnutrition in the elderly person: contributing factors. *Renal Nutr Forum.* 1997; 16(3):insert.
4. Virga G, Mastrosimone S, Amici G, Munaretto G, Gastaldon F, Bonadonna A. Symptoms in hemodialysis patients and their relationship with biochemical and demographic parameters. *Int J Artif Organ.* 1998;21:788–793.
5. Chavez EM, Taylor GW, Borrell LN, Ship JA. Salivary function and glycemic control in older persons with diabetes. *Oral Surg Oral Med Oral Pathol Oral Radiol Endod.* 2000;89:305–311.
6. Chavez EM, Borrell LN, Taylor GW, Ship JA. A longitudinal analysis of salivary flow in control subjects and older adults with type 2 diabetes. *Oral Surg Oral Med Oral Pathol Oral Radiol Endod.* 2001;91:166–173.
7. Meurman JH, Collin H-L, Niskanen L, Töyry J, Alakuijala P, Keinänen S, Uusitupa M. Saliva in non-insulin-dependent diabetic patients and control subjects. *Oral Surg Oral Med Oral Pathol Oral Radiol Endod.* 1998;86:69–76.
8. Moore PA, Guggenheimer J, Etzel KR, Weyant RJ, Orchard T. Type 1 diabetes mellitus, xerostomia, and salivary flow rates. *Oral Surg Oral Med Oral Pathol Oral Radiol Endod.* 2001;92:281–291.
9. Sreebny LM, Yu A, Green A, Valdini A. Xerostomia in diabetes mellitus. *Diabetes Care.* 1992;15: 900–904.
10. Position of the American Dietetic Association and Dietitians of Canada: vegetarian diets. *J Am Diet Assoc.* 2003;103:748–765.
11. Patel C. Results from the vegetarian renal resource questionnaire. *Renal Nutr Forum* 1999;18:15.
12. Kaufman T. Vegetarian diet. Available at: http://www.globalgourmet.com/food/dietsite/0999. Accessed November 6, 2003.
13. International Vegetarian Union. Frequently asked questions, definitions. Available at: http://www.ivu.org/faq. Accessed November 6, 2003.
14. The Vegetarian Resource Group. Frequently asked questions, food ingredients. Available at: http://www.vrg.org/nutshell/faqingredients.htm. Accessed November 6, 2003.
15. Vegetarian Nutrition, A Dietetic Practice Group of American Dietetic Association. Fact Sheets: Vegetarian diets in renal disease. Available at: http://www.vegetariannutrition.net/fact_sheets.htm. Accessed April 2, 2004.

16. Berkoff, N. Vegetarian and vegan meal planning. *Diabetes Self-Management.* 2003;20:56–73.
17. Seventh-day Adventist Dietetic Association. Available at: http://www.sdada.org/GCNC_Position_Statement_on_Veg_Diet.htm. Accessed November 6, 2003.
18. American Dietetic Association. Food Guide Pyramid for Vegetarian Meal Planning. Available at http://www.eatright.org/gifs/adap1197.gif. Accessed November 6, 2003.

Appendix D

Nocturnal Home Hemodialysis

Lesley L. McPhatter, MS, RD

Mortality rates for chronic kidney disease (CKD) patients on dialysis in the United States exceed 20%, more than those of other industrialized countries such as Italy, Japan, and France (1). One reason for the increased mortality rate among people with CKD on dialysis is malnutrition caused by inadequate dialysis. Underdialyzed patients experience decreased taste acuity and anorexia with inadequate dietary calorie and protein intake. In patients who are adequately dialyzed, dietary restrictions and fluid limitations may impair oral intake. Nocturnal hemodialysis provides patients with two to three times more dialysis than the standard three-treatments-per-week hemodialysis (SHD). With frequent nocturnal dialysis (5 to 7 nights per week), dietary and fluid limitations are minimal or unnecessary. Patients eat better, feel better, and report an improvement in quality of life (2–5).

DIALYSIS PRESCRIPTION

Nocturnal hemodialysis is a form of home hemodialysis performed by the patient and/or a partner while the patient sleeps. Most programs do not require a partner due to the safety of dialysis. Decreased blood flow and dialysate flow rates offer hemodynamic stability during treatment. Patients dialyze 5 to 7 nights per week, usually 6 to 10 hours per night, based on their normal preferred sleep cycle. The dialysate flow rate is typically 200 to 300 mL/min and the blood flow rate is 200 to 300 mL/min, but either can be increased based on a particular patient's needs (3,5). The dialysate composition, which is similar to that used in most dialysis units, except for the possible addition of phosphorus, is as follows (3,5):

- Sodium (Na): 137–140 mEq/L
- Potassium (K): 2–3 mEq/L
- Bicarbonate (HCO_3): 28–35 mEq/L
- Calcium (Ca): 2.5–3.5 mEq/L
- Phosphorus (P): 0–4.5 mg/dL. Sodium phosphate (such as unflavored Fleets Phosphosoda) (CB Fleet, Lynchburg, VA 24502) can be added to the acid or the bicarbonate concentrate to maintain predialysis and postdialysis serum phosphate concentrations in the normal range.

Patients can use any size of dialyzer and reprocessing of the dialyzer is possible. Machine choice is facility specific, but the newer simpler machines are preferred for ease of education to the patient.

DIET

Like the diet for any CKD patient on hemodialysis, the recommended diet for NHD patients must be individualized to the patient's dietary needs, preferences, and other medical problems. In the majority of patients, there is no need for restriction of phosphorus (4,5). Patients often need to increase dietary phosphorus when serum levels are less than the normal range (3,6). Patients are encouraged to maintain or increase protein intake to maintain serum albumin within the higher limit of normal range (4). Some, though not all, of the amino acid abnormalities seen during dialysis treatments may be corrected in nocturnal hemodialysis due to more efficient dialysis and improved dietary intake (7).

Energy and protein requirements have yet to be established in this population. Dietitians working with this population currently prescribe 30 to 35 kcal/kg actual or adjusted body weight and 1.2 g protein/kg/actual or adjusted weight (8). Adjustments are made for weight loss or gain and additional protein needs. Weight gain has been seen in this population; therefore exercise is strongly encouraged.

Fluid restriction is not necessary in the majority of patients unless their intake exceeds the maximum they can remove during the treatment regimen (typically about 2.4 to 4.0 L/night). Fluid weight removal goals are individualized based on the patient's intake and dialysis prescription. Fluid removal is limited to promote hemodynamic stability during treatment. A typical restriction is to limit fluid removal to 0.4 kg/hour (4,6). Sodium restriction is guided by the patient's fluid and hypertensive state. Hypotensive patients may benefit from additional dietary sodium, and normotensive patients may need only a healthy dietary limitation of 2,400 mg/day (9). Potassium restriction is rarely needed. In patients who skip 1 night per week and have documented high potassium levels after their longest interdialytic period, a mild restriction can be recommended. Elevated midweek serum potassium levels are rare in the patient who is getting prescribed treatment. Patients who have low serum potassium levels should be encouraged to increase potassium intake to avoid symptoms such as muscle cramping (4,5).

Vitamin needs are increased due to the hemodialysis losses of B vitamins, and all patients should be on a renal multivitamin to ensure adequate vitamin replacement in addition to dietary intake. Presently, vitamin replacement is typically the same as in SHD: 1 to 2 renal vitamins per day after dialysis (10). Recognizing that vitamin losses in nocturnal dialysis are double that of SHD due to dialyzing twice as many days per week, research in this area may ultimately indicate a need to further supplement these patients based on their individual needs.

Increases in cholesterol have been seen in nocturnal hemodialysis patients. Some patients have high triglyceride levels that may be related to the daily glucose absorption from the dialysate. Clinical trials are needed to validate this hypothesis. Dietary counseling using dietary guidelines to limit fat and cholesterol intake may be necessary (9). (See Chapter 10 for more information on hyperlipidemia.)

LABORATORY DATA

Laboratory data are monitored monthly. Desirable levels for most laboratory values are within the normal, nonrenal reference range for the laboratory processing the specimen. Weekly Kt/V and urea reduction rate (URR) are two to three times higher than recommended levels SHD. It is important to note that a single treatment URR will be less than the 65% recommendation of SHD due to the lower pre- and post-BUN levels. Serum sodium, bicarbonate, potassium, calcium, phosphorus, and albumin should be within the normal, nonrenal ranges (3–5).

For patients dialyzing less than 7 days per week, slight increases may be seen in results from laboratory tests conducted after the patient's longest interdialytic period. Although these results do not represent the patient's true steady state, patients with high potassium or phosphorus levels after a skipped treatment should be instructed to limit dietary potassium or phosphorus on the days that the patient does not dialyze (4,5). Midweek laboratory values may indicate low potassium and phosphorus levels and require dietary intervention to improve the levels of these nutrients. Supplementation of phosphorus, either orally or in the dialysate, may be necessary if levels do not improve with dietary intervention (4–6). Intact parathyroid hormone (PTH) and bio-intact PTH levels are reduced, with fewer patients requiring vitamin D therapy for PTH control once they are stabilized on nocturnal dialysis. Patients typically run a higher calcium bath, which may contribute to suppression of PTH levels. Patients on NHD have a calcium × phosphorus product well within the National Kidney Foundation Kidney Disease Outcomes Quality Initiative (K/DOQI) bone disease guidelines of less than 55 and can be treated with vitamin D as needed without the problems associated with hyperphosphatemia. Hypercalcemia can usually be controlled with adjustments in the calcium content of the dialysate (4–6).

Hemoglobin levels are well maintained within K/DOQI guidelines with moderate use of erythropoeitin and intravenous iron replacement (3–6). (See Chapter 17 for more information on anemia management.)

OTHER BENEFITS

Although difficult to quantify, nocturnal dialysis offers a more physiologically normal removal of uremic toxins (4–6). Improvements in hemodynamic stability, decreased hypertension, and fluid removal improve cardiac output. Cardiovascular disease risks are further reduced in this population via the improvement in the calcium/phosphorus balance and reduction of serum homocysteine levels (11). Additionally, one study suggests that removal of middle molecules, such as beta 2–microglobulin, are improved fourfold in the NHD population. Accumulation and tissue deposition of beta 2–microglobulin leads to amyloidosis in long-term SHD patients (12). Additional studies are needed to determine whether these phenomena can be slowed or eliminated with nocturnal hemodialysis.

Finally, the preliminary benefits seem to be a cost savings to Medicare and other health agencies seen as a reduced need for blood pressure medications, phosphorus binders, vitamin D, and erythropoeitin in this population, and a decrease in hospital admissions and length of stay (4–6).

CONCLUSION

Nocturnal dialysis is a growing treatment modality in the United States with programs in at least 15 centers. Medicare reimbursement at adequate levels to support this modality will ultimately lead to another treatment option for all CKD patients and allow better patient care for the CKD patient on dialysis.

REFERENCES

1. Kjellstrand C, Ing T. Daily hemodialysis—history and revival of superior dialysis method and literature review. *ASAIO J.* 1998;44:117–122.
2. Pierratos A, Ouwendyk M, Francoeur R, Vas S, Raj DS, Ecclestone AM, Langos V, Uldall R. Nocturnal hemodialysis: three-year experience. *J Am Soc Nephrol.* 1998;9:859–868.
3. Pierratos A, Ouwendyk M, Francoeur R. Experience with nocturnal hemodialysis. *Home Hemodial Int.* 1997;1:32–36.
4. McPhatter LL, Lockridge RS Jr, Albert J, Anderson H, Craft V, Jennings FM, Spencer M, Swafford A, Barger T, Coffey L. Nightly home hemodialysis: improvement in nutrition and quality of life. *Adv Renal Repl Ther.* 1999;6:358–365.
5. McPhatter L, Lockridge R. Nutritional advantages of nightly home hemodialysis. *Nephrol News Issues.* 2002;16:31–34.
6. Lockridge, R, Spencer, M, Craft, V, Pipkin, M, Campbell, D, McPhatter, L, Albert, J, Anderson, H, Jennings, F, Barger, T. Nightly home hemodialysis: five and one half years of experience in Lynchburg, VA. *Hemodial Int.* 2004;8:61–60.
7. Raj DS, Ouwendyk M, Francoeur R, Pierratos A. Plasma amino acid profile on nocturnal hemodialysis. *Blood Purif.* 2000;18:97–102.
8. National Kidney Foundation K/DOQI Nutrition Work Group. K/DOQI clinical practice guidelines for nutrition in renal failure. Management of protein and energy intake. *Am J Kidney Dis.* 2000;35(suppl):S40–S45.
9. *Dietary Guidelines for Americans 2000.* 5th ed. Washington, DC: US Departments of Agriculture and Health and Human Services; 2000. Home And Garden Bulletin No. 232.
10. Kopple, J, Swenseid, M. Vitamin nutrition in patients undergoing maintenance hemodialysis. *Kidney Int Suppl.* 1975;2:79–84.
11. Friedman AN, Bostom AG, Levey AS, Rosenberg IH, Selhub J, Pierratos A. Plasma total homocysteine levels in patients undergoing nocturnal versus standard hemodialysis. *J Am Soc Nephrol.* 2002;13:265–268.
12. Raj DS, Ouwendyk M, Francoeur R, Pierratos A. Beta 2–microglobulin kinetics in nocturnal hemodialysis. *Nephrol Dial Transplant.* 2000;15: 58–64.

Appendix E

Emergency Meal Planning

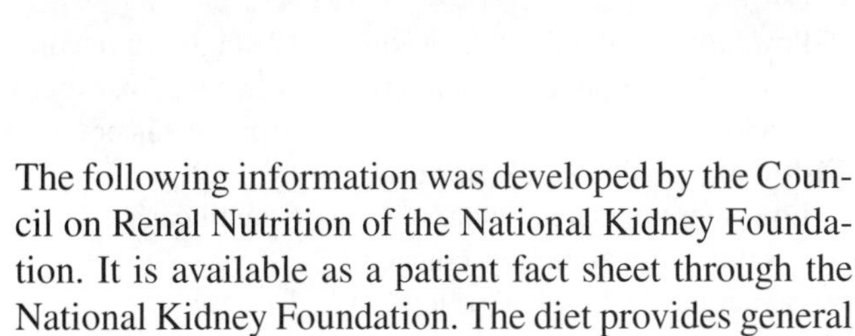

The following information was developed by the Council on Renal Nutrition of the National Kidney Foundation. It is available as a patient fact sheet through the National Kidney Foundation. The diet provides general information on emergency meal planning plus a grocery list and 3–day sample menus for renal and diabetic renal patients.

WHY DO I NEED AN EMERGENCY MEAL PLAN?

This meal plan is for you to use in case of an emergency or a natural disaster when you may not be able to attend dialysis. It is important to follow a limited diet if dialysis has to be missed. A grocery list and a three-day meal plan for an emergency are attached to this fact sheet. This diet is much more strict than your usual diet. This very strict plan is needed to control the build up of toxins such as potassium, phosphorus, urea and fluids that can be life threatening to you if several dialysis treatments are missed due to the emergency.

WHAT SHOULD I EXPECT DURING AN EMERGENCY SITUATION?

Many things we depend on daily may not be working during an emergency. You may be without a telephone. Water and electricity may be cut off, keeping you from cooking your meals in the usual way. You may need to use cold or shelf-stable foods until the crisis is over. Food in your refrigerator will keep safely for up to 12 hours and in the freezer for one to two days, if these appliances are opened *only* when meals are prepared. It is best to eat the foods from your refrigerator and freezer first before using your shelf-stable foods. Distilled water, disposable plates and utensils also should be kept on hand.

HOW DO I PREPARE MYSELF FOR AN EMERGENCY?

As natural disasters may happen without warning, it is good to keep foods with a long shelf-life on hand at all times. If you do stock foods, remember to check dates for freshness and replace regularly.

The following items are important and useful to have on hand in case of an emergency:

- This diet sheet.
- Always have a two-week supply of all medicines and vitamins.
- All of the groceries listed in this guide.
- Diabetics need to have enough insulin and supplies on hand, including extra batteries for the glucometer.

- Emergency phone list with names and phone numbers of your doctor, dialysis unit, and the local hospital.
- Radio with extra batteries
- Flashlight with extra batteries
- Candles and matches
- Measuring cups and scale
- Plastic forks, spoons, knives, plates, bowls and cups
- Napkins
- Hand operated can opener
- 5 gallons distilled water
- Refrigerator thermometer

IS THERE ANYTHING ELSE I SHOULD KNOW?

1. It is *very important* to follow your diet according to the meal plan given.
2. Be careful when eating perishable foods to avoid food poisoning. If a jar or can is opened, do not keep it longer than 4 hours unless refrigerated.
3. Use a refrigerator thermometer to know if food is stored at a safe temperature (under 40 degrees F, 5 degrees C). If your refrigerator temperature is over 40 degrees F, food will only be safe for 4 hrs. After that time—throw it away.
4. Use disposable plates and utensils. Throw away after use.
5. Keep distilled water handy for mixing milk or juice. Mix small amounts of only 4 ounces at a time.
6. Limit intake of fluid to 2 cups or 16 ounces per day. Chew gum to help cope with thirst.
7. *Do not use* salt or salt substitute with your meals. Use salt-free foods when possible.
8. Avoid high-potassium foods. Limit the kinds and portion sizes of fruits and vegetables eaten to those listed in this handout.
9. If you have diabetes, keep instant glucose tablets, sugar, hard candy, low-potassium fruit juices, or sugared soda pop on hand to treat low blood sugars. Avoid high-potassium fruit juices (orange juice).

Three-Day Grocery List for Emergencies

	Amount (per person)
Bread/cereal (use 6–8 servings per day)	
White bread	1 loaf
Dry cereal, unsalted, sweetened or unsweetened puffed wheat or rice, shredded wheat	6 single-serve containers *or* 1 box
Vanilla wafers *or* graham crackers *or* unsalted crackers	1 box
Fruits/juices (limit to 2–4 servings per day)	
Canned or sealed plastic container: applesauce, pears, peaches, pineapple, mandarin oranges, fruit cocktail	12 single-serve containers
Cranberry and apple juice *or* Juice boxes or pouches of premixed fruit punch or lemonade	12 boxes or pouches
or	
Powdered drink mixes: fruit-flavored, fruit punch, or lemonade	12 single-serve containers 2 packages or 1 canister
Fish/meat (limit to 3 oz. per day)	
Low-sodium, canned tuna, salmon, meat, turkey, chicken	6 small cans
Peanut butter, unsalted or low-sodium	1 jar
Milk (limit to ½ cup per day)	
Evaporated milk	3 small cans
Dry milk solids	2 packages
Sweets (use as desired to increase calories)	
Marshmallows	1 large bag
Jelly beans, sourballs, hard candies, butter mints	5 bags total
Honey	1 jar
White sugar	1 small bag
Jelly	1 jar
Fats (use 6 or more servings per day)	
Salad or cooking oil	1 bottle
Mayonnaise (perishable after opening)	Individual packets or 3 small jars
Margarine	1 pound
Other	
Distilled water	5 one-gallon jugs

THREE-DAY MEAL PLAN FOR EMERGENCIES

The sample meal plans given provide about 40–50 grams of protein, 1,500 mg sodium, 1,500 mg potassium and less than 500 mL or 16 ounces of fluid for each of the three days. You may adjust selections to fit your individual taste. These meal plans are stricter than your normal renal diet to keep waste products from building up in your blood during the emergency situation. Fluid is limited to less than 500 mL (2 cups or 16 ounces) each day to prevent you from swelling or having shortness of breath. If the disaster should continue for more than three days the meal plan can be repeated, beginning with Day 1.

Day 1

Breakfast

½ cup milk prepared from dry milk and ½ cup distilled water, or ¼ cup evaporated milk with ¼ cup distilled water
1 single serving of cereal (½–¾ cup)
1 Tablespoon sugar
½ cup pineapple (single serving)

Morning Snack

5 vanilla wafers
Honey or jelly as desired on wafers
10 sourballs

Lunch

2 slices white bread
¼ cup low sodium tuna (open new can daily)
1 Tablespoon margarine or mayonnaise (individual packet or open new jar daily)
½ cup pears (single serving)
Powdered drink mix with ½ cup distilled water

Afternoon Snack

6 unsalted crackers
Honey or jelly as desired on crackers
10 jelly beans

Dinner

2 slices white bread
½ cup (2 oz.) low sodium chicken (open new can daily)
2 Tablespoons margarine or mayonnaise (individual packet or open new jar daily)
½ cup peaches (single serving)
½ cup cranberry juice (from box or pouch)

Evening Snack

3 graham crackers
Honey or jelly as desired on crackers
10 butter mints

Day 2

Breakfast

½ cup milk prepared from dry milk and ½ cup distilled water, or mix ¼ cup evaporated milk with ¼ cup distilled water
1 single serving of cereal (½–¾ cup from box)
1 Tablespoon sugar
½ cup mandarin oranges (single serving)

Morning Snack

3 graham crackers
Honey or jelly as desired on graham crackers
10 hard candies

Lunch

2 slices white bread
¼ cup (1 oz.) low sodium turkey (open new can daily)
1 Tablespoon margarine or mayonnaise (individual packet or open new jar daily)
½ cup fruit cocktail (single serving)
Powdered drink mix with ½ cup distilled water

Afternoon Snack

6 unsalted crackers
Honey or jelly as desired on crackers
10 large marshmallows

Dinner

2 slices white bread
½ cup (2 oz.) low sodium chicken (open new can daily)
2 Tablespoons margarine or mayonnaise (individual packet or open new jar daily)
½ cup pineapple (single serving)
½ cup cranberry juice (from box or pouch)

Evening Snack

5 vanilla wafers
Honey or jelly as desired (use on wafers)
10 sourballs

Day 3

Breakfast

½ cup milk prepared from dry milk and ½ cup distilled water, or ¼ cup evaporated milk with ¼ cup distilled water

1 single serving of cereal (½–¾ cup from box)
1 Tablespoon sugar
½ cup pears (single serving)

Morning Snack

6 unsalted crackers
Honey or jelly as desired on crackers
10 large marshmallows

Lunch

2 slices white bread
2 Tablespoons low sodium or unsalted peanut butter
½ cup peaches (single serving)
Powdered drink mix with ½ cup distilled water

Afternoon Snack

3 graham cracker squares
Honey or jelly as desired on crackers
10 butter mints

Dinner

2 slices white bread
½ cup (2 oz.) low sodium chicken (open new can daily)
2 Tablespoons margarine or mayonnaise (individual packets or open new jar daily)
½ cup mandarin oranges (single serving)
½ cup cranberry juice (from box or pouch)

Evening Snack

5 vanilla wafers
Honey or jelly as desired (use on wafers)
10 sourballs

THREE-DAY *DIABETIC* MEAL PLAN FOR EMERGENCIES

The sample meal plans given provide about 40–50 grams of protein, 1,500 mg sodium, 1,500 mg potassium, 1,800 calories and less than 500 mL or 16 ounces of fluid for each of the three days. You may make changes within a diabetic exchange group to fit your individual taste. These meal plans are stricter than your normal renal and diabetic diet to keep waste products from building up in your blood during the emergency situation. Fluid is limited to less than 500 mL (2 cups or 16 ounces) each day to prevent you from swelling or having shortness of breath. If the disaster should continue for more than three days, the meal plan should be repeated.

Three-Day *Diabetic* Grocery List for Emergencies

	Amount (per person)
Bread/cereal (use 6–8 servings per day)	
White bread Dry cereal, unsalted, unsweetened puffed wheat or rice, shredded wheat	1 loaf 6 single-serve containers *or* 1 box
Vanilla wafers *or* graham crackers *or* unsalted crackers	1 box
Unsweetened fruits/juices (limit to 2–4 servings per day)	
Canned or sealed plastic container of applesauce, pears, peaches, pineapple, mandarin oranges, fruit cocktail	12 single-serve containers
Apple or cranberry juice	12 boxes or pouches
Sugar-free powdered drink mix: fruit-flavored, fruit punch, or lemonade	1 canister or 2 packages
or	
Sugar-free lemon lime or ginger ale soda	6 cans
Fish/meat (limit to 3 oz. per day)	
Low-sodium, canned tuna, salmon, meat, turkey, chicken	6 small cans
Peanut butter, unsalted or low-sodium	1 jar
Milk (limit to ½ cup per day)	
Evaporated milk	3 small cans
Dry milk solids	2 packages
Artificial sweetener	1 box of packets
Sweets (use only to treat low blood sugar)	
Sourballs, hard candies	1 bag
Corn syrup	1 bottle
White sugar	1 small bag
Jelly	1 jar
Sugared lemon-lime or ginger ale soda	3 12-ounce cans; limit use of soda to avoid fluid overload
Fats (use 6 or more servings per day)	
Salad or cooking oil	1 bottle
Mayonnaise (perishable after opening)	Individual packets or 3 small jars
Margarine	1 pound
Other	
Distilled water	5 one-gallon jugs

Day 1

Breakfast

½ cup milk prepared from dry milk and ½ cup distilled water, or mix ¼ cup evaporated milk with ¼ cup distilled water
1 single-serving box of cereal (½ to ¾ cup from box)
2 teaspoons artificial sweetener (optional)
½ cup pineapple in unsweetened juice (single serving)

Morning Snack

6 unsalted crackers
1 Tablespoon margarine spread on crackers

Lunch

2 slices white bread
¼ cup low sodium tuna (open new can daily)
1 Tablespoon margarine or mayonnaise (individual packet or open new jar daily)
½ cup pears in unsweetened juice (single serving)
½ cup sugar-free beverage

Afternoon Snack

5 vanilla wafers

Dinner

2 slices white bread
½ cup (2 oz.) low sodium chicken (open new can daily)
2 Tablespoons margarine or mayonnaise (individual packet or open new jar daily)
½ cup peaches in unsweetened juice (single serving)
½ cup unsweetened apple juice (from box or pouch)

Evening Snack

3 graham cracker squares

Note

- Use 1 Tablespoon peanut butter if you need a protein source at evening snack.
- Continue to monitor blood sugar.
- Follow your protocol for insulin reactions and be sure to keep enough supplies on hand. Best choices for treating low sugars are fluid-free items such as sugar, corn syrup, hard candy, instant glucose, and glucose tablets. Sugared soda and low-potassium juices may also be used but must be counted as part of your 2-cup or 16-ounce daily limit.

Diabetic Plan—Day 2

Breakfast

½ cup milk prepared from dry milk and ½ cup distilled water, or mix ¼ cup evaporated milk with ¼ cup distilled water
1 single-serving box of cereal (½–¾ cup from box)
2 teaspoons artificial sweetener (optional)
½ cup unsweetened applesauce (single serving)

Morning Snack

5 vanilla wafers

Lunch

2 slices white bread
2 Tablespoons low sodium peanut butter
1 Tablespoon margarine or mayonnaise (individual packet or open new jar daily)
½ cup mandarin oranges in unsweetened juice (single serving)
½ cup sugar-free beverage or soda

Afternoon Snack

6 unsalted crackers
1 Tablespoon margarine spread on crackers

Dinner

2 slices white bread
½ cup (2 oz.) low sodium chicken (open new can daily)
2 Tablespoons margarine or mayonnaise (individual packet or open new jar daily)
½ cup pineapple packed in unsweetened juice (single serving)
½ cup unsweetened apple juice (from box or pouch)

Evening Snack

3 graham cracker squares

Note

- Use 1 Tablespoon peanut butter if you need a protein source at evening snack.
- Continue to monitor blood sugar.
- Follow your protocol for insulin reactions and be sure to keep enough supplies on hand. Best choices for treating low sugars are fluid-free items such as sugar, corn syrup, hard candy, instant glucose, and glucose tablets. Sugared soda and low-potassium juices may also be used, but must be counted as part of your 2-cup or 16-ounce daily limit.

Diabetic Plan—Day 3

Breakfast

½ cup milk prepared from dry milk and ½ cup distilled water, or ¼ cup evaporated milk with ¼ cup distilled water
1 single-serving box of cereal (½–¾ cup from box)
2 teaspoons artificial sweetener (optional)
½ cup pears packed in unsweetened juice (single serving)

Morning Snack

6 unsalted crackers
1 Tablespoon margarine

Lunch

2 slices white bread
¼ cup (2 oz.) low-sodium turkey (open new can daily)
1 Tablespoon margarine or mayonnaise (individual packet or open new jar daily)
½ cup peaches packed in unsweetened juice (single serving)
½ cup sugar-free drink or soda

Afternoon Snack

5 vanilla wafers

Dinner

2 slices white bread
½ cup (2 oz.) low-sodium chicken (open new can daily)
2 Tablespoons margarine or mayonnaise (individual packet or open new jar daily)
½ cup fruit cocktail (single serving)
½ cup cranberry juice (from box or pouch)

Evening Snack

3 graham cracker squares

Note

- Use 1 Tablespoon peanut butter if you need a protein source at evening snack.
- Continue to monitor blood sugar.
- Follow your protocol for insulin reactions and be sure to keep enough supplies on hand. Best choices for treating low sugars are fluid-free items such as sugar, corn syrup, hard candy, instant glucose, and glucose tablets. Sugared soda and low-potassium juices may also be used but must be counted as part of your 2-cup or 16-ounce daily limit.

Source: Reprinted with permission from "Emergency Meal Planning Guide," © 2004 National Kidney Foundation, Inc.

Appendix F

Internet Resources

Maureen P. McCarthy, MPH, RD, CSR

The major goal of this appendix is to identify professional resources of value to specialists in renal nutrition. Because so much information is available on the Internet, Web-based resources for the renal nutrition professional will be the focus of this appendix. Of course, the challenge for all information published on the Internet is to be general enough so as not to be quickly outdated and yet detailed enough to be of use to the intended audience. The sites reviewed were active in February 2004.

The pertinent professional organizations for renal dietitians are well known to most of us. They are as follows:

Renal Practice Group (RPG) of the American Dietetic Association

Membership information is available at the American Dietetic Association's Web site: http://www.eatright.org (search "RPG"). RPG also has its own page for members at http://www.renalnutrition.org. This page includes links to discussion groups, archives of *Renal Nutrition Forum,* and other activities for renal dietitians. For patients, there are links to pages that may be appropriate for their needs, although users are advised to consult with health care providers as well as reviewing Internet resources.

Council on Renal Nutrition of the National Kidney Foundation (NKF-CRN)

Extensive information about NKF-CRN, including the "how to" of membership and extensive programs for local and national meetings, is available at http://www.kidney.org/professionals/CRN/index.cfm. NKF patient education handouts are listed. These are available online at http://www.kidney.org (select the menu item "Patient and Family Education" for a list of brochures). Both sites include a list of cookbooks for patients, which is a helpful tool.

Tables F.1 through F.3 identify additional organizations and material of interest to health professionals, patients, and families.

Table F.1. Internet Resources for the Professional

Site Name	*URL*	*Audience*	*Source*	*Contents*	*Accuracy*
Dialysis and Transplantation (D&T)	http://www.eneph.com	Professionals	Creative Age Publications	Index of D&T articles. List of worldwide dialysis centers. Free contact hours. Archive of feature articles	High accuracy
Hypertension, Dialysis, and Clinical Nephrology	http://www.hdcn.com	Professionals	Education site for American Society of Nephrology and the Renal Physicians Association	Current news headlines, current literature. Meeting highlights. Calculators, practice guidelines. Some materials available by subscription only (key zone). Some are free.	High accuracy
Life Options Rehabilitation Program	http://www.lifeoptions.org	Professionals, patients, and family members	Medical Education Institute, Inc.	Bulletin boards to share ideas. Background about the 5 E's.* Materials to support rehabilitation. Extensive links.	Some personal postings must be evaluated case by case. Otherwise high accuracy.
Medline Plus	http://www.nlm.nih.gov/medlineplus/healthtopics.html	Professionals and general public	National Library of Medicine	Built around list of major health topics. Can find nutrition and kidney and urinary health topics. Includes links to news stories, overviews, clinical trials, research reports, and much more.	High accuracy
National Institute of Diabetes and Digestive and Kidney Diseases (NIDDK)	http://www.niddk.nih.gov	Professionals and general public Some materials in Spanish	NIDDK and National Institutes of Health (NIH)	Broad range of materials. Many NIDDK education tools (includes national education programs for diabetes and kidney disease—NDEP and NKDEP). Links to research funding information, clinical trials, NIDDK reports, etc.	High accuracy. Large site size may present problems.
The Nephron Information Center	http://www.nephron.com	Professionals, patients, general public	Steven Z. Fadem, MD, FACP	Top news stories. Comprehensive resources/links for all nephrology professionals and for patients related to CKD and ESRD. Calculators. Legislative stories/links.	High accuracy

Net Nutrition	http://www.satellitehealth.com Go to Satellite Dialysis or Satellite Laboratory Services and select "Net Nutrition" link	Professionals	Satellite Healthcare, Inc.	Tools and guidelines for nutrition assessment, including subjective global assessment. Calculations related to anthropometrics, nutrient requirements, and urea kinetic modeling can be completed.	High accuracy
Pub Med	http://www.ncbi.nlm.nih.gov/entrez/query.fcgi?db=PubMed	Professionals and general public	National Library of Medicine	Free access to MEDLINE search capabilities.	High accuracy
Thomas, Legislative Information on the Internet	http://thomas.loc.gov	Professionals and general public	Library of Congress	Contact information for US senators and representatives. Committee lists. US Congress bill summaries and status.	High accuracy
Tufts Nutrition Navigator	http://navigator.tufts.edu	Health professionals, educators, journalists, general public	Center on Nutrition Information, Friedman School of Nutrition Science and Policy, Tufts University	Reviews of Web pages with nutrition content.	High accuracy
US Department of Agriculture (USDA) Food and Nutrition Information Center (FNIC)	http://www.nal.usda.gov/fnic	Professionals and general public	FNIC of USDA	Links to various food composition databases from USDA. Dietary supplement information. Dietary guidelines. Food Guide Pyramid.	High accuracy
United States Renal Data System (USRDS)	http://www.usrds.org	Professionals	USRDS Coordinating Center	Extensive data reports and reference tables. Slides taken from data reports. Researchers' guide. Related links.	High accuracy

*5 E's = Encouragement, Education, Exercise, Employment, and Evaluation.

Table F.2. Internet Resources For Patients, Family, and the General Public

Site Name	*URL*	*Audience*	*Source*	*Contents*	*Accuracy*
American Association of Kidney Patients (AAKP)	http://www.aakp.org	Patients, family	AAKP	AAKP Patient Plan; RENALIFE online. Washington update.	High accuracy
American Kidney Fund (AKF)	http://www.akfinc.org	Patients, family	AKF	Includes sections on kidney disease facts and healthy lifestyle (includes recipe ideas, not always renal-specific). Online information about Renagel assistance program.	High accuracy, but be prepared to evaluate recipes
Culinary Kidney Cooks	http://www.culinarykidneycooks.com	Patients, family	Sara Colman, RD; Dorothy Gordon, RN; Eric Brooks, PE	Web site for *Cooking For David: A Culinary Dialysis Cookbook.* Weekly recipe and dialysis hints.	High accuracy
Kidney Directions—Inforenal	http://www.kidneydirections.com	Patients, family Allows reader to select language (English, Spanish, Italian, Japanese, Korean)	Baxter	Includes special "KD Kids" recipe of the week, patient of the month, online cookbook. Online support for learning PD at home. Nurses' Corner with online CEUs.	High accuracy
Kidney Options	http://www.kidneyoptions.com	Patients, family, professionals	Fresenius Medical Care, with AAKP	Information about kidney disease, treatment options, nutrition. List of resources with telephone numbers. Bulletin board. Glossary of medical terms.	High accuracy
Kidney School	http://www.kidneyschool.org	Patients, family	Life Options Rehabilitation Program	16 modules ranging from kidney function to treatment options; includes nutrition.	High accuracy

Table F.3. Internet Resources Related to Alternative Care

Site Name	*URL*	*Audience*	*Source*	*Contents*	*Accuracy*
American Botanical Council (ABC)	http://www.herbalgram.org	General public	ABC, publisher of *HerbalGram*	Recent news items. Paid membership reqired for access to many items, including past issues of *HerbalGram* and Herb-Clip (free sample Herb-Clip articles available).	Good to high accuracy
ConsumerLab.com	http://www.ConsumerLab.com	General public and health professionals	ConsumerLab.com, LLC	Some content available by subscription only. Lab testing results for many supplements. Recalls and warnings about products.	High accuracy
National Institutes of Health (NIH) Office of Dietary Supplements—Relevant Links	http://dietary_supplements.info.nih.gov/	General public	NIH	Links to International Bibliographic Information on Dietary Supplements (IBIDS), dietary reference intakes, and recommended dietary allowances. Links to fact sheets on supplements.	High accuracy

Index